Perspectives on Theory for the Practice of Occupational Therapy

D0898359

Perspectives on Theory for the Practice of Occupational Therapy

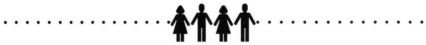

THIRD EDITION

Editors

Kay F. Walker, PhD, OTR, FAOTA
and
Ferol Menks Ludwig, PhD, OTR, GCG

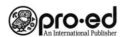

8700 Shoal Creek Boulevard
Austin, Texas, 78757-6897
800/897-3202   Fax 800/397-7633
www.proedinc.com

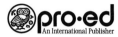
An International Publisher

© 1987, 2004 by PRO-ED, Inc.
8700 Shoal Creek Boulevard
Austin, Texas 78757-6897
800/897-3202   Fax 800/397-7633
www.proedinc.com

Library of Congress Cataloging-in-Publication Data

Perspectives on theory for the practice of occupational therapy / editors,
    Kay F. Walker and Ferol M. Ludwig. — 3rd ed.
        p. cm.
    Includes bibliographical references and index.
    ISBN 0-89079-937-7 (soft cover)
    1. Occupational therapy—Philosophy.   I. Walker, Kay F.   II. Ludwig,
    Ferol M.

RM735.4.P47 2004
615.8'515'01—dc22   2003060209

Printed in the United States of America

1   2   3   4   5   6   7   8   9   10   08   07   06   05   04

We dedicate this third edition
to the memory of
Alice C. Jantzen,
August 17, 1918 – October 22, 1983,
our role model and mentor
who saw potential in us as scholars
. . . and challenged us to become so

And to
students past, present, and future
for inspiring us to realize Alice's challenge

Contents

Preface

Fifteen years after the initial publication of this book in 1987 and 9 years after its revision in 1993, we began work on this third edition to again update information on the theories previously discussed. We also added a chapter with an overview of the burgeoning theoretical developments in occupation-centered and occupation-based practices. The goal of the book remains that of providing a thorough review of selected theorists whose lives and works have influenced the direction and development of clinical practice in occupational therapy. In keeping with this goal, two assumptions have guided our development of this book. First, careful study of existing theoretical material is needed to provide a knowledge base for the refinement of current theories and for the development of new ones. Second, the clinical relevance of a theory can be enhanced when that theory is studied in the context of the individual theorist's attempts to solve clinical problems or address professional issues encountered in his or her own career.

Chapter 1 includes a discussion of the founding ideas of the profession, as well as definitions of theory and its relevance to occupational therapy. This chapter is followed by the core of the book, chapters about seven theorists. Each of Chapters 2 through 8 begins with the biographical sketch of an individual theorist, providing the distinguishing backdrop from which his or her theory evolved. Chapter authors describe factors that influenced and motivated each theorist's professional growth. In this way, the authors enliven each theory through the context of the theorist's personal and professional efforts to solve practical and realistic problems that confront occupational therapists. Following the biographical overview, each theorist chapter includes an objective review of the individual's theory and the use of that theory in occupational therapy. A description of the research and application of the theory by others reveals the impact of each theory on the profession. Comprehensive bibliographies provide a complete listing of each theorist's body of work.

Certainly, many people other than these seven have made and are making significant contributions to occupational therapy's growing theory base. In the last decade, a number of individuals working jointly with others have expressed models and conceptualizations of occupation as the germinal concept in the profession. A new chapter is offered in this third addition to address these developments. Chapter 9 provides an overview of the sociohistorical contexts for occupation-based and occupation-centered theoretical background as well as contemporary theoretical development. This chapter discusses the many advances in occupation-based and occupation-centered practices occurring nationally and internationally. This chapter differs from the preceding ones in that no one particular theorist is selected for in-depth discussion. Instead, some of the major theoretical developments are identified and reviewed to give the reader a schema or framework in which to conceptualize these concepts. Many persons are engaged in this work.

In the final chapter, on theory analysis, the author explores the major themes that run through the individual theories as well as the occupation-based models and occupational science. The organization of this chapter is consistent with that of the individual theory chapters, including discussion of theory development, premises, clinical use, and testing. In this edition, a format for historical context analysis is offered for examining how a theory or an idea developed over time within professional, national, and personal events.

At the time of the first edition's inception in 1987 as *Six Perspectives on Theory for the Practice of Occupational Therapy*, we felt that such a book was needed in the occupational therapy profession for therapists, students, educators, and others. Practicing therapists can use this edition, like its predecessors, to develop a frame of reference for a clinical setting, to review theory related to a new job area, to formulate justifications for practice decisions to other professionals and third-party payers, to establish a rationale for research, or to prepare for continuing education workshops. For the increasing number of therapists returning to school to obtain postprofessional degrees, this book provides an overview of theorists and exhaustive bibliographies for further study. Graduate students also can identify research questions from this theory base. The book is designed to help entry-level students who are in the process of formulating a professional identity. It can assist them to begin to understand the common themes and the differences among the basic theories. Because this book identifies a heritage of outstanding ideas and the exemplary careers of some of the people in the profession, it can ground the student in the ideas of the profession. Educators can use this book to provide a broader conceptual base for course content and curriculum planning, as well as to impart to students an appreciation of the richness of theoretical ideas in the profession. The book also can provide educators with an additional stimulus for their own scholarly research endeavors.

Throughout the writing of the three editions of this book, we have kept in mind Yerxa's statement that "we deal with enormous complexity which we tend to simplify rather than clarify" (1986, p. 211). It has not been possible to address all of the complex issues behind the theories presented, a reality that readers must keep in mind when reading this book. We hope that this work adds more to clarity than to simplification.

We thank Gail Fidler, Lela Llorens, Gary Kielhofner, and Claudia Allen for graciously providing us with updates of their biographies. Our work can only be accomplished in the context of the support and assistance of our families, loved ones, friends, and colleagues, and to you we are grateful. We also appreciate the editors and staff at Aspen Publishers for their assistance in the early development of this edition and at PRO-ED for seeing the project through to publication.

Reference

Yerxa, E. J. (1986). Target tomorrow. In *Occupational therapy education: Target 2000* (pp. 209–213). Rockville, MD: American Occupational Therapy Association.

Contributors

Mary V. Donahue, PhD, OTR
New York University Occupational
  Therapy
35 West 4th St. 11th Floor
New York, NY 10012

Ferol Menks Ludwig, PhD,
OTR, FAOTA, GCG
Professor and Director of Doctoral
  Program
Nova Southeastern University
Health Professions Division
College of Allied Health
Occupational Therapy Department
3200 South University Drive
Ft. Lauderdale, FL 33328-2018

Rosalie J. Miller, PhD, OTR,
FAOTA
Visiting Professor
Department of Occupational Therapy
Florida Gulf Coast University
Ft. Myers, FL 33917

Kay Schwartz, EdD, OTR
Professor
Occupational Therapy Department
San Jose State University
1 Washington Square
San Jose, CA 95192

Patricia Scott, PhD, OTR
Associate Professor and Graduate
  Coordinator
Department of Occupational Therapy
Florida International University
University Park Campus CH-102
Miami, FL 33199

Susan Denegan Shortridge,
MHS, OTR
President
Developmental Health Care
  Services, Inc.
8245 Lake Serene Drive
Orlando, FL 32836

Julia Van Deusen, PhD, OTR,
FAOTA
Professor Emeritus
Department of Occupational Therapy
College of Health Professions
University of Florida
PO Box 100164
596 Museum Road
Gainesville, FL 32610-0164

Kay F. Walker, PhD, OTR,
FAOTA
Professor
Department of Occupational Therapy
College of Health Professions
University of Florida
PO Box 100164
596 Museum Road
Gainesville, FL 32610-0164

About the Editors

Kay F. Walker, PhD, OTR, FAOTA, is a professor in the Department of Occupational Therapy at the University of Florida, Gainsville, and serves as program director of the Internet-based distance learning master's program. She has been an academician in occupational therapy (OT) for more than 30 years. Her research, teaching, presentation, and publication topics include neuroscience, OT theory, anatomy, sensory integration, and early intervention. She serves as a consultant to public schools, a school for students who are blind and deaf, and a state residential facility for adults with developmental disabilities. She enjoys fitness, the beach, golf, and travel, and her two young adult daughters.

Ferol Menks Ludwig, PhD, OTR, FAOTA, GCG, is director of OT doctoral programs and professor at Nova Southeastern University, Ft. Lauderdale, Florida. She is an occupational therapist, occupational scientist, and gerontologist. For over 30 years, she has practiced OT in academic and clinical settings. She has published over 20 articles, given numerous presentations, contributed to several OT texts, and created a simulation board game on aging.

What Is Theory and Why Does It Matter?

1

Rosalie J. Miller and Kay Schwartz

In the practice of occupational therapy, a concentration on individual techniques sometimes obscures the underlying relations between individuals, their function, and their world. An occupational therapist's view of these relationships is theory. Theory explains how some aspect of human behavior or performance is organized, and thus it enables the occupational therapist to make predictions about that behavior. Without a theory of human definition and capability linked to function in the world, occupational therapy as a concept could not exist.

To respond to the question, "What is theory?" we present in this chapter a definition of theory and an explanation of the way it is developed, including the relationship between theory and research. Semantic issues that sometimes confuse are articulated. To address "Why does theory matter?" we discuss the importance of theory in relation to practice, reimbursement, specialization, growth of the profession, and education of competent practitioners. Finally, we describe theory as a unifying foundation. Because theory evolves from the philosophical assumptions made by a profession, we review the assumptions (beliefs) and values that informed the new profession of occupational therapy at the beginning of the 20th century and that provided the underpinnings for the theoretical models that would later be developed by the first and second generations of the profession's theorists, including those discussed in the central chapters of this book.

What Is Theory?

Theory is a way to increase understanding by bridging the gap between concrete experience in the world of observed events, such as falling apples, and "the imagined world of hypothetical concepts, such as gravity" (Folger & Turillo, 1999, p. 742). The major structural components of a theory are *concepts,* which are ideally well defined, and *principles,* or postulates, which explain how the concepts are related to one another.

Concepts

The ability to use symbols through language enables humans to develop concepts. The young child, upon seeing something unfamiliar, asks, "What is that?" and is told, "That's a cow" or "That's a papaya." Through these experiences, categories are formed into which an individual organizes things from the environment. These categories are concepts (Duldt & Giffin, 1985, p. 46).

As one grows, one develops more concept categories, relates more and more things to them, and subdivides levels of concept categories in one's mind. For instance, the large concept category of animals is subdivided into cows, dogs, cats, horses, and others. The child learns that food is subdivided into fruits, vegetables, grains, and so on, which are then further subdivided—fruits into apples, pears, papaya, grapes, and so forth. One learns "to recognize things as belonging to certain categories; thus one develops a notion of concepts" (Duldt & Giffin, 1985, p. 46).

Language orders experience and determines one's perceptions of reality. It enables conceptualization, and because of language, a person can conceptualize things that he or she cannot see, whether because the person is out of sight of the physical thing itself, such as "cow" or "pyramids," or because there is no physical reality to the concept, such as "self-esteem" or "motivation." Concepts such as these latter two that have no physical referent but rather are labels for intangible ideas are often called *constructs.*

Principles

As one learns more about concepts, one also learns about ways in which concepts relate to one another. Relationships between concepts are called *principles* or *postulates*. For instance, once one learns the concepts of "2" and "4," one learns the principle that if 2 is added to 2, the result is 4. Once one has learned the concepts of "cat," "petting," and "enjoyment," one can put together the principle that the cat enjoys being petted. One also learns reverse consequences of principles: 4 minus 2 equals 2; if one strokes the cat against the lay of the fur, it objects; and so on. In all these examples, one is using language symbolically to think about the relationships between concepts, and in so doing, one is deriving principles (Duldt & Giffin, 1985).

Concepts and principles serve two important functions. First, they "help us understand or explain what is going on around us" (Duldt & Giffin, 1985, p. 47). For example, beginning occupational therapy (OT) students are usually somewhat confused about "what occupational therapy is." In the course of their education, they learn new concepts that are used in the field, such as "neurodevelopment" and "occupation," and learn how to categorize other things and ideas (subconcepts) into these major concepts. For example, subconcepts of "activities of daily living," "work," and "play and leisure" are categorized under the major concept of "occupation." Then the student learns principles governing the relationships among concepts—for example, "involvement in occupation is essential to normal neurodevelopment." Through this process of learning concepts and principles, students grow to better understand what occupational therapy is.

Second, according to Duldt and Giffin (1985), established principles also help one to predict future events.

> Some concepts relate to one another so consistently that predictions about future outcomes are relatively simple. For example, when we see dark clouds with lightning and we hear thunder, we know from experience that rain is approaching. We can make this prediction because we understand the relationship between the three concepts—clouds, lightning, and thunder—and because we know they usually combine in such a way that a fourth concept, rain, occurs. Using our knowledge, we can exert some control over the situation by wearing raincoats and using umbrellas. . . . In developing theories, similar relationships are established between concepts. (p. 33)

These relationships can be stated as *correlational* ("dark clouds are often accompanied by rain") or *causal* ("if you stand in the rain without a raincoat or umbrella, you get wet").

From the OT principle stated earlier, one can predict future events. For example, given the principle that involvement in occupation is essential to normal neurodevelopment, one can predict that a child who is in a body cast and kept in an isolated environment for a period of time will suffer setbacks in neurodevelopment. When several related principles of neurodevelopment are logically organized, the outcome can be a theory.

Theoretical Assumptions

Theories provide ways for a profession to organize its knowledge base and to thus guide practice. Related principles, typically organized in a way that ties concepts together to explain and predict a phenomenon, can become a theory.

The principles that explain relationships among concepts often involve assumptions. For instance, the principle that involvement in occupation is essential to normal neurodevelopment is based on assumptions articulated by the founders of the profession. The assumptions that are generally considered basic to the profession influence the type and direction of theories that are introduced. Thus, no theory is totally value free. Every person brings to the task of explaining his or her observations a particular perspective and certain basic values. Certainly most people share the assumption that the world exists and that they can accurately perceive it through their senses. This may or may not be ultimately true, but most theories are based on this assumption.

As Creek and Feaver (1993) stated, "Professional philosophy is the system of beliefs [assumptions] and values unique to each profession which provides its members with a sense of identity and exerts control over theory and practice." (p. 5). It is important to be aware of the assumptions underlying a particular theory so that one may evaluate it thoroughly, rather than accepting it at face value. For instance, a theory may seem quite logical at first, but an examination of the assumptions on which it is based may give one cause to reject it as incompatible with one's own worldview. At the same time, it is important to maintain an attitude of flexibility about one's assumptions and realize that the results of truth seeking might lead one to change an assumption from time to time.

Definition of Theory

Theory is an organized way of thinking about given phenomena. In OT the phenomenon of concern is occupational endeavor. Theory attempts to (1) define and explain the relationship between concepts or ideas related to the phenomenon of interest, (2) explain how these relationships can predict behavior or events, and (3) suggest ways that the phenomenon can be changed or controlled. (Reed, 1998, p. 521)

By helping people understand the unseen relationship(s) between observed or commonly assumed events or concepts, theories advance conceptual development and increase understanding (Beard, 2000). For instance, A. Jean Ayres, in her work with children, gave them controlled sensory input, and observed and recorded their behavioral reaction. To explain the unseen relationship between sensory input and behavior, she posited the theory of sensory integration (see Chapter 5).

Relationship of Research to Theory

The way one determines whether the principles relating concepts in any particular theory are valid is through the process called research. Through research, theories change and develop. The theory of sensory integration and the model of human occupation are two examples of theories in occupational therapy that have evolved significantly through research.

Occupational therapists' research laboratories are the practice settings in which therapists interact with patients and clients. Those therapists who use theoretical principles to make practice decisions and then observe the results are engaging in a process of testing those theories and, in so doing, may also generate new ones.

They also may be engaging in "evidence-based practice," using the most advanced and tested knowledge available to make decisions about the care of their clients (Taylor, 2000). Evidence-based practice draws upon research, as well as the practitioner's cumulative experiences and the client's needs and preferences (Geyman, Deyo, & Ramsey, 2000). "Research is about generating evidence . . . and evidence-based practice is about putting evidence into current practice" (Taylor, 2000, p. 5).

To be valuable and useful, the evidence generated through research needs to be tied back to theory, or it risks becoming "free-floating information of little use in advancing practice" (Giuffre, 1998, p. 36). Therefore, an important cyclical relationship exists between theory, research, and practice, and the development of professional knowledge can begin in any of these places—with theory, which is then tested through research, or through the observations of practice, which then lead to theory (Mosey, 1992).

There are many exciting ways to go about this process of both testing and generating theory. Productive debate about the ways and means by which the theoretical propositions of OT should be generated, investigated, and tested flourished in the late 1980s and early 1990s (Carlson & Clark, 1991; Hasselkus, 1995; Kielhofner, 1992; Mosey, 1992; Ottenbacher, 1992; Yerxa, 1991). Since that time, scholars have devoted more of their energies to the actual generation, investigation, and testing of theories. The development of a solid theoretical and concrete knowledge base of the profession requires that all occupational therapists become more knowledgeable about theory and more conscious and deliberate about the kinds of thinking and problem solving in which they are already engaged, and that they then record and share their findings.

Development of Theory

Stages

Theory is constantly revised as new knowledge is discovered through research. Any new science, according to Lewin (1947), goes through three stages in theory development:

1. *The speculative period*—The field puts forth theoretical models to attempt to explain phenomena.

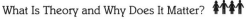

2. *The descriptive period*—The field gathers facts through research to describe what really is happening and to test the theoretical models.

3. *The constructive period*—The field revises old theories and develops new ones that are grounded in facts rather than based on speculation.

Any science must and does go through these stages. Professionals in occupational therapy have developed speculative theories, continue to gather facts through research, and are both revising old theories and developing new ones based on research that uncovers new facts and verifies suspected relationships. This is further evidence that the profession is maturing. The discipline of occupational science has stimulated this process and has speeded the development of theory and research in many of the areas of concern to occupational therapy (Zemke & Clark, 1996).

Process

Theory is generally developed in one of two ways. An individual may have many facts and then develop a theory to explain relationships among them. Charles Darwin, for example, was a scientist who knew the facts that had been gathered up to his time about different species and their description and classification. He posited his theory of evolution as a way of explaining how these many species were related to one another and to human beings (Ostrow, 1980). Alternatively, a person may have a flash of insight that suddenly gives him or her a whole new perspective about the relationship of certain concepts. An example of this type of theory development is Albert Einstein's theory of relativity, which opened up new areas of research and inquiry that had not existed before because no one had ever conceptualized the possibility that energy, matter, and time could be related in the way Einstein suggested.

The way that Jean Ayres's theory of sensory integration (Ayers, 1965) was derived combined these two processes. Ayres saw certain developments in the cognitive, perceptual, and motor functioning of the children with whom she worked. After extensive observation and testing, she presented her theory of sensory integration. Like Darwin, she had accumulated a good deal of knowledge and was a scholar in her area. Also like Einstein, she went beyond the proven, the tested, and the observable to develop her theory. Ayres (1965) stated,

> Exactly how SI occurs in the brain remains elusive, but that lack of knowledge should not be an excuse for avoiding an issue basic to all learning. [Lack of knowledge] must be faced and dealt with in as adequate a manner as possible with full recognition of the limitations involved and with the realization that any conceptual framework is in some aspects erroneous and will require constant revision as new knowledge unfolds. (p. 43)

This willingness to take risks is an essential quality in any theorist. One risk is that of being unpopular when putting forth a theory that contradicts "common knowledge." This has happened throughout history, from Copernicus to Darwin to Ayres (Hull, 1983; Kuhn, 1957; Walker, 1993).

Complexity and Scope

Theories range along a continuum of complexity and scope. At one end lie those that are very broad and complex and attempt to explain major areas within a discipline, and at the other end are those that are narrow in focus and deal with specific phenomena. Parham (1987) defined this continuance as ranging from conceptual frameworks to scientific theories, and said they are

> different kinds of thinking tools for the therapist. An overarching conceptual framework allows the therapist to frame the context for intervention by sketching a general configuration of the situation, while a scientific theory leads the therapist to specify technical details of how to act on a problem once it is selected as a target for intervention. It is likely that, in the best instances of competent clinical practice, both kinds of thinking are involved. (p. 558)

In the nursing literature, this continuum is usually considered to consist of three major levels: grand theories, middle-range theories, and practice theories (Liehr & Smith, 1999; McEwen, 2000).

The model of human occupation (Kielhofner, 1995) is an example of an overarching conceptual framework for the practice of OT that provides a perspective from which the therapist can evaluate and determine areas of function and dysfunction in a given patient or client. Ayres's theory of sensory integration is a scientific theory that guides the therapist's intervention with an individual client once it has been determined that lack of sensory integration is a probable contributor to dysfunction.

The major theories in OT fall at different points along this continuum of complexity and scope, and often in a clinical situation a therapist will use more than one theory. The use of multiple theories is often necessary because of the complexity of the problems faced by many clients; however, one must be certain when using multiple theories that they are based on compatible assumptions and that their concepts fit together logically.

> Often the therapist will have to choose between competing theories that offer different points of view for understanding a single clinical situation. An appreciation of the different kinds of theories available and what each can bring to the understanding of the problem is required if a wise decision is to be made. (Parham, 1987, p. 557)

An obvious example would be a therapist working from a psychoanalytic theory base with a disturbed child, encouraging her to express her anger. It would greatly confuse that child if she were also treated from a behavioral perspective and rewarded for "good" behavior.

Semantic Issues

One of the major difficulties in understanding, analyzing, and comparing theories in OT is that different theorists discuss similar concepts using different labels. The same theorist may even use such terms as "theory," "model," and "paradigm" interchangeably. Mosey (1985) suggested that "the lack of a common vocabulary could mean many things: a disregard for adequate definitions, an attempt to label each idea as new, or a lack of interest in communicating with each other" (p. 507). Whatever the reason, variation in terminology can be confusing to the reader, and efforts need to be made to clarify labels.

A significant attempt to clarify labels was made by Kortman (1994). She reviewed 20 major texts (from 1912 to 1992) and over 100 articles in eight major English-language journals in occupational therapy (from 1976 to 1992). She wrote,

> The fact that there are so many definitions with so little agreement between theorists, suggests that theorists are taking the wrong path by trying to constantly redefine terms. Individual theorists desiring to facilitate order in this terminology have defined meanings for terms which frequently ignore the common use of the words in the English language.
> The terms model, frame of reference, paradigm and approach are all synonyms: words that have the same meaning. Put simply, in common English a model is a frame of reference is a paradigm is an approach; the terms are interchangeable. Of all these terms, the term model appears to be the simplest to use in relation to theory. (p. 116)

One explanation suggested earlier in this chapter, and supported by Kortman (1994), is that there are different levels of theories on a continuum.

Levels of Conceptualization

In her review of the literature, Kortman (1994) found the existence of three types of models, the highest of which was "characterized by a wide description of the role and practice of occupational therapists. This type of model could be applied across many client groups and practice situations and was often described as a professional 'blueprint'" (p. 117). The nursing literature generally labels this level "grand theory" (Chinn & Kramer, 1995). Five of the theorists in this book have presented recommendations for conceptualizing what OT is about. The terms used to describe these overarching conceptualizations differ; consider Fidler's lifestyle performance model (Chapter 2), Mosey's model (Chapter 3), Llorens's schematic (Chapter 4), Reilly's paradigm (Chapter 6), and Kielhofner's paradigm (Chapter 7).

The second level of theory, which nursing titles "middle-range theory" (Chinn & Kramer, 1995), is concerned with describing "principles to be applied in intervention and provides guiding constructs for assessment" (Kortman, 1994, p. 117). Examples of this level are the biomechanical and neurodevelopmental models, which focus on techniques.

The third level for conceptualizing theory is what nursing terms the "practice model" (Chinn & Kramer, 1995) and what Kortman (1994) calls the "application model." "This type of model clearly describes specific assessment and intervention techniques" (Kortman, 1994, p. 118). Ayres's theory of sensory integration (Chapter 5) is one example of this level.

Occupational therapists can and do use several theories at one time. For instance, a therapist might simultaneously use the Canadian model of occupational performance (CMOP; Townsend, 1997) to conceptualize and evaluate an individual's overall situation and needs, and the theory of sensory integration to guide in-depth assessment and intervention if the CMOP evaluation indicates a problem related to sensory processing.

The ongoing process of clarifying and comparing these labels in a way that is consistent and true to theorists' meanings will be a lengthy one. There obviously are very important differences among these concepts that one must take great care not to oversimplify or gloss over. It is imperative, however, that this process continues.

Why Does It Matter?

There are many good reasons why it is important for occupational therapists to become conscious of, interested in, and competent with the use of theory. These reasons are described in the following sections.

To Validate and Guide Practice

The following excerpt from a 1938 editorial in the journal *Occupational Therapy and Rehabilitation* illustrates that the need for theory and research to justify OT practice is not a new concern:

> The following list of questions was recently sent to us by a therapist connected with one of our large state hospitals, [the questions] having been given her by the psychologist connected with that institution. It can be recognized that they are questions

which are often asked by physicians and sometimes we do not have a ready answer for them so that it is desired to hold a symposium upon them in order that all therapists may be prepared.

1. What is the occupational therapist's theory as to how occupational therapy proves of assistance in bringing about recovery?

2. What are the statistics upon which is based the statement that occupational therapy does aid recovery? ("Editorial," 1938, p. 127)

These remain, today, two of the major issues in promoting and explaining the use of occupational therapy. The first question can be addressed by the therapist familiar with OT theories, and the second can be answered by the occupational therapist who is familiar with the knowledge derived from research in the profession.

The theories that guide everyday practice may be used unconsciously. It is critical to bring those theories into the light of consciousness because they may be incomplete, contradictory, or inconsistent. Although it may at first seem threatening to risk discovering that such is the case, concern for providing the best possible care for patients and acceptance of the reality that we are all always learning should provide the necessary motivation to examine the theories one uses in making practice decisions.

As Parham (1987) put it in her classic work on "the reflective therapist,"

> Theory is a key element in problem setting and in problem solving. It is a tool that enables the therapist to "name it and frame it." Both language and logic are needed to identify a problem (name it) and to plan a means for altering the situation (frame it). Theory provides these by giving us words or concepts for naming what we observe, and by spelling out logical relationships between concepts. This allows us to explain what we see and to figure out how to manipulate a situation to cause change. (p. 557)

As the profession moves into wider circles of influence and even more complex arenas of practice, therapists are having to engage in autonomous decision making and problem solving in multifactorial situations. Knowledge of the well-developed theory in the field provides the means to do this and to keep one's focus on occupational therapy. As Creek and Ormstron (1996) warned, "when [occupational therapists] practice without a sound theory base, they are vulnerable to being taken over by the theories of other groups, particularly by powerful, articulate groups such as medicine or psychology" (p. 8).

To Justify Reimbursement

Validation of practice is directly tied to reimbursement. Those who pay for OT services are ever more demanding of substantive justification for what occupational therapists do: They want both an explanation of why something is being done and a demonstration that what is being done works. The explanation is provided through theory, the demonstration through research.

One of the positive outcomes of the recent crisis in OT and health care is that research, into both the effectiveness of interventions and the validity of the theories upon which they are based, is now recognized, supported, and pursued to a greater extent than ever before. The emphasis on what is now called "evidence-based practice" confirms this shift.

To Clarify Specialization Issues

The issue of specialization is related to theory, because occupational therapists need to be able to balance the technical aspects of practice with underlying theoretical explanations that reflect their basic assumptions and identity as occupational therapists. Otherwise, how can one explain the differences between an occupational therapist who specializes in hand therapy and a physical therapist who also specializes in hand therapy? Or, how does one explain the common connections between an occupational therapist who works with adolescent drug abusers and another one who works with elders with Alzheimer's disease?

To Enhance the Growth of the Profession and the Professionalism of Its Members

One of the major attributes of a profession is that it has a distinctive theoretical base. The use of a theory base to guide decision making is much of what distinguishes a professional person from a technician. Although development of a strong theory base will not guarantee that others accept and recognize occupational therapy as a profession, such acceptance and recognition will certainly not come without it.

Along with admonishing that OT is endangered if the field does not accelerate development in a number of areas, including utilization of theory and research by practitioners, Wood (1998) also cited recent positive growth of the body of OT theory and research as cause for celebration. Wood pointed out, for example, the progressive modernization of sensory integrative theory, which has continuously placed at its center the therapeutic power of self-directed play. Wood cited numerous examples of other areas in which OT literature evidences a significant advance in theory and research, along with their application in innovative as well as traditional practice arenas.

What seems most important in the entire controversy about professionalism is that to deliver the best service, both directly to patients and clients and indirectly through communication with other members of the health care system, occupational therapists need to feel confident about what they are doing and about their ability to communicate why they are doing it. This confidence requires a solid theoretical foundation, as well as the ability to apply that theory to facilitating the functional needs of clients.

To Educate Competent Practitioners

The American Occupational Therapy Association (AOTA) document, "Standards for an Accredited Educational Program for the Occupational Therapist," which were adopted in 1998, states that graduates of professional-level programs will understand OT theories, how they are used in evaluation and intervention, and how they influence practice. Graduates will also "be able to apply theoretical constructs to evaluation and intervention with clients, to analyze and effect meaningful occupation," and to understand theory development and its importance for the profession (AOTA, 1998a). These requirements emphasize the importance of theory in enabling a new graduate to engage in independent, critical thinking. Also, to continue to practice with competence, occupational therapists need to keep abreast of new developments in theory and related research throughout their careers. Not only is this a requirement according to the AOTA "Standards of Practice for Occupational Therapy" (AOTA, 1998b, p. 866), but also, as Wood (1998) stated, "It is time to jump into a professional ethic where it would be as unthinkable for occupational therapists to practice without keeping abreast of their field's leading research [and therefore theory] as it would be for one's physician to be similarly outdated" (p. 408).

Theory as a Unifying Foundation

The theoretical base of OT should and can provide major connections among the various aspects of the field. One certainly should be able to explain best those theories that one uses most often. Possessing an understanding of the major theories that influence practice in the field is a goal to which each occupational therapist can aspire, not only in order to be well educated and better able to communicate, but also to be better able to define oneself as an occupational therapist and have confidence that what one is doing with clients and students, as well as in research, is well founded.

One must take care, however, in using any theory without adequate knowledge. Attempts to apply theories with only a cursory understanding of concepts and principles can lead to inaccurate assumptions and potentially harmful practice, with contradictory and confusing outcomes. The words used to describe and explain new theories also can lead to confusion, as different theorists often use different words to name similar concepts. Although there are increasing numbers of theories in the profession, they all directly relate to the field's philosophical assumptions and address OT's common domain of concern, either in whole or in part.

Founding Assumptions and Values

To best understand occupational therapy theories, one needs to know the underlying ideas, values, and beliefs on which the profession was founded. These founding assumptions included a view of occupational therapy that was holistic and humanistic; valued occupation, handcrafts, and habit training; and promoted adaptation, a balance of work and play, and science. The profession proceeded to grow on the basis of these assumptions and values until theorists such as Fidler and Reilly began to move the profession to the next step of theory development in the 1950s and 1960s (see Chapters 2 and 6).

Occupational Therapy Is Holistic

Occupational therapy was envisioned as a profession that would minister to body, mind, and soul. As Meyer (1921/1948b) saw it, "Nothing will replace a simple study of the life factors and the social and personal life problems and their working—the study of the real mind and the real soul, i.e., human life itself" (p. 7). He argued, "Our body is not merely so many pounds of flesh and bone figuring as a machine, with an abstract mind or soul added to it. It is throughout a living organism pulsating with its rhythm of rest and activity" (Meyer, 1922, p. 5). Meyer (1921/1948b) spoke against the medical perspective that reduced the individual to a part or organ. "The great mistake of an overambitious science has been the desire to study [human beings] altogether as a mere sum of the parts, if possible of atoms . . . and as a machine, detached, by itself" (p. 3).

The "Principles of Occupational Therapy," first articulated by a committee chaired by Dunton, explicitly stated that occupational therapists were expected to use a holistic approach to address all aspects of an individual's life: "to arouse interest, courage and confidence; to exercise mind and body in healthy activity; to overcome functional disability; and to re-establish capacity for industrial and social usefulness" (Dunton, Adams, Carr, & Robinson, 1925). Similarly, Johnson (1920) iterated occupational therapy's goal to address the body and the mind in a "rejoining of self-confidence, satisfaction in accomplishment, the direction of thought into wholesome channels, and graded physical exercise producing a healthful tired feeling" (p. 70). Kidner (1930) characterized the holistic approach by citing the novelist John Galsworthy's speech to a post–World War I Conference on the After-Care of Disabled Men:

> Restoration is a matter of spirit as well as of body, and must have as its central truth: body and spirit are inextricably conjoined. To heal the one without the other is impossible. . . . To

carry the process of restoration to a point short of this is to leave the cathedral without spire. (p. 41)

Occupational Therapy Is Humanistic

Occupational therapy was founded on the belief that human beings—their values, capacities, and achievements—were the fundamental concern of the occupational therapist and should be the focus of the therapeutic process. "A respect for [the individual's] dignity as a starting point and central issue, and each 'human' as the resultant democratic person, is something to work on and to work for" (Meyer, 1943/1948e, p. 629). This belief was based on the doctrine of humanism, which held that the individual "is the most important issue that civilization today should consider its concern, if we are to [have] . . . a livable society" (Meyer, 1934/1948d, p. 318).

Dunton (1917) traced the historical roots of occupational therapy back to the humanistic movement known as moral treatment. Moral treatment began in the 19th century with Philippe Pinel (1809), a French physician and scholar who proposed a "revolution morale" (p. 260) in which persons with mental illness would be treated according to humane principles, which included occupation, in place of the approach that viewed persons with mental illness as unredeemable beings to be hidden away and chained to their beds. As a 20th-century psychiatrist, Dunton proposed that moral treatment remained the best approach for occupational therapists to use in the treatment of persons with mental illness.

Occupation Is Essential

Occupational therapy was founded on the assumption that engagement in occupation was an essential part of life—the way to gain and maintain health. Dunton (1931) asserted, "No matter what may be the environment, occupation of some sort is a necessity for men, women, and children" (p. 6). Meyer (1895), one of the earliest proponents of using occupation in treatment, declared, "Occupation is, with good right, called the most essential side of hygienic treatment" (p. 59). According to Barton (1920), occupation strengthened the body, clarified the mind, and offered "a new life upon recovery" (p. 307). Johnson (1920) emphasized occupation's ability to "divert the mind from destructive tendencies, substitute normal interests and constructive activity, and crystallize them into right mental habits" (p. 69). Hall (1913) documented the changes that took place when a patient was engaged in occupation: "After a few weeks of work . . . observe the change in facial expression, in precision and skill of movement and in the morale of the patient" (p. 10).

Meyer (1934/1948d) advocated that, to effectively treat patients, occupational therapists should examine all aspects of occupation within a person's life:

> We take up a survey of functions of the person beginning with the full-fledged performances and achievements and attempts that give an idea of the individual; the personal care, the jobs and hobbies . . . family, sociability, public life, education, religious activity, etc. . . . [all] interests and ambitions, one's perceptive life (sensual and esthetic gratifications), dreaming, thinking, acting. (p. 319)

Once this analysis is completed, the occupational therapist engages the patient in therapeutic occupations chosen specifically for that individual based on interest and purpose.

> Occupational therapy should be of interest, therefore a certain amount of variety is necessary . . . [and] useful, not aimless. Occupational therapy must be individualistic. Each patient is a law unto himself and the occupational therapy should be given which is best fitted to meet the peculiar conditions of the case. (Dunton, et al., 1925, pp. 278–279)

Johnson (1920) warned that when the right occupations were not selected by the therapist, the patient was at risk of becoming demoralized from "routine occupations which provide exercise for muscles only and call forth little or no mental activity or self expression" (p. 70).

Handcrafts Have Therapeutic Value

The profession's founding coincided with a surge in popularity for the creative arts and crafts in the United States. This was in large part due to the arts and crafts movement that originated in England with William Morris and John Ruskin. The movement was established as an attempt to ameliorate the negative effects of industrialization by advocating that people return to a simpler life, a time when hand-crafted objects were created by individuals rather than by machines and factories (Boris, 1986).

Early occupational therapists recognized the therapeutic value in having their patients engage in creative, pleasurable handcrafts and used them for diversion, prevocational interest, and curative value. The occupation classes that Dunton supervised at Sheppard-Pratt Hospital used leatherwork, weaving, art, and bookbinding (Fields, 1911). Under the supervision of Eleanor Clarke Slagle at Phipps Clinic, groups of patients worked with "rafia and basket work, or with various kinds of handiwork and weaving and bookbinding and metal and leatherwork" (Meyer, 1922, p. 3). According to a committee formulated by AOTA, "The [occupation] shop should be equipped with large and small looms . . . [and] equipment for metal work, basketry, and other handcrafts" (Dunton et al., 1925, p. 283). Johnson (1920), a former arts and crafts teacher, eloquently described the therapeutic effect of handcrafts:

> The regaining of self-confidence, satisfaction in accomplishment, the direction of thought into wholesome and normal channels, and graded physical exercise producing a healthful tired feeling without overstrain which in turn brings its demand for relaxation, rest and sleep, are all factors within the therapeutic value of handcrafts. (p.70)

Habit Training Is Critical

At the time of the founding of occupational therapy, many new theories were being proposed in the psychiatric community for the cause and treatment of persons with mental illness. Some professionals hypothesized that genetics was the important factor; others emphasized environmental factors; still others supported Freud's ego construct. In contrast, Meyer spent his career advocating what he called his "commonsense" approach. Although he admitted that genes, environment, and ego could all be important, Meyer (1905/1948a) asserted that an understanding of habits was also critical:

> It will be our duty to define in actual cases what sets of habits
> we find interwoven and with what effect. This directs the
> attention to the investigation of matters which are open to in-
> fluence in education, and to a more rational management of
> dementia praecox, as well as many other mental disorders.
> (p. 180)

He further argued that it was necessary to distinguish "various
types of habit disorganization, to study the working of the various sets of activities and habits in the patient, determine their
relative value by accurate observation . . . and shape our therapeutic measures in accord with these principles" (p. 181).

Meyer (1905/1948a) proposed that "habit-disorder is to be
treated by habit training" (p. 180) and hired Slagle to help im-
plement such a program in occupational therapy at Phipps
Clinic.

> The first point is development of habits which can be thor-
> oughly satisfied in harmony with the environment and with
> ample opportunity for satisfaction. . . . There must be habits of
> work for which there is a market and call, habits of care of one-
> self in keeping with the probable opportunities, habits of recre-
> ation easily enough dovetailed with life, habits of melioristic
> self-culture—social, educational, civil and religious habits and
> contacts." (Meyer, 1922/1948c, p. 486)

Slagle applied habit training to the most profoundly involved patients. She designed programs for small groups of patients
which followed a strict schedule that included self-care and personal hygiene, walks and other physical activities, occupation
classes, and meals.

> To visualize the picture more clearly, let us consider a group of
> sixteen untidy, destructive, assaultive, abusive and rapidly de-
> teriorating young women who were selected. . . . These patients
> were placed on a twenty-four hour program which had been
> drawn up by the director of occupational therapy. . . . At the
> end of considerably less than a year's intensive work fifteen of
> this group are entirely retrained in decent habits of living and
> are now being trained in carefully graded tasks. (Slagle, 1924,
> p. 100)

Adaptation Requires a Balance of Work, Play, and Rest

In his paper "The Philosophy of Occupation Therapy," Meyer (1922) conceptualized mental illness as a disorder of adaptation, and he defined successful adaptation as "being and living and acting in time and harmony with [one's] nature" (p. 5). He described the many rhythms of life to which we must be attuned: "the larger rhythms of night and day, of sleep and waking hours, of hunger and its gratification, and finally the big four—work and play and rest and sleep" (p. 6). He proposed that the only way an individual learned to achieve balance was through "actual doing, actual practice" (p. 6). According to Meyer, people learn to organize time in the context of doing things, "and one of the many good things [they do] between eating, drinking, and wholesome nutrition . . . we call work and occupation . . . and proper use . . . of time with its successions of opportunities" (pp. 9–10).

Meyer (1922) proposed that occupational therapists were the professionals most suited to assist individuals in gaining mastery over their use of time and achieving a balance of work, play, and rest.

> The awakening to a full meaning of time as the biggest wonder and asset of our lives and the valuation of opportunity and performance as the greatest measure of time; those are the beacon-lights of the philosophy of the occupation worker. (p. 9)

Meyer suggested that occupational therapy would help each individual to structure a treatment program that created an "orderly rhythm . . . the sense of a day simply and naturally spent, perhaps with some music and restful dance and play, and with some glimpses of activities which one can hope to achieve and derive satisfaction from" (p. 6). It would be the occupational therapist's responsibility to engage the patient in occupations that were of personal interest and within the individual's capability. This was particularly important because

> a large proportion of our patients present inferiority feelings, often over a sense of awkwardness and inability to use the hands to produce things worth while, i.e., respected by themselves or others. To get the pleasure and pride of achievement

and use of one's hands and muscles, the feeling of worth-while-ness of a little effort and of a well fitted use of time, is the basic remedy. (pp. 6–7)

Scientific Research Is Important but Restrictive

At the time the profession was founded, a popular belief was that science could reform all of society's problems, including health care (Wiebe, 1967). This belief was justified by the many scientific discoveries in the 20th century that resulted in vastly improved medical care. The founders recognized the importance of science as a way to gain knowledge about occupations and to justify the profession. Hall (1913) established Devereux Mansion as an experimental laboratory to study occupations for "invalids." Barton (1916/1917) proposed that time and motion studies provided an excellent model for the study of occupations. Dunton (1928) led an effort to systematically analyze occupations.

One problem with scientific inquiry in occupational therapy was that the prevalent scientific models and attitudes did not easily support analysis that took into account the full complexity of the individual and his or her engagement in occupation. Meyer (1943/1948e), for example, was concerned with a scientific perspective that was too reductionistic in viewing human beings. He advocated a "concept of a science of the whole person in his pluralistic nature and settings" (p. 628). He (1934/1948d) argued that we need to "change the arbitrary dogma of science and study [the individual] with, and as, a living soul and full-souled body" (p. 318). Thus, although the founders acknowledged the importance of scientific inquiry and promoted the study of occupations, they also recognized the limitations of the scientific models that were in use at that time.

Beyond These Foundations

The assumptions and values articulated by the individuals who helped to establish the profession of OT emphasized a humanistic, holistic approach that recognized the multifaceted nature of the individual, as well as the complexity of the process that stimulated engagement in occupation. Meyer (1922) wrote that successful adaptation required a balance of work, play, and rest, and that the occupational therapist was best suited to design a therapeutic program that could engage the individual in the occupations that would best achieve adaptation. Two primary modalities for achieving this were through habit training and handcrafts. The following chapters in this book describe how these founding assumptions evolved into OT theories.

From 1950 to 1990, each theory developed in occupational therapy was identified with one individual. In each of the next seven chapters, the life and work of one of these major theorists are described. Each chapter begins with a biographical sketch of the theorist in an effort to place the person in social and professional context, to identify influences on his or her theory development, and to "demystify" by presenting the person behind the ideas. We hope that this will both enlighten the reader as to the theorist's perspective and inspire the reader to see his or her own practice and potential within a broader historical and professional context.

Beginning in the late 1980s, new theories began to be developed by pairs or groups of individuals working together, and occupational therapists in countries outside the United States became more active and influential in theory development. Also during this time, the academic discipline of occupational science was founded and began to influence OT toward greater consensus that occupation was the central concept around which OT theories should be built. The most influential of these issues and theories are addressed in Chapter 9. In the final chapter, theorists and the central ideas from their theories are compared and contrasted within the context of the political, social, and professional events of their times.

References

American Occupational Therapy Association. (1998a). *Standards for an accredited educational program for the occupational therapist*. Retrieved July 5, 2003, from http://www.aota.org/nonmembers/area13/links/LINK31.asp

American Occupational Therapy Association. (1998b). Standards of practice for occupational therapy. *American Journal of Occupational Therapy, 52*, 866–869.

Ayres, A. J. (1965). Sensory integrative processes and neuropsychological learning disability. In J. Hellmuth (Ed.), *Learning disorders* (Vol. 3, pp. 41–58). Seattle, WA: Special Child Publication.

Barton, G. E. (1917). The movies and the microscope. Occupational therapy: The papers of George Edward Barton. (*Trained Nurse and Hospital Review, 62,* 193–197. (Original work published 1916)

Barton, G. E. (1920). What occupational therapy may mean to nursing. *Trained Nurse and Hospital Review, 64,* 304–310.

Beard, M. T. (2000). Theory development in a new millennium. *The Journal of Theory Construction and Testing, 4,* 5–6.

Boris, E. (1986). *Art and labor: Ruskin, Morris, and the craftsman ideal in America.* Philadelphia: Temple University.

Carlson, M. E., & Clark, F. (1991). The search for useful methodologies in occupational science. *American Journal of Occupational Therapy, 45,* 235–241.

Chinn, P. L., & Kramer, M. K. (1995). *Theory and nursing: A systematic approach.* St. Louis, MO: Mosby.

Creek, J., & Feaver, S. (1993). Models of practice in occupational therapy: Part 1, Defining terms. *British Journal of Occupational Therapy, 56,* 4–6.

Creek, J., & Ormstron, C. (1996). The essential elements of professional motivation. *British Journal of Occupational Therapy, 59,* 7–10.

Duldt, B. W., & Giffin, K. (1985). *Theoretical perspectives for nursing.* Boston: Little, Brown.

Dunton, W. R. (1917). History of occupational therapy. *The Modern Hospital, 8,* 380–382.

Dunton, W. R. (1928). The three "R's" of occupational therapy. *Occupational Therapy and Rehabilitation, 7,* 345–348.

Dunton, W. R. (1931). Occupational therapy. *Proceedings of the Congress on Medical Education, Medical Licensure and Hospitals* (pp. 1–6). Chicago: American Medical Association.

Dunton, W. R., Adams, J. D., Carr, B. W., & Robinson, G. C. (1925). Outline of lectures on occupational therapy to medical students and physicians. *Occupational Therapy and Rehabilitation, 4,* 277–292.

Editorial. (1938, April). *Occupational Therapy and Rehabilitation, 17,* 127.

Fields, G. E. (1911). The effect of occupation upon the individual. *The American Journal of Insanity, 8,* 103–109.

Folger, R., & Turillo, C. J. (1999). Theorizing as the thickness of thin abstraction. *Academy of Management Review, 24,* 742–758.

Geyman, J. P., Deyo, R. A., & Ramsey, S. D. (2000). *Evidence-based clinical practice: Concepts and approaches.* Boston: Butterworth Heinemann.

Giuffre, M. (1998). Science and theory. *Journal of PeriAnesthesia Nursing, 13,* 35–38.

Hall, H. J. (1913). *The systematic use of work as a remedy in neurasthenia and allied conditions.* Boston: W. M. Leonard.

Hasselkus, B. R. (1995). Beyond ethnography: Expanding our understanding and criteria for qualitative research. *Occupational Therapy Journal of Research, 15,* 75–84.

Hull, D. L. (1983). *Darwin and his critics: The reception of Darwin's theory of evolution by the scientific community.* Chicago: University of Chicago Press.

Johnson, S. C. (1920). Instruction in handcrafts and design for hospital patients. *Modern Hospital, 15,* 69–75.

Kidner, T. B. (1930). *Occupational therapy: The science of prescribed work for invalids.* Stuttgart, Germany: W. Kohlhammer.

Kielhofner, G. (1992). *Conceptual foundations of occupational therapy.* Philadelphia: F.A. Davis.

Kielhofner, G. (1995). *A model of human occupation: Theory and application* (2nd ed.). Baltimore: Williams & Wilkins.

Kortman, B. (1994). The eye of the beholder: Models in occupational therapy. *Australian Occupational Therapy Journal, 41,* 115–122.

Kuhn, T. S. (1957). *The Copernican revolution: Planetary astronomy in the development of western thought.* Cambridge, MA: Harvard University Press.

Lewin, K. (1947). *Principles of topological psychology.* New York: McGraw-Hill.

Liehr, P., & Smith, M. J. (1999). Middle range theory: Spinning research and practice to create knowledge for the new millennium. *Advances in Nursing Science, 21,* 81–91.

McEwen, M. (2000). Teaching theory at the master's level: Report of a national survey of theory instructors. *Journal of Professional Nursing, 16,* 354–361.

Meyer, A. (1895). Treatment of the insane: A report to the governor of Illinois. In *The commonsense psychiatry of Dr. Adolph Meyer: Fifty-two selected papers* (pp. 53–60). New York: McGraw-Hill.

Meyer, A. (1922). The philosophy of occupation therapy. *Archives of Occupational Therapy, 1,* 1–10.

Meyer, A. (1948a). The role of habit-disorganizations: Paper for the New York Psychiatrical Society. In A. Lief (Ed.), *The commonsense psychiatry of Dr. Adolph Meyer: Fifty-two selected papers* (pp. 178–183). New York: McGraw-Hill. (Original work published 1905)

Meyer, A. (1948b). The contributions of psychiatry to the understanding of life problems: An address at the celebration of the 100th anniversary of Bloomingdale Hospital. In A. Lief (Ed.), *The commonsense psychiatry of Dr. Adolph Meyer: Fifty-two selected papers* (pp. 1–15). New York: McGraw-Hill. (Original work published 1921)

Meyer, A. (1948c). Normal and abnormal repression: Address to the Progressive Education Association. In A. Lief (Ed.), *The commonsense psychiatry of Dr. Adolph Meyer: Fifty-two selected papers* (pp. 479–490). New York: McGraw-Hill. (Original work published 1922)

Meyer, A. (1948d). The birth and development of the mental-hygiene movement: A paper for the 25th anniversary dinner of the National Committee for Mental Hygiene. In A. Lief (Ed.), *The commonsense psychiatry of Dr. Adolph Meyer: Fifty-two selected papers* (pp. 312–319). New York: McGraw-Hill. (Original work published 1934)

Meyer, A. (1948e). Respect of self and others and equity for peace: A paper for the fourth symposium of the Conference on Science, Philosophy and Religion. In A. Lief, (Ed.), *The commonsense psychiatry of Dr. Adolph Meyer: Fifty-two selected papers* (pp. 628–636). New York: McGraw-Hill. (Original work published 1943)

Mosey, A. C. (1985). The Eleanor Clarke Slagle Lecture, 1985: A monistic or a pluralistic approach to professional identity? *American Journal of Occupational Therapy, 39,* 504–509.

Mosey, A. C. (1992). *Applied scientific inquiry in the health professions: An epistemological orientation.* Rockville, MD: American Occupational Therapy Association.

Ostrow, P. C. (1980). The foundation: The care and feeding of theories. *American Journal of Occupational Therapy, 34,* 272–273.

Ottenbacher, K. J. (1992). Confusion in occupational therapy research: Does the end justify the method? *American Journal of Occupational Therapy, 46,* 871–874.

Parham, L. D. (1987). Toward professionalism: The reflective therapist. *American Journal of Occupational Therapy, 41,* 555–561.

Pinel, P. (1809). *Traite medico-philosophique sur l'alienation mentale* (2nd ed.). Paris: J. A. Brosson.

Reed, K. L. (1998). Theory and frames of reference. In M. E. Neistadt & E. B. Crepeau (Eds.), *Willard and Spackman's occupational therapy* (9th ed.; pp. 521–524). Philadelphia: Lippincott.

Slagle, E. C. (1924). A year's development of occupational therapy in New York State hospitals. *Occupational Therapy and Rehabilitation, 22,* 98–104.

Taylor, M. C. (2000). *Evidence-based practice for occupational therapists.* London: Blackwell Science.

Townsend, E. (Ed.), (1997). *Enabling occupation: An occupational therapy perspective.* Ottawa, Ontario: Canadian Association of Occupational Therapists.

Walker, K. F. (1993). A. Jean Ayres. In R. J. Miller & K. F. Walker (Eds.), *Perspectives on theory for the practice of occupational therapy.* Gaithersburg, MD: Aspen.

Wiebe, R. H. (1967). *The search for order: 1877–1920.* New York: Farrar, Straus and Giroux.

Wood, W. (1998). It is jump time for occupational therapy. *American Journal of Occupational Therapy, 52,* 403–411.

Yerxa, E. J. (1991). Nationally speaking: Seeking a relevant, ethical and realistic way of knowing for occupational therapy. *American Journal of Occupational Therapy, 45,* 199–204.

Zemke, R., & Clark, F. (Eds.). (1996). *Occupational science: The evolving discipline.* Philadelphia: F.A. Davis.

Gail Fidler

Ferol Menks Ludwig

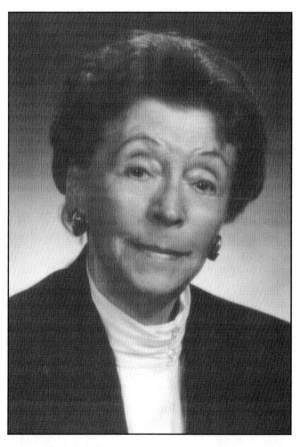

I urge that occupation be understood as the science of doing—an art and science that explains the meaning and defines the uses of occupation. (Fidler, 2000, pp. 99–100)

This sentence by Gail Fidler characterizes her central pursuit throughout her 60-year career in occupational therapy, which is to explain the processes involved in matching the characteristics of the activity with the person, and the dynamics of these processes in "triggering and sustaining motivation" (2000, p. 100). In this chapter, I attempt the awesome task of reviewing her works. I begin with Gail Fidler's biographical sketch, which is helpful for appreciating her as an individual as well as a leader in the field.

Biographical Sketch

Gail Fidler was born in Spencer, Iowa, in 1916. The first of four children, she lived with her family in South Dakota and later in Lebanon, Pennsylvania. Her father was a high school teacher and coach who fostered her avid interest in sports. She played varsity basketball and field hockey in high school and college, and later used her certification as a basketball referee to help support herself during occupational therapy school. Other activities in high school and college included being on the debating team, writing poetry for the college paper, doing art illustrations, and performing with her local church's drama club and choral group.

Educational Background

Gail Fidler earned her bachelor of arts degree from Lebanon Valley College in 1938 with a double major in education and psychology. After graduation she worked for 6 months as a high school history teacher, but she found the school system to be too constricting for her (G. Fidler, personal communication, May 13, 1982). At that time, limited financial resources prevented her from pursuing graduate work in psychology or attending medical school to become a psychiatrist. To earn the money for tuition, she worked as a hospital attendant at Wernersville State Hospital, where she discovered occupational therapy (OT). She described the director of OT as an interesting and well-educated person with whom she felt that she could connect, and she appreciated the normalizing, pleasant atmosphere of the OT clinic.

I was impressed by the change in patients' behavior while they were in occupational therapy. They seemed almost like different persons when they were engaged in productive activity. Working as an attendant on the back wards of the state hospital was an incredible learning experience for me. It was extremely difficult, challenging and exciting, all at the same time. (G. Fidler, personal communication, July 1992)

She enrolled in the OT certificate program at the University of Pennsylvania in 1940 and, while attending the program, was employed as a group worker at Smith Memorial Settlement House in Philadelphia until her graduation in 1942. During a summer break, she returned to work at the Wernersville State Hospital, where she met a medical student, Jay Fidler, who was to become her husband in 1944.

Always stimulated by the questions raised in practice, Fidler sought more answers by attending the William Alanson White Institute of Psychiatry and Psychology in New York City from 1947 to 1951. During this time, she was significantly influenced by the work of Harry Stack Sullivan (1953), particularly his interpersonal theory and hypotheses regarding ego development, self-esteem, and competence. Gail Fidler wanted to pursue graduate education in occupational therapy, but at the time no such program existed. She enrolled in the graduate clinical psychology program at New York University but withdrew after one semester because she felt it was not relevant to the questions that she had or to what she wanted to do. Several years later she enrolled in social work and discontinued that for similar reasons.

Professional Roles

Gail Fidler has explored many career roles and made many contributions in all of them and continues to do so. The following sections describe her accomplishments.

Clinician

Her first position as an occupational therapist was in 1942 at the Norristown State Hospital in Pennsylvania. She described this experience:

It was quite different than my experiences with OT as a student. I had high expectations and what I was seeing in practice was certainly different. I suddenly had to confront reality in comparison to my expectations, knowing that I could not stay in OT if it was no more than I was seeing. It was quite upsetting to suspect that I had made an error in choosing occupational therapy as a career. (G. Fidler, personal communication, May 13, 1982)

In retrospect the department of OT at Norristown was probably the most comprehensive and best organized one that I have seen. It was highly respected and acknowledged as a valuable service to patients. What was lacking, and disturbing to me, was a rationale for practice. The whys were not being asked and the challenge of hypotheses—of theoretical explanation—was simply not being faced. (G. Fidler, personal communication, November 3, 1987)

She decided, however, that it was not wise to make a decision on the basis of sheer emotion, so she entered into a year's contract with herself to study and explore thoroughly the potential of OT in psychiatry. She clearly defined the procedures that she would follow to answer the question, "Is this all that there is to OT?" She decided that if at the end of a year she discovered that occupational therapy was no more than what was reflected in current practice, she would leave the field. During the following year, she methodically attempted to find some rationale for what her 60 patients were doing and how the activities were or were not helpful. It was during this time that she conceived the idea of her activity analysis, which is described in more detail later in "Theoretical Concepts."

Midway through my searches I was hooked and felt that at this time I could not pursue medical school or any other career. I had hold of this idea and I needed to see it through. It has been almost 40 years of seeing it through. (G. Fidler, personal communication, May 13, 1982)

During that year she also had the opportunity to learn from Dr. Alfred Noyes, a renowned psychiatrist and superintendent of Norristown State Hospital. "It was a rare privilege to see this man in action and my commitment to psychiatry and to the pursuit of a rationale for occupational therapy was reconfirmed" (G. Fidler, personal communication, May 1, 1987). She also stated,

> Mainly my motivation has come from a very fundamental itch that began during that first year of inquiry. This thesis is that there has to be some relationship among what people do, their interests, how they occupy their time, their state of health, and their characteristic personality patterns. (G. Fidler, personal communication, May 13, 1982)

Early in her career, Fidler also worked as an occupational therapist at Walter Reed Army Hospital, Washington, D.C.; chief occupational therapist at the Army Hospital in Fort Story, Virginia; and as a staff therapist at the Veterans Hospital in Lyons, New Jersey.

Educator

Throughout her career, Fidler has displayed a strong dedication and enthusiasm for the education of the young professional. From 1952 to 1955, she was an instructor with the Pennsylvania Department of Mental Health Training Programs. In that capacity, she assumed a major teaching and consultant role in implementing an ongoing series of training institutes for program staff throughout the Pennsylvania mental health system. She has contributed to many educational programs for occupational therapists. She taught a summer session at the Philadelphia School of Occupational Therapy. While working at the New York State Psychiatric Institute and Hillside Hospital, Fidler directed the master's degree programs in psychiatric occupational therapy at New York University and at Columbia University. She introduced occupational therapists to supervision as a tutorial learning process and offered the first workshops in supervision at Columbia University in the 1950s. During the 1970s, she was a visiting professor at the University of California at San Jose, Kean College, the University of Pennsylvania, and Boston University. In the summer of 1990, Fidler was asked by College Misericordia to assume the position of interim program director of occupational therapy. With almost 300 students in three different tracks at the school, the college found itself suddenly without a program director and with only two faculty members. She commented,

> I was indeed surprised at their request for me to help them out, since academic administration was something that I had never done. Although I had taught students, part time teaching is a far cry from academic administration and being enmeshed in the system of higher education. However, I have always looked for challenge in any position that I have ever taken; the challenge of problems, and the challenge of learning. What I discovered as Interim Program Director, very rapidly, was that there were plenty of both! (G. Fidler, personal communication, July 1992)

From 1991 to 1995, she was a "scholar in residence" at College Misericordia. It was here that she began her association with Beth Velde, and they continue to work together to develop further the lifestyle performance model. She also continues to meet with students and looks forward to these opportunities to mentor.

Administrator and Consultant

From 1959 to 1968, Fidler served as director of professional education for the Department of Occupational Therapy at the New York State Psychiatric Institute. In that position she developed and directed clinical field work study for occupational therapists and students; provided in-service education to physician residents, social workers, and nurses; supervised OT staff; initiated prevocational and work rehabilitation programs; developed patient evaluation and diagnostic measures; and collaborated with the sociology department to research and measure the nature and effect of change within institutional systems.

Next, Fidler became director of the Activities Therapy Department at Hillside Hospital, where she was responsible for administration, coordination, and management of a staff consisting of occupational therapists, vocational counselors, therapeutic recreators, secondary school teachers, music and dance therapists, and volunteers. She designed and implemented new service programs for the day hospital, aftercare center, and acute admission center. She served as liaison between the city school system and the school at Hillside Hospital and planned in-service education for teachers on working with adolescents with emotional disturbances. She also developed undergraduate and graduate fieldwork experiences with 10 curricula and collaborated to develop a community outreach rehabilitation grant.

Fidler also served as a consultant to several state and hospital programs. During the 1970s and 1980s, she continued her consultative services to several psychiatric hospitals, where she planned and organized OT services and activity therapy programs and coordinated these services with vocational rehabilitation. The Department of Rehabilitation Services that she developed at Springfield Hospital Center in Maryland was subsequently used as a model for service delivery in mental health hospitals throughout the state.

During the 1980s, Fidler served as the assistant hospital administrator for programming at Greystone Park Psychiatric Hospital in New Jersey. She was a consultant in curriculum development to the New York University Department of Occupational Therapy, and was appointed rehabilitation consultant to the New Jersey Division of Mental Health Hospitals. During her tenure as rehabilitation consultant, she developed and had approved state standards for rehabilitation programs in mental health facilities and agencies and established staffing standards and quality assurance monitoring.

From 1984 to 1988, she was chief executive officer of the Hagadorn Center for Geriatrics, a New Jersey state facility. In 1987, she completed a major reorganization of the center from a long-term nursing care facility to a geropsychiatric rehabilitation center that provides community-based day treatment and housing programs to sustain the elderly in the community. According to Fidler, "Hagadorn Center operates on those fundamental constructs of occupational therapy which emphasize and prioritize the meaning and value of human performance and the ability 'to do' as the quality of life and as characterizing health" (G. Fidler, personal communication, May 1, 1987).

National Association Positions

From 1955 to 1957, Fidler was the coordinator of the American Occupational Therapy Association (AOTA) Psychiatric Study Group, which was funded by a National Institute of Mental

Health (NIMH) grant to examine, assess, and define the current concepts and practice of OT in psychiatry and to find ways to improve the preparation of future occupational therapists in this specialty area. This study culminated in the Allenbury Workshop Conference on the Function and Preparation of the Psychiatric Occupational Therapist. The proceedings of this workshop conference were published in the book *Changing Concepts and Practices in Psychiatric Occupational Therapy,* which was edited by Wilma West (1959). Fidler served as one of the editorial consultants for this book.

Fidler served as member-at-large for the AOTA board of management from 1957 to 1963. In January 1971, she served as associate executive director, managing the practice, education, and research divisions. She wrote grants that enabled AOTA to offer a series of training institutes for practitioners and educators. She was instrumental in obtaining a grant to support graduate traineeships, and she helped AOTA secure grants totaling over $500,000 to conduct several major studies.

Fidler served as interim executive director of AOTA from March 1975 until that October, when she became coordinator of AOTA's Educator Training Institutes. In that capacity, she planned, organized, and implemented regional institutes for OT academic and clinical faculty from all of the professional and technical programs. These institutes focused on curriculum design, teaching methods, and competency-based learning. An outgrowth of these educator institutes was the project to revise the certified occupational therapist and the certified occupational therapy assistant registration examinations to emphasize competency-based outcomes in preference to the accumulation of knowledge.

Volunteer Professional Organization Leader

Because of her firm commitment to the development of OT as a profession, Fidler has been very active in volunteer professional activities from the beginning of her career. She has chaired numerous task forces within AOTA and has served on many of its committees. She also has been on the board of directors of the AOTF and on the advisory board of the *American Journal of Occupational Therapy.* Fidler is also a member of a number of professional organizations. She has served on the advisory board of Kean College, on the board of the Coalition for the Reform of the

New Jersey Mental Health System, and on the board of directors of the Union County Mental Health Association and its professional advisory committee. She was also a member of the New Jersey Rehabilitation Committee and was the chair of the monitoring committee in the Office of the Public Advocate for the State of New Jersey.

Honors

Fidler has received the highest honors awarded by the OT profession. In 1965 she was the Eleanor Clarke Slagle Lecturer (Fidler, 1966a), and in 1980 she was presented the AOTA Award of Merit. She is also a Fellow of the AOTA. She has received many other honors and rewards for her work with states, universities, and colleges.

Author

Fidler has written over 30 articles and chapters, has authored or coauthored six books, and is still writing.

Civic Involvement

Fidler's civic activities included involvement with the League of Women Voters, United Fund Council, Visiting Nurse Association Homemakers Program, Education Committee for Teachers and Parents, Plainfield Public Schools, and Union County Aftercare Program. In her work with this latter group, she was instrumental in developing the state's first psychiatric aftercare program.

Personal Roles

Fidler is the very proud mother of two children, a daughter Dagny and a son Eric, and she has two grandchildren. She and her husband, Jay, reside in Fort Lauderdale, Florida.

Looking back over her many contributions in a myriad of roles, one cannot help but be impressed by the perseverance and the contributions of a feisty leader who has influenced the lives and careers of countless health professionals. She continues to give presentations, institutes, and workshops, and to engage in independent practice.

Reflections on the Profession

Fidler believes that some of the obstacles to theory development in OT stem from the profession's minority position in the health care system and its subsequent difficulty influencing the medical model with its own concepts and constructs. She commented,

> I've always said that what we really have to deal with is double jeopardy. What we theorize and practice is not in the top priority of the medical and health care delivery system structure. It is so "mundane" and seemingly obvious that it carries very little glamour, and it is hard to convince people of the value of something that is part of their everyday life. It is hard to maintain one's professional self-respect when references are continually made to psychology, the psychiatrist, the nurse, the social worker and "others." I was an "and others" for so long it became difficult to maintain a level of ego strength and self-respect in the practice arena. (G. Fidler, personal communication, May 13, 1982)

Any success or contributions that Gail Fidler made were often credited to her personally rather than to the profession. This angered her because she experienced it as a criticism of the profession.

Another barrier to the development of the OT profession involved attitudes about its predominantly female composition, which tend to perpetuate its minority status and are the other half of the "double jeopardy" concept.

> We are many times our own worst enemy and there is a critical need to develop more assertive behaviors and attitudes among our members. We need to state what we do, write it, and publicize it. We need to educate and socialize students into professional behaviors, rather than reinforcing female stereotypical behaviors. (G. Fidler, personal communication, May 13, 1982)

To address this concern, Fidler saw the need to recruit young, bright, and ambitious women and men and to stimulate them by providing an assertive career role model within the profession. Fidler also has offered workshops across the country to teach skills for negotiating the system and to facilitate the development of leadership skills, behaviors, and attitudes based on awareness of self and on interpersonal competence. At the 1992 AOTA conference, her presentation titled "Our Search for Efficacy" dealt with these issues.

More recently, Fidler (personal communication, June 2001) stated that OT today had lost a pool of bright and intelligent women who are now able to become physicians, executives, and lawyers. Furthermore, many women in the profession still think of having a job and not a career and accept a job that accommodates their lifestyle instead of making a career commitment.

Because occupational therapy is a very complex profession, Fidler has long believed that a master's degree should be a prerequisite for entry-level positions in the field. To understand the constructs of the art and science of the field requires a longer term of educational socialization than is provided by baccalaureate programs. Other bona fide professions are built on graduate-level work, and their entry into practice is at the graduate level (G. Fidler, personal communication, May 13, 1982).

In 1982 (personal communication), Fidler expressed being disturbed by the devaluation of activities in OT practice and their replacement with "talking groups" in mental health and with physical therapy modalities in physical dysfunction. She felt that the mimicking of other professions brought the field very close to losing essential and critical aspects of occupational therapy.

Eighteen years later, her concerns about the profession's fit with the medical model continue, especially in regard to the manner in which our narrow identity as a remedial rehabilitation service has "hindered our discovery and validation of the rich and broad dimensions of occupation" (Fidler, 2000, p. 99). She has decried the markedly reduced and narrow range of occupations and activities used by occupational therapists in medical and health care settings.

> I believe that the demands, priorities, and operational philosophy of the medical and health care systems of today are such that our identity and survival as a unique, emerging profession is at high risk if these environments remain our principal focus. (Fidler, 2000, p. 99)

According to Fidler, "To survive in the medical model we must buy into it" (personal communication, September 2001). She does not propose that the profession abandon these settings, but rather that it widens the scope and practice and gives priority to environments "that will make it possible for society and systems to benefit from the practice of authentic occupational therapy" (Fidler, 2000, p. 99).

Balancing out the challenges to her work in OT is the support she has received from others in and outside the profession.

> I was indeed fortunate to have been able to work with and learn from so many very talented and famous persons in the field of psychiatry, such as Nathaniel Apter, Elvin Semiad, Alfred Noyes, and Lawrence Kolb. Another strong incentive has been the positive, challenging responses of the many young, bright occupational therapists with whom I've been privileged to work. Certainly the most positive force has been the interest and support of my husband. He has continued to be my finest advocate, teacher, and friend. (G. Fidler, personal communication, September 24, 1984)

Fidler states that many persons influenced her thinking and motivation (G. Fidler, personal communication, May 1, 1987). She credits her father with teaching her the values and attitudes of critical thinking and creative and logical problem solving. He taught her to understand that only she can be responsible for herself. Her husband, Jay Fidler, immeasurably shaped her thinking, sparked her motivation, and "clarified realities with loving care" (G. Fidler, personal communication, May 1, 1987). She credits Helen Willard with teaching her about "integrity and dignity without ever once threatening the spontaneous fun in me" (G. Fidler, personal communication, May 1, 1987). She mentioned Elizabeth Ridgway, whose understanding and sensitivity about the schizophrenic patient impressed her and taught her much.

She described her viewpoint on occupational therapy in 1984 as follows:

> I have not become disenchanted nor have I had any questions about the fundamental concept of OT. The longer I have looked and worked with it, the more convinced I am that there is a

credibility and relevance to this perspective of human functioning that is unique and different from any other perspectives about human behavior. I have no question about that. I do have a question about how we pursue development and how we do not pursue it. (G. Fidler, personal communication, September 24, 1984)

This last statement was of great concern to her. She felt that the fundamental concept underlying occupational therapy was viable, and that if the profession did not develop it and use it, other professions would. When she was asked if she still agreed with her statement from 1984, she stated, "Absolutely, I have continued to pursue this and am disappointed that the profession has let HMOs influence our thinking and education of OTs to such an extent" (G. Fidler, personal communication, September 5, 2001).

She (Fidler & Velde, 1999) has become increasingly concerned with the role of environment and has raised some interesting questions on environment and activity. She thinks that occupational therapists need to study the influence of activity on the environment and vice versa. "Activities shape societies and reflect cultures and by altering occupations we can change culture and vice versa. This is an important idea for occupational therapists to grasp" (G. Fidler, personal communication, September 5, 2001).

Theoretical Concepts

Since entering the field of occupational therapy in 1942, Fidler has consistently believed that purposeful planned activity is the very core of the field's therapeutic process. Although her theoretical constructs were derived initially from psychoanalytic concepts and were mainly applicable to psychosocial function and dysfunction, she has continued to expand them to include new knowledge and developments in related basic and applied sciences and in occupational therapy and occupational science. Her theory concerning activity addresses physical, cognitive, psychological, and sociocultural aspects of the individual, and how purposeful activity and objects in the human and nonhuman environment might best match the needs of the individual. She believes that the meanings of activities cannot be reduced to one or two factors, but instead interact in complex dynamics. Throughout her career, Fidler has continued to further articulate and refine these dynamics. The following subsections examine these processes and their hypothesized relationships, beginning with Fidler's earlier works and progressing through their evolution, culminating with the books *Activities: Reality and Symbol* (Fidler & Velde, 1999), which provides a sequential and experiential learning process to examine the characteristics of activities and their meaning in a person's life, and *Lifestyle Performance: A Model for Engaging the Power of Occupation* (Velde & Fidler, 2002).

Nonhuman Environment and Object Relations

Searles's (1960) psychoanalytic work on the human and nonhuman environment strongly supported Fidler's early formulations of the meaning of activity and environmental context. Persons develop object relationships with the nonhuman environment from infancy through adulthood. These interactions serve many functions. Symbolically and realistically, they are a means of communicating feelings, needs, and ideations; they mediate between the inner and outer world; and they help one achieve a sense of self. One uses object relations to differentiate self from oneself and to learn more about both. The nonhuman environment is a source of need gratification. Ego functions are developed and strengthened by realistic encounters with objects.

Object relations and their symbolic meaning and unconscious processes (Azima, 1961; Azima & Azima, 1959; Wittkower & Azima, 1958) were key elements of Fidler's early theories. She and Susan Fine (1962) outlined procedures for evaluating and measuring clients' responses to objects, which included responses to the therapist, the activity, and the group. Such responses provided diagnostic information regarding clients' basic needs, whether and how these needs were being gratified, and clients' development of adequate ego defenses and strengths (Fidler & Fidler, 1954, 1963; Fidler & Fine, 1962). Fidler and Susan Fine created the Object History around 1970 as a guideline to explore a person's attachment to and engagement with meaningful objects throughout his or her growth and development. They believed that reflecting on and describing one's own engagement with objects increases awareness of the significance of these in one's development. Fidler and Fine (1970) expanded this history to detail further the process of how one's engagement with a valued object shapes, behavior, feelings and attitudes, interpersonal potential, and cultural differences (Fidler & Velde, 1999).

Communication Process

Another of Fidler's early ideas was that the purpose of activity was to express thoughts and feelings nonverbally. "Occupational therapy is in effect another language for communication with the patient" (Fidler & Fidler, 1963, p. vi). In their 1954 and 1963 texts, Gail and Jay Fidler described this language as an expression of needs, attitudes, and emotion, and explained their reasoning behind this application. "As a communication process occupational therapy is concerned with action, the meaning of action, its use in communicating feelings and thoughts, and the use of such nonverbal communication for the benefit of the patient" (Fidler & Fidler, 1963, p. 19). Action of the patient involved in occupational therapy was more likely to reveal the unconscious. The therapist would use techniques such as uncovering, supporting, or directing to help the patient to communicate.

More recently, Fidler and Velde (1999) wrote about the importance of consensually validating activity experiences and promoting communication. Activities and objects convey meanings through their own inherent qualities. Components of activity analysis provide a "qualitative dialog" (p. 54).

Activity Analysis

A central theme of Fidler's work throughout her career has been the analysis of the components of activities and the correlation of these components with the client's specific needs, interests, and abilities in order to provide action-oriented learning experiences to facilitate needed skill acquisition. Her early activity analysis (Fidler, 1948; Fidler & Fidler, 1954, 1963) focused mainly on the psychodynamic properties of activities as a guide for the therapist in evaluation and treatment. She urged therapists to examine motion, procedures, materials, creativity, symbols, hostile and aggressive components, control, predictability, narcissism, sexual identification, dependence, reality testing, and group relatedness because she felt that these factors provide valuable clues to what emotional needs and drives might be encouraged by particular activities. She believed that activities should be selected that correlate with the client's specific needs, and then the performance of those activities should be controlled and guided to increase their therapeutic value.

Subsequently, Fidler expanded the analysis of activities to include motor, sensory integrative, psychological, sociocultural, cognitive, and interpersonal skills (Fidler, 1958, 1981a, 1982a). According to Fidler, activities need to be matched to the individual's readiness to learn or to receive stimuli, to personal characteristics, to interests and abilities, and to sociocultural values and norms. The real and symbolic meanings of activities used to promote acquisition of these essential skills also need to be explored (Fidler, 1981a). This concept is further developed in the Fidlers's construct of "doing" (Fidler & Fidler, 1978). Fidler expanded this into an experiential process called the multimedia "activity workshop" to explore the complex meanings and dimensions of occupation (Fidler & Velde, 1999).

Fidler has assembled and integrated much of her work on the study and potential of activities in *Activities: Reality and Symbol* (Fidler & Velde, 1999). In this book, the authors describe the content and processes for discovering social, cultural, and personal meanings inherent in activities and the potential of activities to represent, reflect, and infer social, cultural, and personal meanings and to elicit physical, cognitive, and affective responses. This text is intended to serve as a guide in exploring more about these dynamics and the potential power of activities and responses most frequently educed. This is accomplished by organizing the contents to provide carefully planned experiential learning experiences. This book provides many exercises for analysis and reflection of a wide variety of occupational choices. Fidler feels that it is essential to develop an understanding and deep appreciation for the meanings of activities and their related objects and action processes before one is able to use activities therapeutically to facilitate health, wellness, and quality of life.

Doing

Fidler and Fidler (1978) used the term *doing* to connote performing, producing, or causing purposeful action in order to (a) test a skill, (b) clarify a relationship, or (c) create an end product. The process of doing enables the development and integration of the sensory, motor, cognitive, and psychological systems; is a socializing agent; and verifies one's efficacy as a competent, contributing member of one's society. Thus, the occupational therapist uses doing to enable patients to learn the performance skills that they will need to care for and maintain themselves more independently, to satisfy their personal needs for intrinsic gratification, and to contribute to meeting the needs and enhancing the welfare of others within an appropriate cultural context.

At any given point in time, the level and type of performance skills and the balance among them are determined by the individual's age, developmental level, unique biology, and culture. The balance among these skill clusters is critical to a lifestyle that is health sustaining and satisfying to oneself and to significant others (Fidler & Fidler, 1978).

According to Fidler and Fidler (1978), the acquisition of skills needed to perform one's life tasks and roles is influenced both by factors in the external environment and by internal systems. Such variables as culture, economics, family constellation, social class, housing, geographic surroundings, and architectural structures affect the external environment. They can inhibit or facilitate performance skill development. Internal systems refer to the individual's unique biology—that is, his or her sensory, motor, physical, cognitive, and psychological systems. Maturational or developmental delays or deficits caused by trauma affect these systems and thereby influence the development of performance skills learning (Fidler & Fidler, 1978). Thus, new learning is integrated through "relevant doing experiences" (Fidler & Velde, 1999, p. xii).

Competence and Mastery

Gail Fidler's hypotheses concerning the relationship of purposeful activity to competence were influenced by the works of Sullivan (1953), Arieti (1962), White (1959, 1971), and other ego psychologists who proposed an innate drive to master and explore the environment that results in survival and a sense of competence from direct successful encounters with it. The reward is intrinsic, and reinforcement from others is not necessary. According to Fidler (1981a; Fidler & Fidler, 1983), the more experiences of mastery one has, the stronger one's sense of competence becomes. Each success then reinforces more attempts to develop skills and competencies further. Thus, "doing" facilitates one's sense of competence and efficacy by creating experiences with human and nonhuman objects in one's environment. One learns about one's potential and limitations through these direct, action-oriented experiences.

Fidler (1981a) believed that the profession of occupational therapy must work to relate competence, mastery, adaptation, and self-esteem to OT practice. She views competence, mastery, achievement, self-esteem, self-value, and self-worth as interrelated states that are derived from direct encounters with and successful management of elements in the environment. When each of these experiences is verified both by the resulting intrinsic gratification and by positive feedback from significant others, one's value is enhanced (Fidler, 1981a, 1981b). She emphasizes that the feedback one receives from the process of doing is essential to learning about the realities of the self and the world. People learn about reality and test their perception of reality from predictable learned interactions with it (Fidler, 1981a; Fidler & Fidler, 1983). Until one acts on an idea or thought, there can be no distinction between reality and nonreality. It is necessary to test one's ideas and thoughts through action or doing in order to ascertain their validity, efficacy, and relevance to one's life.

According to Fidler (Fidler & Fidler, 1978), the social feedback from "doing" is important because it provides consensual validation of masteries and competencies by their value to others. A related hypothesis that Fidler offers—that the values and norms of a society place higher status on certain tasks and activities than on others—is germane to the meaning and use of activities and their social relevance. Some activities may have high social significance and priority, whereas others may be less important or even be seen as having negative significance or value (Fidler, 1981a). Thus, when one successfully performs an activity valued by society, one's sense of esteem and value as a human being is enhanced. Likewise, when one senses a risk of failure, doing in the presence of others is threatening and may be inhibited. Activities that are not valued by society may adversely affect one's sense of worth and competence (Fidler & Fidler, 1983). Fidler has continued to expand upon this theme and further conceptualize the role of the environment on activities and the person, as well as of activities and the person upon the environment.

Fidler's advocacy of the use of task groups in occupational therapy was based on the hypothesis that the task selected within a group context would meet the social, developmental, and learning needs of the participants by providing feedback on the efficacy of the action within sociocultural norms. By working within the context of a task group, the patient has a chance to learn constructive and rewarding behavior patterns. Opportunities arise for the development of several different roles, and a variety of individual needs can be met simultaneously (Fidler, 1969). The client learns to use his or her existing integrative assets and capacities to develop and improve skills necessary for the assumption of successful economic and social roles in everyday life outside the hospital. Age-appropriate social skill development remains a critical component of performance and is facilitated or impaired both by factors in the external environment and by internal processes.

Integrative Process

Fidler (1982a) hypothesized that activities are an integral part of human development, represent real-life situations, and are valuable and realistic vehicles for acquiring or redeveloping skills necessary to fulfill life roles and provide a source of satisfaction. The acquisition of these functional skills is a developmental process and progresses hierarchically. Certain behaviors are prerequisites to more mature and complex performance skills. Specific actions of an activity or task elicit distinguishable and measurable sensory integrative, motor, cognitive, psychological, and social behaviors. When these are matched with the individual's needs and capacities, opportunities are provided to learn skills and develop more functional abilities in sensorimotor integration, self-maintenance, task behaviors, and leisure skills. Thus, by engaging in purposeful activity, the development and integration of internal sensory, motor, cognitive, and psychological processes are facilitated (Fidler, 1982a).

Health and Illness

Fidler views health as the ability to perform those roles and tasks of living throughout the life cycle that are essential to care for and to maintain the self independently, to satisfy one's personal needs and thus provide intrinsic gratification, and to contribute to the welfare of others within a socially and age-appropriate context (Fidler, 1981a, 1981b, 1982a; Fidler & Fidler, 1978, 1983). A sense of competence and social efficacy is basic to the ability to cope and adapt. This sense of the self as competent is achieved largely through successful doing experiences that carry social value and indicate mastery and achievement. The lifestyle performance model emphasizes the quality of a person's life in terms of the establishment, maintenance, and interplay of healthy activity patterns (Fidler, 1996).

Dysfunction results when physical, social, cognitive, or psychosocial problems or trauma impedes development or impairs functions and adaptations that are fundamental to daily living skills for self-maintenance, work, and leisure (Fidler, 1984; Fidler & Fidler, 1978, 1983). Thus, domains of a person's lifestyle performance are deficient enough to produce distress in the person or in significant others (Fidler, 1996).

Application to Occupational Therapy

Application to Occupational Therapy Practice

Fidler's theories and hypotheses were derived from and directed toward clinical practice. This section describes their application to OT assessment and treatment, which culminate in the lifestyle performance model for practice (Fidler 1996; Velde & Fidler, 2002). This model is a conceptual framework for both the study and application of occupation in persons' lives, institutions, and society. Central to this model are "those tenets that affirm the power of occupation in human existence" (Velde & Fidler, 2002, p. 9).

Assessment

Fidler developed several useful assessment tools to explore the meaning and use of activities and the quality of the processes in occupational therapy. She created an activity analysis initially to examine the psychodynamics of activity (Fidler, 1948; Fidler & Fidler, 1963). She wrote that practitioners needed a thorough understanding of each component of the OT experience to become more skilled in its use. "We believe that the nature or characteristics of the action experience are of primary importance. Involvement in an activity can be either therapeutic or damaging to the patient" (Fidler & Fidler, 1963, pp. 72–73). Thus, the purpose of the activity analysis was to guide the understanding of the basic psychodynamics of an activity. The focus was on assessment of the activity, not the person (Fidler & Velde, 1999). This structured analysis was further developed to include sociohistorical and sociocultural dimensions for a fuller understanding of the many dimensions of an activity.

> The purpose of an activity analysis is to arrive at an understanding of the activity's inherent qualities and characteristics, its meaning in and of itself, irrespective of a performer. Only after such an analysis has been made can one begin to discern the probable impact of an activity on an individual or group. (Fidler & Velde, 1999, p. 47)

The activity analysis is an essential first step in matching an activity and person. "Thus, the learner's own experience should precede gathering information and impressions from others" (Fidler & Velde, 1999, p. xii). Fidler and Velde (1999, pp. 54–57) provide a very detailed and comprehensive outline of questions to analyze the activity in terms of the form and structure, properties, action processes, outcome, and actual and symbolic meaning.

Fidler's Outline for Evaluation (Fidler & Fidler, 1963, pp. 104–107) guided the therapist by raising questions about the psychodynamics manifested by the patient in relation to the therapist, activity, and group. For example, "What is the nature of the patient's overt behavior toward the therapist?" "What feelings are expressed in the content and in the way he handles the material, the process?" This tool is psychoanalytically oriented, as was most of her work until the early 1970s.

The Diagnostic Battery, a projective test (Fidler, 1968), consisted of a drawing, a finger painting, and a clay sculpture. The therapist observed the client's approach to the task; response to examiner; use of space, lines, form, and color; perspective; mode of handling objects and materials; content; and organization. The client was asked to comment on each end product after it was completed. These creations and the client's responses were interpreted and used in total team treatment planning.

Fidler further refined the Diagnostic Battery, adapting it for use within a group context. The result, the Activity Laboratory (Fidler, 1982a, pp. 195–207), consists of five tasks (stencil cutout and crayon, finger painting, collage, obstacle course, and circle ball tag game) and has been used since 1965 with a variety of clients, with numerous students, and with interdisciplinary staffs. During that time, Fidler has made many refinements to the instrument to more effectively enable its tasks to elicit important areas of skill components and performance. Fidler does not propose using this as the only evaluation instrument to determine treatment planning. Rather, it is intended as an "initial tentative behavioral profile" (Fidler, 1982a, p. 196). It also explores how strengths and characteristic styles of organizing and responding can be maximized in treatment intervention. How the individual handles the five tasks in the Activity Laboratory indicates his or her predominant sensory, motor, cognitive, psychological, and social behavior needs (Fidler & Velde, 1999).

Fidler and Fine (1970) developed the Object History to help people learn about and understand the importance of objects. Fidler feels that every occupational therapist should complete the Object History as part of his or her education. This instrument provides a descriptive account of the ways in which certain nonhuman objects are significantly linked with phases of an individual's growth and development. The participant selects an object that has had or continues to have special meaning during a particular part of his or her life. Objects might be toys, animals, household items, nature objects, clothing, or food. The participant is then asked to describe the object, how it came to be his or hers, how it was used, what meaning and importance it has, how family and friends were aware of or involved with the object, and how the object relationship was ended (Fidler & Velde, 1999).

Fidler's Play/Activity History, developed in 1971 (Fidler & Velde, 1999), is intended to develop an individual's appreciation for cultural and sexual differences in his or her play history and to help him or her understand better the real and symbolic meanings of these activities. The person is asked to identify and briefly describe those games or activities in which he or she engaged during childhood and adolescence. Then the person is asked to identify who taught him or her the game, what he or she most enjoyed about the game, with whom he or she most frequently shared it, and to what extent it was part of his or her family's culture. Next, the person describes the specific practice or learning that the game provided in such areas as sensory–perceptual, motor, self-identity, reality orientation, cognition, dyadic interactions, and group skills. Aspects felt to be most and least enjoyable are then explored. Another section examines the strategies involved, the game's aesthetic elements, and the role played by chance in determining the game's outcome. Competitive elements and the game's symbolic, creative, structured, and unstructured properties also are analyzed. Finally, the individual identifies three hobbies or activities important in his or her present lifestyle, compared with activities from earlier years and compared with one's present job or career choice (Fidler & Velde, 1999).

Fidler developed the Lifestyle Performance Profile (1982b) as part of a conceptual framework that described adaptive performance as a fundamental concern of OT practice, building on her concepts of "doing" and competence. According to Fidler, OT practice is concerned primarily with skill development and the achievement of a satisfying, health-sustaining lifestyle. To achieve these goals, the occupational therapist has to evaluate the individual's existing strengths and skill deficits, developmental levels, and external barriers and resources (Fidler, 1982b). The Lifestyle Performance Profile provides a structure for identifying and organizing the person's sensorimotor functions and cognitive, psychological, dyadic, and group social skills within the context of his or her sociocultural milieu and characteristic response patterns and management of life tasks. It also identifies sociocultural and environmental resources that support skill development or interfere with and impede it. The therapist must assess which work, play, and self-care skills are required of this individual in his or her given environment and which of these are intact or dysfunctional. This information may be obtained from existing records, interviews, standardized tests, and observations of the patient in specifically planned tasks and activities that involve sensorimotor, cognitive, and social behaviors.

> The profile was expected to provide both the patient and therapist with a view of the patient's characteristic activity patterns of daily living and the harmony and disharmony or balance among them and then serve as a guide in defining occupational therapy interventions. (Fidler, 1996, p. 139)

Further exploration of these tenets in practice in mental health, geriatrics, and physical disabilities led to the development of the lifestyle performance model, which is discussed in more detail in a later section.

Intervention

Patient evaluations and assessments are fundamental means of gathering data needed to plan and set priorities among treatment goals, to measure progress, and to plan for discharge. From the evaluation and assessment information, the therapist obtains an overview of the patient's strengths and deficits in managing the everyday tasks of his or her world and of performance patterns and related functional deficits that impair coping and adaptation (Fidler, 1984, pp. 33–36; 1996; Velde & Fidler, 2002).

Fidler's early theories about intervention and application were derived mainly from a psychoanalytic frame of reference. According to that perspective, the occupational therapist was a valuable contributor to the psychotherapeutic process because of his or her use of the combination of activities, the dyadic relationship, and groups. Specific treatment guidelines, rationale, and case histories were described in several publications (Fidler, 1958; Fidler & Fidler, 1954, 1963, 1978). In their 1954 book, the Fidlers explained that nonverbal techniques and the use of objects and object relationships were effective treatment methods to incorporate into the total treatment regimen for many patients. In their 1963 book, the Fidlers developed these concepts further, describing OT as a communication process in terms of the action itself, objects used in the action process, and the end products of those actions and interpersonal relationships. The therapeutic process, goals, and case examples are described in that book as consistent with the psychodynamic theoretical constructs described earlier in this chapter.

The idea of the dyadic or therapeutic relationship (discussed as "therapeutic use of self" by Fidler) was based on Harry Stack Sullivan's (1953) work on interpersonal theory. Therapeutic use of self involved the therapist's use of actions that would be helpful to the patient. According to the Fidlers, "The problem in therapy is to anticipate the degree and type of response that will help the patient" (Fidler & Fidler, 1963, p. 41).

Group phenomena in OT are an essential part of intervention. The group leader is responsible for the emotional atmosphere of the group. He or she sets the tone and the expectations for group behavior. Important social roles and behaviors are learned in the context of task-oriented group activity (Fidler, 1969; Fidler & Fidler, 1963).

Fidler's conceptualization of the rehabilitative process is built on her theories of meanings, both real and symbolic; of activity; and of involvement with objects. Activities were initially used to explore and express the unconscious, provide gratification of needs, teach adaptive ego defenses and functional skills, provide a base for reality testing, and explore interpersonal relationships (Fidler, 1948, 1957, 1966b; Fidler & Fidler, 1963; Ridgway & Fidler, 1955). Activities also may be used to sustain and protect intact functions and abilities and to prevent further disability. The therapist selects activities that provide experiences to enable the individual to use existing interests and skills for personal growth, to experience intrinsic gratification, and to meet needs for acceptance, achievement, creativity, autonomy, and social relationships. Activities and tasks are also chosen that will promote and enhance work skills and habits and teach and encourage independent functioning in activities of daily living. The therapist also introduces new activities that will provide compensatory learning and practice for the skills the patient needs to assume for his or her roles in community life. The individual is able to develop new interests and explore potentials because of his or her new experiences with activities. The client comes to see himself or herself as the "doer," and the end product as tangible evidence of his or her ability to achieve (Fidler, 1981a).

As Fidler developed her theory further to include new developments in the art and science of occupational therapy, more implications for practice emerged. Purposeful activity is an organizing construct for practice and the distinguishing characteristic of OT (Fidler, 1981b). Purposeful activity, as expanded into the concepts of "doing" and competence, became an essential link in the treatment process. The Fidlers relinquished the term *treatment* because it connoted changing and altering pathology and adopted instead the terms of *habilitation* or *remediation* (activity workshop, Galveston, Texas, September 22–23, 1983).

According to Fidler, when pathology is identified, "doing" must be used in the service of personality integration via performance skill development and reinforcement with treatment modalities that are adaptive and relevant to the performance skill demands and expectations of the home setting. An understanding of the nature and complexity of these performance skills and their interrelationship with internal and external processes is required. These skills are needed to enable one to feel that one is a productive, contributing, and needed member of society (Fidler & Velde, 1999). Action is directed toward (a) testing a skill, (b) clarifying a relationship, or (c) creating an end product. As discussed earlier, activities and doing experiences must be analyzed and matched to the individual's developmental needs and skill readiness in motor, sensorimotor integration, cognitive, psychological, and interpersonal components in ways that are relevant and significant to the needs and values of the person's sociocultural group and satisfying to the self (Fidler & Fidler, 1983, pp. 267–280). The fit between the individual and an activity is crucial (a) if integration of these systems and an adaptive response are to occur and (b) if choices of leisure, work, and self-maintenance activities are to result in intrinsic gratification, pleasure, and social efficacy of the individual (Fidler & Fidler, 1978).

Fidler's future goals for her theory development are to reach a sophisticated understanding of the nonhuman environment and nonhuman objects, the complex process of engagement with and manipulation of the environment, and the "doing" process as a facilitative process. Fidler encourages occupational therapists to go out into the community and create environments that are less stressful and more supportive of the individual. She is convinced that the field's future is dependent on fuller development of these constructs through doctoral and postdoctoral studies and research.

Gail Fidler wrote *The Design of Rehabilitation Services in Psychiatric Hospital Settings* (1984) as a result of her work as a consultant with the Mental Hygiene Administration of the Maryland State Department of Health and Mental Hygiene at Springfield Hospital Center and at Greystone Park Psychiatric Hospital in New Jersey. The book is a comprehensive guide to program design of rehabilitation services primarily for public psychiatric hospitals, but it is also relevant to private hospitals and community mental health centers. It shows how rehabilitation services can be integrated into the program of a psychiatric hospital by describing policies and procedures for rehabilitation services, clarifying the rationale and focus of the program design, and giving guidelines for practice and administration of a rehabilitation program. The goal of rehabilitation services is to develop and support functional skills that patients need to perform basic everyday living tasks and social roles as independently as possible so that they can cope with their environmental demands in ways that are satisfying to themselves and to significant others. Fidler described in detail how to organize a number of specialized services to achieve this goal, focusing on program principles, staffing and supervisory patterns, referral guidelines, evaluations and assessments, program evaluation, budget, planning, and task and activity group programs and protocols.

In *Recapturing Competence: A System's Change for Geropsychiatric Care*, Fidler and Bristow (1992) present their efforts to apply Fidler's theoretical constructs and concepts to an entire institutional system. This was a significant development in her work in that she moved beyond a treatment focus on the individual to application and validation with larger environments such as the large institution. The book is a case presentation of her 3 years as chief executive officer at Hagadorn Center, a 188-bed long-term nursing care facility for elders with chronic mental illness. After 3 years, the Hagadorn Center had evolved into a comprehensive treatment and rehabilitation hospital.

> This endeavor involved the generation of fundamental changes in the institution's organization and administrative functions, its clinical policies and practices, its definition of patient needs, intervention strategies, and priorities. These alterations finally brought about significant change in both patient and

staff expectations regarding autonomy, achievement, and productivity. (Fidler & Bristow, 1992, p. 1)

Lifestyle Performance Model

Fidler's work for the past 30 years has evolved from the Lifestyle Performance Profile, which was conceptualized in the mid-
1970s, into the lifestyle performance model (Fidler, 1982b, 1996;
Velde & Fidler, 2002). "It differs from all other OT models I'm
certain, because it is the only model that takes as its priority, the
strengths and skills and abilities and interests of the client; not
what is wrong with the client" (Fidler, personal communication,
May 2001). It is concerned with functional deficits or disabilities
only if they seriously interfere with the pursuit of a healthy
lifestyle and quality of life for the individual.

> My thesis is that if you enhance and develop and reinforce an
> individual's strengths and skills and interests, . . . that this is
> going to add to the quality of his or her life and compensate for
> any deficit he or she may have. (G. Fidler, personal communi-
> cation, May 2001)

The primary concern is with what a person has going for him or
her, and deficits are secondary. Theoretical bases for this model
also include dynamic systems, nonlinearity, and self-organization
concepts as used in chaos theory and complexity theory (Velde &
Fidler, 2002).

The lifestyle performance model provides a conceptual
framework for discovering and understanding a person's complete activity repertoire that is situated within his or her human
and nonhuman environment (see Figure 2.1). This lifestyle web
conceptualizes a dynamic interrelatedness of the person, environment, activity profile, and quality of life. This holistic view
uses relevant and meaningful occupations that facilitate the
planning of interventions that "hold maximum potential for elic-
iting and sustaining a person's intrinsic motivation to pursue an
evolving lifestyle optimally satisfying to self and significant others" (Fidler, 1996, p. 139). This is achieved and maintained by
age-specific, culturally relevant synergy among the following
four primary domains of performance: (a) self-care and self-
maintenance, (b) intrinsic gratification, (c) social contribution,

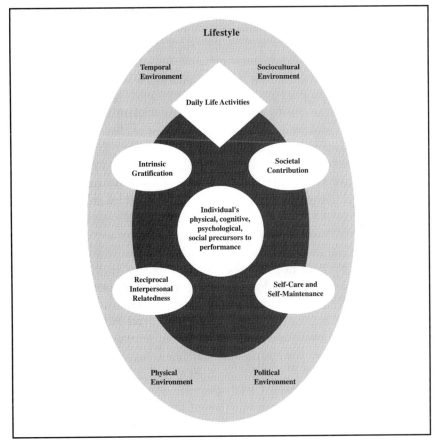

Figure 2.1. The lifestyle web. *Note.* From Lifestyle Performance: A Model for Engaging the Power of Occupation (p. 27), by B. P. Velde and G. S. Fidler, 2002, Thorofare, NJ: SLACK, Inc. Copyright 2002 by SLACK, Inc. Reprinted with permission.

and (d) interpersonal relatedness. In her earlier conceptualizations, Fidler used terms such as work and self-care for what are now conceptualized as the four domains of living (Fidler, personal communication, May 2001). Terms such as work and leisure and self-care were difficult to operationalize and define. These domains of living are Velde and Fidler's (2002) resolution of the definition and classification dilemma regarding occupations as work, play, and self-care. This classification scheme was also an attempt to explain daily activity living patterns in more personally meaningful terms. These domains comprise the structure of the Lifestyle Performance Profile. Fidler defines lifestyle as "a configuration of activity patterns" (Fidler, 1996, p. 140). Thus, these domains are interrelated parts of a lifestyle that express a personal and social identity and self-concept.

One of the four domains, self-care and self-maintenance, involves taking care of oneself at a level that is more self-dependent than dependent on others. It involves self-care and self-management in terms of maintaining one's identity and link with others. Thus, one's ways and manner of caring for and maintaining the self play out the paradox of the need for individuality and affiliation with others (G. Fidler, 1996, p. 144). The second domain is "what I call intrinsic gratification. You do it because it feels good and you thoroughly enjoy it" (Fidler, personal communication, May 2001). The third domain, social contribution, encompasses activities that an individual engages in for the sake of contributing to others and to fulfill societal responsibilities. Social roles such as homemaker, wage earner, and caregiver are examples. The fourth domain, interpersonal relatedness, involves activities aimed at creating and sustaining reciprocal relationships with others. This domain involves parts of the person's activity repertoire that enable friendships, intimate relationships, and peer group affiliations. As an example of how Fidler is continually expanding and refining her ideas, she added, "I see now even a fifth domain as the environment because it is essential to the nature of the kinds of activities that are possible and that are responsive in meeting human needs" (G. Fidler, personal communication, May 2001).

Assessment involves discovering and understanding the individual's lifestyle and how this does or does not reflect personal and social expectations and needs.

> Data-gathering processes that are most relevant to the Lifestyle Performance Model use methodologies that engage the person in reflecting on and developing his or her story about what has been, what is, and what might be the activity patterns that comprise his or her living and the meaning of these for self and significant others. (Velde & Fidler, 2002, pp. 55–56)

Data are gathered collaboratively in a client-centered manner to develop an activity-based Lifestyle Performance Profile within each of the model's four domains. The Lifestyle Performance Interview is used to develop the person's unique Lifestyle Performance Profile, which illuminates the current and previous typical lifestyle activity pattern. Skill strengths and limitations relative to each of the four activity domains are assessed. Balance and imbalance among domains within the context of age, social and cultural norms and interests, and social resources and constraints are also explored.

Intervention is indicated when one or more domains of the individual's lifestyle performance are assessed to be inadequate to "a degree that produces distress in that person or in those who are part of that person's social matrix" (Fidler, 1996, p. 140). Thus, the goal of intervention is to help the person to establish or reestablish a lifestyle configuration of activities that will enhance his or her quality of life and satisfaction. Therefore, this practice model provides a framework composed of both remedial and wellness-generating interventions. The occupational therapy treatment plan is created in response to five fundamental questions:

1. What does the person need to be able to do, and what performance skills are essential?

2. What is the person able to do in terms of strengths, capacities, interests, and external environment?

3. What is the person unable to do as a result of internal and external factors?

4. What interventions are indicated and in what priority so that the person can progress toward fulfilling relevant lifestyle performance needs and expectations?

5. What characteristics of activity patterns and the environment will enhance the quality of living for this person?

The model extends the parameters of occupational therapy beyond reducing disabilities, shifts the focus of practice beyond the realm of our traditional daily living activities, and establishes as a top priority the development of an individualized life-style profile as both a first step in defining intervention goals and an outcome focus of practice. (Fidler 1996, p. 140)

This practice model is consistent with Fidler's continuous belief that intrinsic motivation is elicited and sustained when there is congruence between the characteristics of an activity and the biopsychosocial characteristics of the person.

> The Lifestyle Performance Model is the outgrowth of all of my work to date. It is important not to deal only with dysfunction. It is more than that. If we are to discover a science of occupation we must move beyond a technology of treatment and of course . . . discover the multi-faceted role of activities in societies, cultures, and persons. (G. Fidler, personal communication, September 5, 2001)

Application to Occupational Therapy

Gail Fidler has posed many hypotheses and raised numerous questions about OT. She commented,

> I have always believed that defining the question and pursuing the question is far more important than coming up with an answer. The writing that I have done has pushed for clarifying the question because I think that once the question is clarified, this will inevitably lead to answers. (G. Fidler, personal communication, May 13, 1982)

Fidler has spent most of her professional life pursuing these questions through her writings, grants, workshops, seminars, and clinical, administrative, and educational activities. She has taught and challenged others to clarify and search out the questions and answers. She has influenced the practice and education of occupational therapists in their everyday activities, as well as the work of other theorists, by her relentless search for the meaning of activities and their application in occupational therapy. With her husband, she wrote the first major texts for occupational therapists in psychiatric settings. For almost 20 years, these works remained as the only texts. She educated therapists about object relationships and developed several assessment tools and guides for treatment planning. Her conceptualization of "doing" further supported the importance of activities as therapeutic agents and their relationship to competence, mastery, self-worth, and achievement.

Fidler has led a charge to explore ways for seeking under-standing of the nature and meaning of occupations, as activities in their own right and as complex entities in themselves. She has advanced person–activity congruence in practice and has carried this over to use with organizations, agencies, and insti-tutions. She encourages occupational therapists to go into the community and create environments that are less stressful and more supportive of the individual. She is convinced that OT's fu-ture is dependent on fuller development of these constructs through doctoral and postdoctoral studies and research.

Fidler has integrated the contextual aspects of "doing" into a practice model that transcends focus on disability and limita-tions and focuses on meaningful and client-centered perfor-mance and wellness. Wellness and well-being are priority out-comes. She has been a catalyst and leader in the field, and many of those she touched can remember her questioning, her chal-lenging and provocative discussions, and their experiential en-counters with activities that connected with and reinforced the essence and power of occupational therapy. Her influence has reached out across the world, and some of her books have been translated into Japanese.

Fidler (2001) encourages occupational therapists to reach beyond the medical model and to include other services in their practice and to enlarge their concept of community. She wrote about OT's future as being "beyond the therapy model" (Fidler, 2000, p. 99).

In my vision of tomorrow that stretches beyond our here and now, beyond our therapy model, I can envision an occupational scientist who will have a number of options for specialized study, research, and practice across a broad spectrum of opportunities. These options will include domains of at least the following:

- Services and programs of wellness, of prevention, of learn-ing enhancement, and lifestyle counseling

- Community planning and design

- Organizational, agency, and institutional design and operations

- Treatment, restorative interventions, and rehabilitation (Fidler, 2000, p. 101)

Theory Validation and Research

Thirty years ago, Gail Fidler wrote,

> To date, there has been very little effort to study activities with a standardizing process to list the most common types of response. It is possible to give people a variety of activities and have them express their subjective experience while they are involved in the activity. (Fidler & Fidler, 1963, p. 36)

Fidler's Activity Laboratory is perhaps the most studied and applied aspect of her work. Since 1965, she and her students and others have collected data on the use of the Activity Laboratory experience with many people in a variety of settings.

> Its broad use over these many years with both client and professional groups has made it possible to compare responses, clarify differences in the characteristics and sociocultural significance of activities, demonstrate agreement on the nature of these characteristics, and consensually validate the thesis that an activity does indeed have a "character," a language of its own. (Fidler & Velde, 1999, p. 29)

The researchers have described their results—for example, how one responds to unstructured materials and consensually validated use of materials. There remains a strong need to conduct cross-cultural studies, as well as studies with persons of varying ages. Fidler readily acknowledges that she has experience only with a Western culture (G. Fidler, personal communication, September 5, 2001). She has contacted Suzuki and colleagues in Japan suggesting they do a similar work to describe the social, cultural, and symbolic activities of an Asian culture.

Although informal surveys done during Mental Health Focus workshops in the 1980s indicated that many occupational therapists based their practice on her work, very little research has ensued. Much of Fidler's work is highly abstract, and the conceptualizations do not readily lend themselves to empirical research, especially quantitative research. Much of her work needs to be translated into researchable questions and systematically developed and pursued.

Fidler's book with Beth Velde, *Activities: Reality and Symbol* (1999),

> was perhaps the most gratifying, joyful achievement of my career. It was unfolding in my mind over many many years. I believe that it is the tip of an iceberg in the science of occupation. It needs to be further developed and researched. (G. Fidler, personal communication, September 5, 2001)

Anne Hiller Scott (2000, p. 351), in a review of the book, stated, "This material is to be savored and relished for it truly acknowledges and celebrates the complexity and diversity of activities."

Fidler suggests areas and raises hypotheses for further investigation. She wrote, "Our uniqueness of OT is in what we know and need to know about the history, the sociology, the culture, and psychology of occupations, and the dynamic dimensions of their performance imperatives" (Fidler, 2000, p. 99). She urges that occupational therapists analyze and scrutinize these areas further.

> To understand occupation, we must seek to explain the match between the characteristics of person and characteristics of activities and the force of this dynamic in triggering and sustaining motivation. I believe that this phenomenon comprises the essence of what occupation is all about and what the occupational scientist in our future will know and continue to explore. (Fidler, 2000, p. 100)

Other areas for research include Fidler's hypothesis that wellness and well-being are optimally satisfying to the self and significant others and that "such satisfaction is gleaned from personally and socially relevant activities that focus on and maximize individual strengths, capacities, and interests" (Fidler, 1996, p.140), and her hypothesis that "intrinsic motivation is elicited and sustained when there is congruence between the characteristics of an activity and the biopsychosocial characteristics of the person" (p. 140). Fidler (1996, p. 142) raises another interesting question for research: "how doing or being occupied relates to the dimensions of physical integrity, psychologic structure, and social relatedness." Also, the match of activities to larger bodies such as social institutions is a powerful construct that needs further examination.

Gail Fidler has continuously incorporated new information and, in her recent work with Beth Velde (Velde & Fidler, 2002), is advancing the construction, cohesion, and integration of the theory of the lifestyle performance model. This model has emerged from practice and been applied in practice settings. A variety of case studies using the lifestyle performance model in clinical practice are included in *Lifestyle Performance: A Model for Engaging the Power of Occupation* (Velde & Fidler, 2002). Former students and faculty have been very helpful in both using and illustrating their use of the model in practice, and some have contributed to the text through these case examples. College Misericorda developed an OT master's program on this model, and several students have applied it to their clinical practice and have written case studies. Suzuki and her colleagues are examining the cross-cultural application in Japan.

Hocking and Whiteford (1997, p. 154) critiqued Fidler's 1996 presentation of the lifestyle performance model and argued that its construction was "flawed" for several reasons. First, they commented that the four domains neither resolve nor avoid the problems with the terms *work, play, self-care,* and *leisure*. They also took issue with the universality of the theory. Third, they criticized the theory for not defining key terminology. Fourth, they stated that relationships of concepts to cited cross-disciplinary theories were incorrect or not evident. Fifth, they said the model lacked "clarity of central concepts" (p. 154). Velde, Gerney, Trompetter, and Amory (1997) rebutted Hocking and Whiteford's critique. They traced the long history over which Fidler developed the concepts, components, and theoretical construction of the model. They argued that the model is a "template with which to view an individual candidate for occupational therapy services" (p. 784). They also wrote, "Because the model is individually referenced, it can be applied to any person, despite age, culture, or health status" (p. 785), and commented that environment is considered an important and highly individual and variable context. They concluded their rebuttal with the following statement urging more discourse on theory building and practice:

> To continue the dialogue regarding the use and value of models, and for occupational therapy to grow, the intellectual en-

gagement must continue. This common commitment to inquiry may not result in a single ideology that passes for truth but a continuation of the discourse that leads to an understanding of the manner in which human beings construct and live the reality they define. It can only strengthen the profession of occupational therapy. (pp. 786–787)

Fidler's work with Velde (Velde & Fidler, 2002) has further developed the lifestyle performance model and made many of the concepts clearer and more structured. Fidler (personal communication, May 2001) is encouraging others to do cross-cultural study and applications of her work and is looking forward to the work being done by Suzuki and her colleagues in Japan. Using ethnographic techniques, other researchers are also studying cultural groups and how culture influences lifestyle and how the model does or does not fit. Velde and Fidler (2002, p. 28) state that their theory is "grounded in the philosophy of phenomenology, [and] research regarding the model is based in grounded theory and ethnographic traditions." The authors continue to collect data and analyze it using grounded theory methodology to further refine the model.

Although Fidler's work is still quite abstract and neither intricately nor copiously woven, it is becoming more specific and amenable to research, as indicated by the researchable topics and questions listed in previous paragraphs. Fidler has contributed valuable means to explore and study activity that has direct application to practice. However, her theory is very individualistic and relies heavily on subjective experience. What are needed are more systematic investigations of her findings and use of qualitative research methods to study this subjective individual experience, which is an area of inquiry in which she has made the most contributions. It is necessary to formulate quantitative research questions and constructs to test hypotheses generated by her work in order to make predictions. Her work has not lent itself particularly to positivistic quantitative research.

Throughout her 60 years in OT, Fidler has demonstrated a dedicated and focused pursuit of knowledge about "doing" in order to develop a clearer understanding of occupation and its relation to health and well-being. She has expanded her theoretical base, from psychoanalytic theory, to include new knowledge and other theories and contexts. Fidler's lifestyle performance model also has expanded and has become increasingly integrated and cohesive. She remains true to her central theme that purposeful planned activity is the very core of the OT therapeutic process and to the importance of the complex process of matching the activity characteristics with the person. She urges occupational therapists to include wellness, lifestyle counseling, and community and institutional planning and design into their practice, and to expand beyond the medical model. She continues to develop and refine her work and disseminate her knowledge through publications, speaking engagements, mentorship, and independent practice. Further research, however, is needed to validate these constructs and to develop measurements.

Bibliography

1948

Fidler, G. S. (1948). Psychological evaluation of occupational therapy activities. *American Journal of Occupational Therapy, 2,* 284–287.

1953

Fidler, G. S. (1953). Comments on a study of a task directed and a free choice group. *American Journal of Occupational Therapy, 7,* 124, 130.

1954

Fidler, G. S., & Fidler, J. W. (1954). *Introduction to psychiatric occupational therapy.* New York: Macmillan.

1955

Ridgway, E. P., & Fidler, G. S. (1955). Occupational therapy: Laboratory for living. *Mental Health Views, 3*(3).

1957

Fidler, G. S. (1957). The role of occupational therapy in a multidisciplinary approach to chronic illness. *American Journal of Occupational Therapy, 11,* 8–12.

1958

Fidler, G. S. (1958). Educational experiences for the occupational therapist. *Journal of the South African Occupational Therapy Association.*

Fidler, G. S. (1958). Some unique contributions of occupational therapy in the treatment of the schizophrenic. *American Journal of Occupational Therapy, 12,* 9–12.

1962

Fidler, G. S., & Fine, S. B. (1962). The occupational therapist and psychotherapy. In R. Morehouse (Ed.), *Transitional programs in psychiatric occupational therapy* (pp. 14–20). Dubuque, IA: William Brown.

1963

Fidler, G. S., & Fidler, J. W. (1963). *Occupational therapy: A communication process in psychiatry*. New York: Macmillan.

1964

Fidler, G. S. (1964). A guide to planning and measuring growth experience in the clinical affiliation. *American Journal of Occupational Therapy, 18,* 240–243.

1966

Fidler, G. S. (1966). Learning as a growth process: A conceptual framework for professional education. The Eleanor Clarke Slagle lecture. *American Journal of Occupational Therapy, 20,* 1–8.

Fidler, G. S. (1966). A second look at work as a primary force in rehabilitation. *American Journal of Occupational Therapy, 20,* 72–74.

1968

Fidler, G. S. (1968). Diagnostic Battery—Scoring and summary. In *Final report* (Rehabilitation Services Administration Grant No. 123-T-68 for Field Consultant in Psychiatric Rehabilitation). Washington, DC: U.S. Government Printing Office.

Fidler, G. S. (1968). The task-oriented group as a context for treatment. In *Final report* (Rehabilitation Services Administration Grant No. 123-T-68 for Field Consultant in Psychiatric Rehabilitation). Washington, DC: U.S. Government Printing Office.

1969

Fidler, G. S. (1969). The task-oriented group as a context for treatment. *American Journal of Occupational Therapy, 23,* 43–48.

1970

Fidler, G. S., & Fine, S. B. (1970). *Object history*. Unpublished manuscript.

1971

Fidler, G. S. (1971). *Play / activity history*. Unpublished manuscript.

1977

Fidler, G. S. (1977). From plea to mandate. *American Journal of Occupational Therapy, 31,* 653.

1978

Fidler, G. S. (1978). Professional or non-professional. In *Occupational therapy: 2001 AD* (pp. 31–36). Rockville, MD: American Occupational Therapy Association.

Fidler, G. S., & Fidler, J. W. (1978). Doing and becoming: Purposeful action and self-actualization. *American Journal of Occupational Therapy, 32,* 305–310.

1979

Fidler, G. S. (1979). Specialization. *American Journal of Occupational Therapy, 33,* 34.

1981

Fidler, G. S. (1981). From crafts to competence. *American Journal of Occupational Therapy, 35,* 567–573.

Fidler, G. S. (1981). *Overview of occupational therapy in mental health*. Prepared by the American Occupational Therapy Task Group of the American Psychiatric Association on Psychiatric Therapies.

1982

Fidler, G. S. (1982). The activity laboratory: A structure for observing and assessing perceptual, integrative, and behavioral strategies. In B. Hemphill (Ed.), *The evaluation process in psychiatric occupational therapy* (pp. 195–207). Thorofare, NJ: Charles B. Slack.

Fidler, G. S. (1982). The Lifestyle Performance Profile: An organizing frame. In B. Hemphill (Ed.), *The evaluative process in psychiatric occupational therapy* (pp. 43–47). Thorofare, NJ: Charles B. Slack.

1983

Fidler, G. S., & Fidler, J. W. (1983). Doing and becoming: The occupational therapy experience. In G. Kielhofner (Ed.), *Health through occupation: Theory and practice in occupational therapy* (pp. 267–280). Philadelphia: F.A. Davis.

1984

Fidler, G. S. (1984). *The design of rehabilitation services in psychiatric hospital settings.* Laurel, MD: Ramsco.

1988

Fidler, G.S. (1988). *The Lifestyle Performance Profile. In focus: Skills of assessment and treatment.* Rockville, MD: American Occupational Therapy Association.

1990

Fidler, G. S. (1990). Reflections on choice. *Occupational Therapy in Mental Health, 10,* 77–84.

1991

Fidler, G. S. (1991). The challenge of change to occupational therapy practice. *Occupational Therapy in Mental Health, 11,* 1–10.

1992

Fidler, G. S., with Bristow, B. J. (1992). *Recapturing competence: A system's change for geropsychiatric care.* New York: Springer.

1993

Fidler, G. S. (1993). The quest for efficacy. *American Journal of Occupational Therapy, 47,* 583–586.

1995

Fidler, G. S. (1995). *The psychosocial core of occupation: A position paper.* American Occupational Therapy Association.

1996

Fidler, G. S. (1996). Life-style performance: From profile to conceptual model. *American Journal of Occupational Therapy, 50,* 139–147.

1999

Fidler, G. S., & Velde, B. (1999). *Activities: Reality and symbol.* Thorofare, NJ: SLACK.

2000

Fidler, G. S. (2000). Beyond the therapy model: Building our future. *American Journal of Occupational Therapy, 54,* 99–101.

2001

Fidler, G. S. (2001). Community practice: It's more than geography. *Occupational Therapy in Health Care, 3*(3/4), 7–9.

2002

Velde, B. P, & Fidler, G. S. (2002). *Lifestyle performance: A model for engaging the power of occupation.* Thorofare, NJ: SLACK.

References

Arieti, S. (1962). Psychotherapy of schizophrenia. *Archives of General Psychiatry, 6,* 232–239.

Azima, H. (1961). Dynamic occupational therapy. *Diseases of the Nervous System Monograph Supplement, Section 2, 22*(4), 138–142.

Azima, H., & Azima, F. (1959). Outline of a dynamic theory of occupational therapy. *American Journal of Occupational Therapy, 13,* 215–221.

Fidler, G. S. (1948). Psychological evaluation of occupational therapy activities. *American Journal of Occupational Therapy, 2,* 284–287.

Fidler, G. S. (1957). The role of occupational therapy in a multidisciplinary approach to chronic illness. *American Journal of Occupational Therapy, 11,* 8–12.

Fidler, G. S. (1958). Some unique contributions of occupational therapy in the treatment of the schizophrenic. *American Journal of Occupational Therapy, 12,* 9–12.

Fidler, G. S. (1966a). Learning as a growth process: A conceptual framework for professional education. The 1965 Eleanor Clarke Slagle lecture. *American Journal of Occupational Therapy, 20,* 1–8.

Fidler, G. S. (1966b). A second look at work as a primary force in rehabilitation. *American Journal of Occupational Therapy, 20,* 72–74.

Fidler, G. S. (1968). Diagnostic Battery—Scoring and summary. In *Final report* (Rehabilitation Services Administration Grant No. 123-T-68 for Field Consultant in Psychiatric Rehabilitation). Washington, DC: U.S. Government Printing Office.

Fidler, G. S. (1969). The task-oriented group as a context for treatment. *American Journal of Occupational Therapy, 23,* 43–48.

Fidler, G. S. (1971). *Play/activity history.* Unpublished manuscript.

Fidler, G. S. (1981a). From crafts to competence. *American Journal of Occupational Therapy, 35,* 567–573.

Fidler, G. S. (1981b). *Overview of occupational therapy in mental health.* Prepared by the American Occupational Therapy Task Group of the American Psychiatric Association on Psychiatric Therapies.

Fidler, G. S. (1982a). The Activity Laboratory: A structure for observing and assessing perceptual, integrative, and behavioral strategies. In B. Hemphill (Ed.), *The evaluation process in psychiatric occupational therapy* (pp. 195–207). Thorofare, NJ: Charles B. Slack.

Fidler, G. S. (1982b). The Lifestyle Performance Profile: An organizing frame. In B. Hemphill (Ed.), *The evaluation process in psychiatric occupational therapy* (pp. 43–47). Thorofare, NJ: Charles B. Slack.

Fidler, G. S. (1984). *The design of rehabilitation services in psychiatric hospital settings.* Laurel, MD: Ramsco.

Fidler, G. S. (1996). Lifestyle performance: From profile to conceptual model. *American Journal of Occupational Therapy, 50,* 139–147.

Fidler, G. S. (2000). Beyond the therapy model: Building our future. *American Journal of Occupational Therapy, 54,* 99–101.

Fidler, G. S. (2001). Community practice: It's more than geography. *Occupational Therapy in Healthcare, 3*(3/4), 7–9.

Fidler, G. S., with Bristow, B. J. (1992). *Recapturing competence: A system's change for geropsychiatric care.* New York: Springer.

Fidler, G. S., & Fidler, J. W. (1954). *Introduction to psychiatric occupational therapy*. New York: Macmillan.

Fidler, G. S., & Fidler, J. W. (1963). *Occupational therapy: A communication process in psychiatry*. New York: Macmillan.

Fidler, G. S., & Fidler, J. W. (1978). Doing and becoming: Purposeful action and self-actualization. *American Journal of Occupational Therapy, 32*, 305–310.

Fidler, G. S., & Fidler, J. W. (1983). Doing and becoming: The occupational therapy experience. In G. Kielhofner (Ed.), *Health through occupation: Theory and practice in occupational therapy* (pp. 267–280). Philadelphia: F.A. Davis.

Fidler, G. S., & Fine, S. B. (1962). The occupational therapist and psychotherapy. In R. Morehouse (Ed.), *Transitional programs in psychiatric occupational therapy* (pp. 14–20). Dubuque, IA: William Brown.

Fidler, G. S., & Fine, S. B. (1970). *Object history*. Unpublished manuscript.

Fidler, G. S., & Velde, B. S. (1999). *Activities: Reality and symbol*. Thorofare, NJ: SLACK.

Hocking, C., & Whiteford, G. (1997). What are the criteria for development of occupational theory? A response of Fidler's Life Style Performance Model. *American Journal of Occupational therapy, 51*, 154–157.

Ridgway, E. P., & Fidler, G. S. (1955). Occupational therapy: Laboratory for living. *Mental Health Views, 3*(3).

Scott, A. H. (2000). Book review: Activities: Reality and symbol. *American Journal of Occupational Therapy, 54*, 350–351.

Searles, H. (1960). *The nonhuman environment*. New York: International University Press.

Sullivan, H. S. (1953). *The interpersonal theory of psychiatry*. New York: Norton.

Velde, B. P., & Fidler, G. S. (2002). *Lifestyle performance: A model for engaging the power of occupation*. Thorofare, NJ: Charles B. Slack.

Velde, B., Gerney, A., Trompetter, L., & Amory, M. A (1997). The issue is—Fidler's Life Style Performance Model: Why we disagree with Hocking and Whiteford's critique. *American Journal of Occupational Therapy, 51*, 784–787.

West, W. L. (Ed.). (1959). *Changing concepts and practices in psychiatric occupational therapy*. New York: American Occupational Therapy Association.

White, R. W. (1959). Motivation reconsidered: The concept of competence. *Psychiatric Review, 66*, 297.

White, R. W. (1971). The urge toward competence. *American Journal of Occupational Therapy, 25*, 271–274.

Wittkower, E. D., & Azima, H. (1958). Dynamic aspects of occupational therapy. *Archives of Neurology and Psychiatry, 79*, 706–711.

Anne Cronin Mosey

Ferol Menks Ludwig

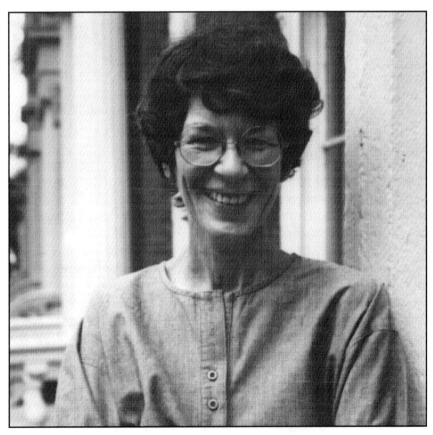

I have attempted to plead a case for the conscious use of theoretical frames of reference as the basis for the treatment of psychosocial dysfunction. (Mosey, 1970b, p. v).

Anne Cronin Mosey (1970b) expressed this concern over 30 years ago in the preface to *Three Frames of Reference for Mental Health*. This was clearly a springboard from which she continued to develop her conceptualizations about the knowledge base of the profession of occupational therapy (OT). Throughout her works, readers can see a copious progression and detailing of thought that leads from the frames of reference to an examination of the epistemology of practice and her unswerving support for positivist applied scientific inquiry.

Biographical Sketch

Anne Cronin Mosey was born in 1938, the third of seven children, and was raised in Minneapolis, Minnesota. As a child, she read extensively, helped with cooking for nine people, and had long talks with her father about the state of the world. She asserts that "life picked up" when she discovered boys and began to date (A. C. Mosey, personal communication, August 4, 1985).

Educational Background

After graduation from high school, she attended the University of Minnesota, where she pursued a double major in sociology and psychology. Her Irish family background did not permit young ladies to work, so during the summer of her junior year she volunteered at the Veterans Hospital in Minneapolis. At the suggestion of the coordinator of volunteer services, she worked in the OT department on the psychiatric unit.

Although she had not really understood what OT was about, she had enjoyed the work, so she changed her major to OT when she returned to college. In 1961, she earned her bachelor of science degree in occupational therapy from the University of Minnesota School of Medicine. Mosey credits Marvin Lepley, her adviser at the University of Minnesota, with playing an important role in her professional development through his confidence in her and his encouragement (A. C. Mosey, personal communication, October 4, 1984; Richert, 1989).

Professional Career

After graduation, Mosey worked for several months at Glenwood Hills Hospital in Minneapolis. She then moved to New York City to work with and learn from Gail Fidler. She joined the OT department at New York State Psychiatric Institute, where she remained for 5 years until August 1966. As her supervisor, Fidler encouraged Mosey to think, read, and broaden her horizons about clinical practice and to focus on patient needs.

Mosey decided after a few years that she wanted to be an educator. She began graduate studies in occupational therapy at New York University and earned her master's degree in 1965. She then enrolled in Human Relations and Community Studies, also at New York University, and was awarded her doctorate in 1968. Lloyd Barenblatt, one of her instructors and chair of her dissertation committee, helped her "to refine skills in critical thinking" (A. C. Mosey, personal communication, October 4, 1984).

From 1966 to 1968, Mosey was an instructor in OT at Columbia University. During this period, she (a) realized that "teaching is something one must learn how to do and is a difficult task" (A. C. Mosey, personal communication, May 3, 1987), (b) developed the idea and structure of the frame of reference, (c) wrote *Three Frames of Reference for Mental Health* (1970b), and (d) completed her dissertation. She then joined the OT faculty at New York University and moved upward through the academic ranks to professor with tenure. She served as department chair from 1972 to 1980 and as acting head of the Division of Health in 1977.

Mosey has served The American Occupational Therapy Association (AOTA) in several leadership capacities on the state and national levels. Since 1979, she has been a continuous reviewer of proposed presentations for AOTA annual conferences. She was a member of the Panel of Experts of the AOTA Continuing Education Program in Mental Health from 1984 to 1988. She was a member of the Scholars Group for the Directions for the Future Project of AOTA and the American Occupational Therapy Foundation (ATOF) (1988–1991). She is a member of the Panel for Review of Research Proposals of AOTF and is an AOTF research consultant. She also served on the editorial board of the journal *Occupational Therapy in Mental Health*. Mosey participated in the development of the AOTA Self Study Series on Cognitive Rehabilitation (A. C. Mosey, personal communication, September 20, 1992).

Mosey also has shared her experience and knowledge by serving as a consultant to several hospitals and state mental health systems. From 1966 to 1969, she was a consultant for the Massachusetts Department of Mental Health. She was a faculty member for the AOTA Regional Institutes from 1966 to 1967. As an invited participant, she was involved with the Theory Building Seminar for AOTA in 1967. She also served as consultant to the Division of Rehabilitation Education at New York University, Hillside Hospital Professional Examination Services, the Family Centered Research Project, the Institute of Pennsylvania Hospital, the Greater Trenton Mental Health Center, and Christopher House.

Mosey has published 17 papers and seven books and has given numerous presentations and workshops. One of her articles is a collection of four poems about the thoughts of an occupational therapist arriving home late on a dark winter night after a long and exhausting day (Mosey, 1976). As the therapist looks out the window at the blinking city lights below, she tries to put into words the thoughts and feelings of four patients. These sensitive and insightful poems demonstrate empathy, understanding, and caring.

Numerous students and therapists have learned from Mosey and sought her guidance. She supervised master's and doctoral research projects since 1968 until her recent retirement. She taught international students, a task that she found to be "a tough, fun, insightful, and interesting learning experience" (A. C. Mosey, personal communication, August 4, 1985).

Her profession honored her in 1973 by naming her a fellow of the AOTA. In 1975 she received the Distinguished Service Award from the National Association of Activity Therapy, and in 1985 she was awarded the AOTA's Eleanor Clarke Slagle Lectureship. Her lecture, "A Monistic or a Pluralistic Approach to Professional Identity?" spoke to issues regarding theoretical frames of reference for practice.

Mosey lives in Greenwich Village. She is divorced and has a grown son whom she considers to be her best critic (A. C. Mosey, personal communication, May 3, 1987). She is interested in history and anthropology and enjoys the theater, concerts, being with friends, and being alone to think, read, and "contemplate the nature of the world" (A. C. Mosey, personal communication, August 4, 1985). Her most recent professional interest has been examining and attempting to identify what areas need to be addressed in the philosophical study of health professions, and constructing a philosophy of applied science (A. C. Mosey, personal communication, September 20, 1992). She is currently preparing for retirement and New York University has named a lectureship in her honor.

Theoretical Concepts

Throughout her career, Mosey has been concerned with laying the theoretical groundwork for the OT evaluation and intervention process. She has searched for answers to the questions of where occupational therapists are now, how they got there, and how they know what they know. She has investigated the theoretical building blocks of the profession in a scholarly manner and has organized them into a taxonomy of the profession, and delved further to describe an epistemology of practice. Three main themes can be seen in her work: (a) the translation of theories of psychosocial dysfunction into frames of reference to apply to OT practice in mental health, (b) the development of a taxonomy and configuration that identifies the various elements and structure of the profession and their relationship to each other, and (c) an interpretation of the epistemology of practice and the importance of positivistic applied scientific inquiry. Each of these is discussed in the following sections.

Major Theme 1: Frames of Reference for OT Practice in Mental Health

This section traces Mosey's early conceptualization of frames of reference for OT practice in mental health from "recapitulation of ontogenesis" through subsequent additions of the analytic and acquisitional frames of reference, then with wider application and "doing" processes.

Recapitulation of Ontogenesis

One of the three main strands of Mosey's work, that of developing and articulating frames of reference for OT in mental health, began with her proposal, in "Recapitulation of Ontogenesis: A Theory for the Practice of Occupational Therapy" (1968b), of a developmental frame of reference for evaluation and treatment. Its theoretical base was derived from a variety of personality and developmental theories proposed by Sullivan (1953), Piaget (Flavell, 1963), Bruner (1966), Sigmund Freud (1949), Anna Freud (1965), Llorens (Llorens & Beck, 1966), Schilder (1950), Searles (1960), Sechehaye (1951a, 1951b), Ayres (1958, 1961, 1963, 1964), and Hartman (1958). Her clinical work with Fidler also was influential in the development of this frame of reference. The biological term *ontogenesis,* referring to the biological development of an individual organism, is used by psychologists to denote the individual's progression through developmental stages. It denotes a hierarchical pattern of maturation. Mosey's frame of reference is concerned with the development of basic adaptive skills that build on each other and must be learned in proper sequence, beginning with the most elementary components and moving to the more complex in a hierarchical manner (Mosey, 1968b, 1986).

Mosey (1968b) proposed that the individual seeks equilibrium. Disequilibrium results from changing psychological and physical needs and new environmental demands. It motivates one to develop the adaptive skills needed to reestablish equilibrium. Mosey describes seven adaptive skills, each of which has component subskills, in the sequential order in which they are expanded:

1. Perceptual-motor skills
2. Cognitive skills
3. Drive object skills
4. Dyadic interaction skills
5. Primary group interaction skills
6. Self-identity skills
7. Sexual identity interaction skills

When all of the component subskills of a given skill have been integrated, the person has achieved full maturity in that skill.

A function–dysfunction continuum exists. A state of function is characterized by the integration of those adaptive skill components needed for successful participation in the social roles expected of the individual in his or her usual setting. One's cultural group usually sets minimal and maximal limits. Adaptive skill performance enables one to obtain gratification and meet environmental demands.

Dysfunction results when necessary skill components are not acquired because of (a) abnormalities or lack of maturation of physical structures, (b) severe environmental stress, or (c) lack of environmental elements necessary for the development of these skill components. Failure to develop skill components needed for the fulfillment of social roles may result in unproductive interactions with the social system or maladative patterns such as depression or hyperactivity (Mosey, 1968b).

To evaluate the patient, an occupational therapist must observe the patient in roles and activities that will elicit adaptive skills and then identify whether particular skill components are present or absent. The therapist needs to collaborate with the patient and other staff to learn more about what skills are needed in the patient's expected environment.

Patients can move from a state of dysfunction to a state of function through activities that are similar to those object interactions responsible for normal skill development. The therapist selects these activities and helps the patient grow from where normal development ceased by providing experiences that take the patient through the developmental stages of skill acquisition and facilitate development of the needed skills. Thus, therapy recapitulates ontogenesis, the normal sequence of individual development, and enables the patient to complete that sequence. Activities are interactive, and the objects with which the patient interacts vary according to the component that needs to be built up. Symbolic activities may be used, but reality and the here and now are stressed. In particular, the more mature skill components must employ reality-oriented activities (Mosey, 1968b).

The long-term goal of this developmental approach is to help the person participate fully in his or her expected social roles and environment. The short-term goal is to develop the skill component.

Developmental Groups

In her next publication (1969), Mosey provided a psychoanalytic developmental frame of reference, consistent with her recapitulation of ontogenesis frame of reference (1968b), for the evaluation and treatment of pathological distortion of body image. What is particularly notable about this publication is her inclusion and description of the use of developmental groups in OT practice. Her conceptualization of these groups had a huge impact on practice in mental health. In keeping with her recapitulation of ontogenesis frame of reference, Mosey proposed the use of developmental groups for persons who lack primary group interaction skills (1970a). The position of a client on the function–dysfunction continuum is determined by his or her achievement of primary group interaction skills and skill components.

Developmental groups are defined as groups that are structured to simulate the various types of nonfamilial groups usually experienced in the normal developmental process. Mosey described a progression through five levels of developmental groups: (a) parallel group, (b) project group, (c) egocentric group, (d) cooperative group, and (e) mature group. Learning occurs as the person experiences the consequences of his or her behavior in the structured group setting. The type of behavior to be learned is clearly spelled out; adaptive behavior is reinforced and maladaptive behavior is not. Developmental groups can be used to treat deficiencies in other adaptive skill components that can be either partially or completely learned through nonfamilial groups. The group must be structurally similar to the type of group in which these components are normally acquired. Developmental groups can also be used to satisfy mental health needs (Mosey, 1970a, 1986).

Three Frames of Reference

Mosey continued work on her frames of reference, which led to the publication in 1970 of *Three Frames of Reference for Mental Health*. She stated that this was written "to plead a case for the conscious use of theoretical frames of reference as a basis for the treatment of psychosocial dysfunction" (1970b, p. v), and it has served for many years as a basic text on the subject. The three frames of reference that it considers are analytical, developmental, and acquisitional.

The *analytical* frame of reference is concerned with concepts of need fulfillment, expression of primitive impulses, and control of inherent drives. It is based on the theories of Sigmund Freud (1949), Anna Freud (1965), Maslow (1962), Erikson (1950), and Jung (1933, 1964).

Mosey's *developmental* frame of reference was based on "Recapitulation of Ontogenesis: A Theory for the Practice of Occupational Therapy" (Mosey, 1968b). In this frame of reference, Mosey incorporates Sigmund Freud's stages of psychosexual development and Erikson's eight stages, whereas development that is learned or acquired is relegated to the acquisitional frame of reference. Skills in the developmental frame of reference are interdependent, qualitative, and stage specific. They are usually acquired in the normal developmental process in growth-facilitating environments.

The *acquisitional* frame of reference, in contrast to the developmental frame of reference, concerns skills and abilities that are independent of each other, quantitative, and not stage specific. They do not rely on maturation, but rather on learning; that is, they are acquired. This perspective is based on learning theories, such as those of Bandura (1969), Wolpe and Lazarus (1966), Dollard and Miller (1950), and ego theories, such as that of Sullivan (1953). It is also based on the work of such occupational therapists as Diasio (1968), Sieg (1974), and Smith and Tempone (1968).

Mosey regarded these three frames of reference as the major current frames of reference in OT in psychosocial dysfunction at the time. In her book *Psychosocial Components of Occupational Therapy* (1986), she refined the frames of reference and developed their application further. She also analyzed the work of other OT researchers, such as Fidler and Fidler (1963), King (1978), Llorens (1976), Reilly (1962, 1974), and Kielhofner (1977), and integrated their thinking into the frames of reference. Thus, she considers Reilly (1962, 1974), Banus (1979), Llorens (1976), Kielhofner (1977, 1983), Margaret Rood, Signe Brunnstrom, and Karel and Berta Bobath to be contributors to the developmental frame of reference, and she has included the biomechanical and rehabilitative approaches of Trombly and Scott (1977) in her acquisitional frame of reference.

Activities Therapy

In Mosey's (1973a) *Activities Therapy,* the sequence, principles, and case examples of the evaluation and treatment process are consistent with her *Three Frames of Reference for Mental Health* (1970b). In *Activities Therapy,* Mosey also described the kinds of psychiatric treatment centers in which this type of treatment might be applicable. The book was written to show how therapy that uses immediate, action-oriented interactions can help persons with mental illness learn to be a part of their community and to cope with the stresses of daily life.

Activities Therapy is based on the assumption that psychosocial dysfunction is due to a lack of one or more of the following abilities:

Planing and carrying out a task

Interacting comfortably in a group

Identifying and satisfying needs

Expressing emotions in an acceptable manner

Attaining a fairly accurate perception of the self and the human and nonhuman environment

Establishing a value system that allows the person to meet his or her needs without infringing on the rights of others

Performing activities of daily living skills

Working at a relatively satisfying job

Enjoying avocational and recreational activities

Interacting comfortably in relationships with family and friends

Any deficits in these abilities limit one's effective performance in the community. Deficit learning or learning of inappropriate behaviors can be treated by teaching more effective behaviors.

As in her earlier works, Mosey (1973a) stressed the importance of learning through doing in the here and now. Activities provide realistic situations to help participants learn new skills, identify faulty patterns of behavior, and recognize the feelings and values that support these maladaptive patterns. The therapist is concerned with the (a) greater understanding of self and (b) development of skills.

According to Mosey (1973a), human beings have three facets: basic skills, the private self, and the public self. Basic skills are those that a person must have to function satisfactorily in the community with others. They include task and group interaction skills. The private self is composed of those aspects that cannot be directly seen or experienced by others, such as cognitive processes, needs, emotions, and values. The public self involves aspects of the individual that can be observed by others and can be a point of contact. Activities of daily living, work, recreation, and intimacy are essential components of the public self (1973a). The teaching–learning process and group dynamics that use action-oriented experiences help the client learn necessary skills.

Major Theme 2: Structure and Taxonomy

Initially, Mosey was concerned with developing a structure for theoretical frames of reference for OT practice in mental health. Later, she developed a biopsychosocial model that led her on a quest to develop characteristics and structure of a professional model. This led to her development of a configuration of the OT profession. This section covers these developments.

Theoretical Frame of Reference

Mosey's second major theme has been to explore the structure of a frame of reference for use in practice. In *Three Frames of Reference for Mental Health* (1970b), she defined theory as a set of statements that describes the relationship among events and makes predictions about these events. A theoretical frame of reference is derived from theory and makes use of concepts, definitions, and postulates from a theory or theories. It is composed of principles to guide action that are derived from scientific postulates regarding change. Whereas a theory is merely descriptive, a theoretical frame of reference provides principles for action and is prescriptive. It applies to daily situations and can guide the practitioner's decisions.

Mosey (1970b) used a four-part structure for a frame of reference that she derived from Ford and Urban (1963; see Table 3.1). The first component is a theoretical base that is drawn from theory or theories from such fields as psychology, sociology, and neuroscience. It specifies the nature of human beings, the environment, and their relationship to each other, and identifies the parameters of the frame of reference. It is the basis from which all other parts are deduced.

The second part is made up of function and dysfunction continua and operational definitions of verbal and nonverbal behaviors that are indicative of function or dysfunction. These are derived from the assumptions of the theoretical base concerning health and dysfunction, and vary according to the frame of ref-

Table 3.1
Components of a Theoretical Frame of Reference

1. Statement of the Theoretical Base

    a. Statement of the nature of man and environment

    b. Statement of relation between man and environment

2. Delineation of Function and Dysfunction Continua

    a. Identification and definition of the areas of concern

    b. Listing of behaviors indicative of function and dysfunction in these areas

3. Evaluation

    a. Identification and description of tools and techniques

    b. Procedural information

    c. Rules for interpretation of data

    d. Reliability and validity

4. Postulates Regarding Change

    a. Deduced from theoretical base

    b. Statements about alteration of dysfunction

    c. Identification and description of techniques to be used

    d. Guidelines for selecting techniques

    e. Step-by-step sequence of treatment process

Note. Adapted from *Three Frames of Reference for Mental Health* (p. 13), by A. C. Mosey, 1970, Thorofare, NJ: Charles B. Slack, Inc. Adapted with permission.

erence selected. The behaviors are what the therapist assesses in the evaluation process.

Evaluation, the third part of the frame of reference, is the process of identifying whether an individual is in a state of function or dysfunction. It is used as a basis for treatment. Evaluation tools and techniques serve as stimuli to elicit observable and measurable behaviors that differentiate between function and dysfunction. Procedures and rules to interpret the data are determined by the frame of reference selected.

Prescriptive statements derived from the postulates of the theoretical base make up the fourth part of the frame of reference. They state the principles by which an individual is aided in moving from a state of dysfunction to one of function. They guide the therapist in arranging his or her interaction with the client and the nonhuman environment. Ideally, these postulates have been empirically tested. Similar activities may be used with different frames of reference or postulates, but they will differ in the ways they are structured and used. For example, both analytical and developmental task groups might use finger painting; however, the analytical group might be using finger painting to express primitive impulses, whereas the developmental group might be working on primary social skill interaction.

Treatment is aimed at effecting predetermined change in the patient's limitations so that he or she may be a more productive member of a social system. It is a planned, collaborative interaction between the patient, therapist, and nonhuman environment (Mosey, 1970b).

The criteria for a frame of reference are stringent and are a statement of the ideal rather than the actual. Mosey has painstakingly synthesized theories and developed them into three frames of reference according to this four-part structure. She does not consider them to be complete, but has proposed them to stimulate thinking about frames of reference and what they should and should not include, to identify a goal for continued work in the area, and to give an orientation for classification of frames of reference that are currently available.

Structure of the Profession

Mosey's position as program director of the OT curriculum at New York University led her to widen her focus to the profession of OT as a whole. She began to search for its common elements so she could describe and analyze the profession's form and structure and the ways in which its parts relate to one another (A. C. Mosey, personal communication, October 4, 1984). This pursuit led her to pose a biopsychosocial model for the profession. This was meant not as a frame of reference, but rather as a professional model. Her subsequent work in this vein focused on the configuration of a profession. Thus, she developed a taxonomy or classification system and developed a model of the profession as a whole. After this, the third theme developed, with her delving into the epistemology of the field, which is the study of how humans know what they know, and how they develop knowledge.

Biopsychosocial Model

In 1974, Mosey developed a biopsychosocial model as an alternative to the medical or health models for OT. She argued that the medical model was not relevant to the OT process because occupational therapists are not concerned with diagnosis of disease or elimination of pathology. The health model was too vague; because it focused primarily on assets rather than limitations or dysfunction, the model was useful for prevention and community practice but too limiting for remediation. Neither model permitted the complete organization of the theoretical base of occupational therapy.

Mosey's biopsychosocial model, in contrast, focused on the individual's body, mind, and environment. It viewed the individual as a physical being who suffered the effects of illness and injury; a person with thoughts, emotions, needs, and values; and a player of many and varied social roles. This model is concerned with the skills, knowledge, abilities, and values that the individual must learn to function productively with others in his or her expected environment. The therapist effects change in the individual primarily by identifying learning needs and guiding the teaching–learning process. The teaching–learning process, as described in Mosey's earlier works (1968b, 1970b, 1973b) and in her 1981 book *Occupational Therapy: Configuration of a Profession,* may be based on any of a variety of theories about learning, such as operant conditioning and social learning theory. The therapist, as the teacher, begins where the learner is and moves at a rate that is comfortable for the learner. The therapist provides opportunities for trial and error, imitation, repetition, and practice in different situations so that the learner can observe and experience the consequences of an action. The learner needs to understand both what is to be learned and the rationale for learning.

Mosey (1974) initially felt that this biopsychosocial model would be useful for practice because it (a) provides a method to systematize OT knowledge, (b) provides a holistic statement of the profession's goals and theories of change, (c) is oriented to the development of skills needed by the client or patient for fuller participation in the community setting, (d) helps clarify the role of OT in relation to medicine and the other health-related professions, and (e) is well suited to community-based programs and the meeting of health needs. However, 6 years after presenting the biopsychosocial model, she wrote that "it became evident that the biopsychosocial model did not provide sufficient structure and content to give a holistic view of occupational therapy" (1980, p. 11). She continued with her quest for a model for the profession, refining the biopsychosocial model in an attempt to provide a holistic or generic approach to the philosophical and scientific foundation for the practice of occupational therapy. In 1980, she wrote, "My goal was and remains the identification of those factors which give unity to the profession and a firm base for the further development of areas of specialization" (p. 11).

Characteristics of a Professional Model

Mosey further researched the OT literature and primary sources most frequently cited by occupational therapists, and discussed with faculty, students, and clinicians factors that give unity to a profession and professional models. Based on this further study, and on philosophical and sociological literature of what constitutes a profession, she defined and described the structure, function, and characteristics of a model for professions in general and one specific to occupational therapy (1980, 1981, 1986). A model for a profession describes the way in which a profession perceives itself, its relationship to other professions, and its relationship to society, as well as its responsibility to society, methods, and rationale. A model applies to the entire profession rather than to any particular area of specialization. A model defines and delineates the nature of the profession and is accepted by its members and by society. It is dynamic, and its content is continually changing. Some of the changes result from changes in the body of knowledge and expertise of the profession, the domain of concern of other professions, and the needs, mandate, or acceptance of society. Each part of the model is interrelated, and a change in one part affects change in others. Mosey cautioned that a profession takes great risks in expanding its model beyond the limits of its present theoretical foundation and domain of concern. More may be claimed than can be delivered, and this may result in a loss of respect for the profession (Mosey, 1981, pp. 52–57).

The structure and characteristics of a model seem to be similar for all health professions. Some content, such as theories of human growth and development, may be shared by several professions. However, each profession's model has its own specific content. Mosey stated that a profession's model comprises the following six elements: philosophical assumptions basic to practice, ethical code, theoretical foundation (later referred to as a body of knowledge), domain of concern, nature of and principles for sequencing the various aspects of practice, and legitimate tools. Mosey (1980, 1981, 1986) described each of these components in detail in terms of its composition, structure, and relation to and influence on other components.

▶ 1. Philosophical Assumptions of a Professional Model

In Mosey's model for occupational therapy, the first element—philosophical assumptions—contains seven basic beliefs about the individual, his or her relationship with the human and nonhuman environment, and the profession's goals or purpose. They are as follows:

1. Each individual has the right to a meaningful existence; to an existence that allows one to be productive; to experience pleasure and joy; to love and be loved; and to live in surroundings that are safe, supportive, and comfortable.

2. Each individual is influenced by stage-specific maturation of the species, the social nature of the species, and the cognitive structure of the species.

3. Each individual has inherent needs for work, play, and rest that must be satisfied in a relatively equal balance.

4. Each individual has the right to seek his or her potential through personal choice within the context of some social constraints.

5. Each individual is only able to reach his or her potential through purposeful interaction with the human and nonhuman environment.

6. Each individual is only able to be understood within the context of his or her environment of family, community, and cultural group.

7. OT is concerned with promoting functional independence through intervention directed toward facilitating participation in major social roles (occupational performances) and the development of the physical, cognitive, psychological, and social skills (performance components) that are fundamental to these roles. The extent to which intervention is focused on occupational performances or performance components is dependent on the needs of a particular client at any given point in time. (Mosey, 1986, p. 6)

▶ 2. Ethical Code

The profession's ethical code comprises principles of human conduct regarding what is moral behavior toward clients, students, and colleagues. Mosey (1981, pp. 64–70) refers the reader to AOTA's Code of Ethics.

▶ 3. Profession's Body of Knowledge

The profession's body of knowledge, which is also referred to as its theoretical foundation, contains the scientific basis for the profession. It is derived from an ordered set of selected theoretical systems from a variety of different disciplines, as well as from the profession itself. Although professions may share some knowledge with other fields, each profession selects from outside its boundaries knowledge of particular relevance to it and develops its own unique combinations and adaptations of this knowledge. Occupational therapy's body of knowledge comes from the biological sciences, behavioral sciences, the arts, medicine, and OT (Mosey, 1980, 1981, 1986).

▶ 4. Domain of Concern

The domain of concern delineates the profession's areas of expertise. Although the concept of domain of concern and the subconcepts of performance components and areas of occupational performance had been identifed and labeled by an AOTA task force, Mosey conducted her own survey of the literature, including the writings of Reilly (1962, 1974), Llorens (1976; Llorens & Beck, 1966), Kielhofner (1977, 1983), and many others, to identify those areas of human function that occupational therapists believed they could successfully influence (see Figure 3.1). She lists the components of performance as motor function, sensory integra-

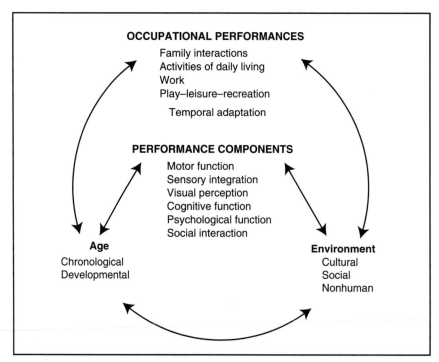

Figure 3.1. Domain of concern for occupational therapy. *Note.* Adapted from *Occupational Therapy: Configuration of a Profession* (p. 75), by A. C. Mosey, 1981, New York: Raven Press Ltd. Copyright 1981 by Raven Press Ltd. Adapted with permission.

tion, visual perception, cognitive function, psychological function, and social interactions. Occupational performances include family interactions, activities of daily living, school–work, play–leisure–recreation, and temporal adaptation. The clients' chronological and developmental age and cultural, social, and physical environment all interact with performance components and occupational performances.

▶ **5. Nature and Principles**

The nature of and principles for sequencing the various aspects of practice (Mosey, 1980, 1981, 1986) describe the problem-identification and problem-solving processes used to evaluate and treat clients. Mosey wrote about these in her earlier works (1970b, 1973a) mainly as applicable to frames of reference. In *Occupational Therapy: Configuration of a Profession* (1981) and in *Psychosocial Components of Occupational Therapy* (1986), she built on and integrated these principles into the larger concept of a model.

▶ **6. Legitimate Tools**

Legitimate tools are the modalities that the profession uses to achieve its goals. From her review of the OT literature, Mosey identified the following six tools: nonhuman environment, conscious use of self, the teaching–learning process, purposeful activity, activity groups, and activity analysis and synthesis (Mosey, 1981, 1986).

Models and Frames of Reference

Because frames of reference are derived from a theoretical base, they may be said to derive from the model of the profession that includes that base. In 1986, Mosey provided an expanded definition of frame of reference:

> It is a set of interrelated, internally consistent concepts, definitions, and postulates derived from or compatible with empirical data that provide a systematic description of, or prescription for, a practitioner's interaction within a particular aspect of a profession's domain of concern for the purpose of facilitating evaluation and effecting change. (p. 376)

The professional model provides the linkages among the various frames of reference to the profession as a whole.

Frames of reference are more limited than models. They link theory and practice in only a small area of the profession's body of knowledge and domain of concern, whereas a model defines the whole profession. A model is almost universally accepted by the profession and the society to which it is responsible. In contrast, a frame of reference has more limited acceptance by practitioners, and more than one frame of reference may be applied to the same portion of the domain of concern in the profession. The conflict and disagreement that may ensue can lead to clarification of concepts and further research. Whereas a frame of reference guides the practitioner in his or her daily interaction with clients, a model gives overall direction to the profession.

Professional Configuration

According to Mosey (1981, 1986), both a profession's model and its frames of reference are basic elements of a larger professional configuration. This configuration is a loop with six parts: philosophical foundation, model, frames of reference, practice, data, and research (see Figure 3.2). Philosophical assumptions, ethics, art, and science are basic elements of all professions. From each profession's particular philosophical foundation, a unique professional model develops. Various frames of reference are deduced from this model and serve as a guide for practice. Practice then produces data that enable one to evaluate their effectiveness and to refine the profession's body of knowledge. Thus, the arrows flow in two directions among data, research, and model. In Mosey's configuration, there is no direct relationship between research and practice or between research and frames of reference. Research only directly influences the body of knowledge component of the model by modifying or supporting its theoretical base. When a theory is altered by research findings, changes are effected in frames of reference that utilize that research base. These in turn lead to changes in practice. Thus, research can influence practice only after it is integrated into the professional model and relevant frames of reference. The professional model also influences research because a theoretical foundation should be evaluated continually (Mosey, 1981, 1986).

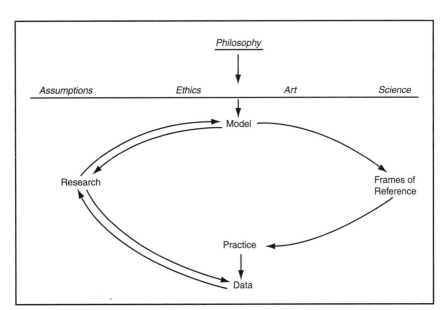

Figure 3.2. Occupational therapy loop. *Note.* From *Occupational Therapy: Configuration of a Profession* (p. 42), by A. C. Mosey, 1981, New York: Raven Press Ltd. Copyright 1981 by Raven Press Ltd. Adapted with permission.

Major Theme 3: Epistemology

The third theme that Mosey copiously worked on is the epistemology of the profession. The first and second editions of *Applied Scientific Inquiry in the Health Professions: An Epistemological Orientation* (Mosey, 1992a, 1996) are even more focused, esoteric, and detailed than any of her other work to date. The 1996 edition was clearer but still unique to her style of conceptualizing. These works delve into the realm of philosophies about knowledge, or epistemology. In the first edition, Mosey (1992a) articulated existing points of view about knowledge generation and presented the neopositivistic orientation as the one most relevant for the health professions. She argued that applied scientists, such as occupational therapists, need to understand theory both to determine which theories are suitable for their use and to apply them; therefore, she devoted a chapter to explaining how theory is developed and tested.

Mosey explained that whereas basic scientific inquiry has as its sole purpose the generation of theory and the discovery of new knowledge, applied scientific inquiry is concerned with immediate practical ends. She also distinguished two types of applied scientific inquiry: Type I, the goal of which is to develop guidelines for practice, and Type II, the goal of which is to determine the best answer to a particular practical problem. Examples from OT illustrate how guidelines for practice, or frames of reference, are formulated (1992a). Her purpose in writing this book was to facilitate the study and discussion of the epistemology of practice. In 1996, she published the second edition for the following two reasons. The first was to provide more depth about applied Type II scientific inquiry, especially the research associated with this type of scientific investigation. She carefully distinguished Type II scientific inquiry from basic scientific inquiry. The second reason was to address the "astounding number of myths about scientific inquiry that I encountered subsequent to publication of the first edition" (p. v). In the second edition, she provided "corrective additional information" about the most common myths and addressed them.

Application to Occupational Therapy

Application to Occupational Therapy Practice

Mosey (1973b, 1992a, 1996) regarded clinical practice as the process of using science and applying theories. In her opinion, the therapist must consciously select theories and use them as a guide for action. Although the therapist's actions may be guided by more than one theory, the postulates need to be logically compatible. Mosey objects to therapists' doing what they feel is right intuitively without reference to any particular theoretical system. Thus, a major contribution of hers has been to advocate for the use of coherent theory-based treatment.

Until more refined techniques of measurement are developed and researched, no one frame of reference can claim authority. Therefore, Mosey encourages therapists to select their own individual frame of reference and techniques for patient care to suit their style of practice. The frame of reference selected needs to be appropriate to the client's cultural norms and background. She suggests that the beginning therapist study and use a variety of frames of reference with a nonjudgmental attitude. Initial efforts to apply frames of reference should be made under competent supervision.

Mosey (1971) stated that without the conscious application of a theoretical base, therapists function primarily as technicians rather than as professionals. She was concerned that the emphasis was placed on technique, not on theory. To remedy this state of affairs, she encouraged researchers to systematically organize the considerable practice-relevant knowledge, which would enable practitioners to eliminate the irrelevant and help them identify what knowledge was lacking and what was available, thereby facilitating the organization of theory and research. Mosey began this work in her book *Psychosocial Components of Occupational Therapy* (1986), which reviewed, synthesized, and systematized the literature basic to psychosocial OT from within the field and from related disciplines and professions. Mosey wrote that the book's "purpose is to provide an overview of the psychosocial components—both the body of knowledge and approaches to evaluation and intervention" (Mosey, 1986, p. vii).

Mosey said that psychosocial components are applicable to all areas of specialization because they are "fundamental to the understanding of our clients, ourselves as therapists, and the tools that we use in practice" (Mosey, 1986, p. vii). Consistent with her thinking was the pluralistic approach and use of a variety of frames of reference. Through Mosey's painstaking synthesis of the theoretical base of the profession as a whole and her taxonomy and configuration of its specific parts, the therapist is provided with a structure needed to make the transition from theory to practice. Mosey (1986, 1992a, 1996) also described the essential role of research in practice and for the building of theories.

Application to the Occupational Therapy Profession

Much of Mosey's work has focused on developing and articulating occupational therapy's theoretical basis and professional identity, and exploring how these influence practice. Mosey argues that this kind of professional self-questioning is a natural and necessary process that "occurs in cycles and provides a healthy means for reexamination, revitalization, and change"

(1981, p. 120). In her book *Psychosocial Components of Occupational Therapy* (1986), a chapter titled "Historical Perspective" traces a history of changes in types of intervention, frames of reference, and techniques employed by occupational therapy, and discusses the profession's "search for identity" from its initial reliance on medicine to its development of frames of reference.

In her Eleanor Clarke Slagle Lecture in 1985, Mosey explored monism and pluralism as two approaches that professions can take to form their identity. Monism is an attempt to define a profession by one of its elements or a facet of an element that is considered primary and that governs all other elements. A pluralistic approach is much broader and takes into consideration all of the elements of a profession. The whole is defined by the totality of its parts, and each of these parts is distinct and different.

A monistic approach usually takes the form of a comprehensive theory (Mosey, 1985). According to such an approach, the profession has one theoretical base and one method for applying it to its domain of concern. Some of the approaches that Mosey considered for a comprehensive theory for OT were developmental theory as proposed by Llorens (1976), occupational behavior as described by Reilly (1962, 1974), purposeful activity as discussed by Fidler and Fidler (1978), King's (1978) theory of adaptive response, and the model of human occupation as proposed by Kielhofner (1983). Although there would be more approaches now, these were the ones she identified at the time. Mosey (1985) stated that a monistic approach may exclude important facts, ignore important social needs, and discourage creative, divergent thinking. A comprehensive theory may oversimplify the profession's body of knowledge, domain of concern, and practice, or it may be too complex and intricate to be easily understood. It may also inhibit research if the concepts cannot be operationalized and made into variables for empirical testing to assess the theory's validity or the effectiveness of interventions derived from that theory.

Therefore, Mosey has consistently advocated a pluralistic approach in her development of frames of reference. The pluralistic approach regards all the elements of a profession as being of equal importance. The legitimate tools of the profession are as important as the theories that underlie their application and vice versa. Mosey feels that the pluralistic model is more flexible and can more readily allow for change as new ideas, knowledge, and beliefs emerge to meet the changing needs of society. Diversity in orientations is healthy and potentially more adaptive (Mosey, 1985, 1986).

Mosey (1985) suggested a taxonomy for the articulation of a pluralistic identity. She said that each of the elements of the profession—philosophical assumptions, ethical code, theoretical foundation, domain of concern, principles for sequencing various aspects of practice, and legitimate tools—needs to be clearly defined and the various contents outlined. By making clear the content of each element, this taxonomy and configuration would allow researchers to readily identify incongruence among elements. It would also enable occupational therapists to recognize what their many specialties have in common. Content could be added or deleted as appropriate. Professional identity would be derived from all of the elements. This pluralistic approach would provide a structure that would make it easier for occupational therapists to analyze their philosophical assumptions critically, select or develop new theories, make changes in their domain of concern, consider alternative legitimate tools, and formulate more definitive and additional frames of reference. Mosey argued that an important part of this effort must be the exploration of current theories generated by other disciplines, such as neurophysiology, and their integration into occupational therapy.

Mosey's steadfast commitment to applied scientific inquiry as the method of scientific inquiry for OT is again clearly demonstrated in her articles "Partition of Occupational Science and Occupational Therapy" (1992b) and "Partition of Occupational Science and Occupational Therapy: Sorting Out Some Issues" (1993). She argues that occupational science be kept completely separate from occupation therapy financially, epistemologically, scientifically, and professionally. This opened a lively debate between her and some occupational scientists (Carlson & Dunlea, 1995; Clark et al., 1993) regarding whether occupational therapy is better served by complete separation, whether there is a continuous and nondichotomous relationship between basic and applied scientific inquiry, and what roles basic scientific inquiry and applied scientific inquiry have in occupational therapy. Her position is clear and unwaveringly in support of applied scientific inquiry.

Theory Validation and Research

Mosey's work has contributed immeasurably to an understanding of the profession's parts and wholeness. However, because her major work has been to develop a taxonomy and configuration, and more recently an epistemology of a profession, it is difficult to evaluate subsequent research and application of her work. Mosey's pluralistic model has received support, but whether researchers and practitioners will actually adopt it remains to be seen.

Mosey's view of her own influence is modest:

> It takes a long time for professions to change and I present my ideas and people can accept or not accept them. I have no driving need for people to accept my ideas. I am not a public person. The thrill and reward come from playing with ideas and putting ideas together and knowing that eventually it will help our patients. (A. C. Mosey, personal communication, August 4, 1985)

Mosey has repeatedly emphasized that occupational therapists need to test the theories and theoretical foundations that they have and use them as a basis for practice, translate them into frames of reference, and evaluate their effectiveness (1968a, 1968b, 1970b, 1980, 1981, 1986, 1992a, 1996). She has painstakingly given the OT profession the framework with which to do this. Through the research process, data generated from practice can systematically lead to tentative hypotheses that will refute, develop, refine, or verify the theoretical bases. This can help researchers evaluate frames of reference and their theoretical base. According to Mosey (1986, 1992a, 1996), when the theoretical base is altered by research findings, changes in frames of reference result, and these in turn lead to changes in practice. Researchers who wish to engage in this process will find Mosey's works an invaluable tool.

Bibliography

1968

Mosey, A. C. (1968). *Occupational therapy: Theory and practice.* Medford, MA: Pothier Brothers Press.

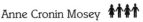

Mosey, A. C. (1968). Recapitulation of ontogenesis: A theory for the practice of occupational therapy. *American Journal of Occupational Therapy*, 22, 426–432.

1969

Mosey, A. C. (1969). Treatment of pathological distortion of body image. *American Journal of Occupational Therapy, 23*, 413–416.

1970

Mosey, A. C. (1970). The concept and use of developmental groups. *American Journal of Occupational Therapy, 24*, 272–275.

Mosey, A. C. (1970). *Three frames of reference for mental health*. Thorofare, NJ: Charles B. Slack.

1971

Mosey, A. C. (1971). Involvement in the rehabilitation movement 1942–1960. *American Journal of Occupational Therapy, 25*, 234–236.

1973

Mosey, A. C. (1973). *Activities therapy*. New York: Raven Press.

Mosey, A. C. (1973). Meeting health needs. *American Journal of Occupational Therapy, 27*, 14–17.

1974

Corry, S., Sebastian, V., & Mosey, A. C. (1974). Acute short-term treatment in psychiatry. *American Journal of Occupational Therapy, 28*, 401–406.

Mosey, A. C. (1974). An alternative: The biopsychosocial model. *American Journal of Occupational Therapy, 28*, 137–140.

1976

Mosey, A. C. (1976). The night of January twenty-seven. *American Journal of Occupational Therapy, 30*, 648–649.

1980

Katz, G. M., & Mosey, A. C. (1980). Fieldwork performance, academic grades and preselection criteria of occupational therapy students. *American Journal of Occupational Therapy, 34*, 794–800.

Mosey, A. C. (1980). A model for occupational therapy. *Occupational Therapy in Mental Health, 1*, 11–32.

1981

Mosey, A. C. (1981). The art of practice. In B. C. Abreu (Ed.), *Physical disabilities manual* (pp. 1–3). New York: Raven Press.

Mosey, A. C. (1981). *Occupational therapy: Configuration of a profession*. New York: Raven Press.

1985

Mosey, A. C. (1985). A monistic or a pluralistic approach to professional identity? Eleanor Clarke Slagle lecture. *American Journal of Occupational Therapy, 39*, 504–509.

1986

Mosey, A. C. (1986). *Psychosocial components of occupational therapy*. New York: Raven Press.

1989

Mosey, A. C. (1989). The proper focus of scientific inquiry in occupational therapy: Frames of reference. *Occupational Therapy Journal of Research, 9*, 195–201.

1991

Mosey, A. C. (1991). Letter to the editor: Common vocabulary. *Occupational Therapy Journal of Research, 11*, 67–68.

1992

Mosey, A. C. (1992). *Applied scientific inquiry in the health professions: An epistemological orientation*. Rockville, MD: American Occupational Therapy Association.

Mosey, A. C. (1992). The issue is—Partition of occupational science and occupational therapy. *American Journal of Occupational Therapy, 46*, 851–853.

1993

Mosey, A. C. (1993). Partition of occupational science and occupational therapy: Sorting out some issues. *American Journal of Occupational Therapy, 47*, 851–853.

1996

Mosey, A. C. (1996). *Applied scientific inquiry in the health professions: An epistemological orientation* (2nd ed.). Rockville, MD: American Occupational Therapy Association.

Mosey, A. C. (1996). *Psychosocial components of occupational therapy* (2nd ed.). Philadelphia: Lippincott-Raven.

References

Ayres, J. (1958). The visual-motor function. *American Journal of Occupational Therapy, 12*, 130–139.

Ayres, J. (1961). Development of body scheme in children. *American Journal of Occupational Therapy, 15*, 99–102.

Ayres, J. (1963). The development of perceptual motor disabilities. *American Journal of Occupational Therapy, 17*, 221–225.

Ayres, J. (1964). Tactile function. *American Journal of Occupational Therapy, 18*, 6–11.

Bandura, A. (1969). *Principles of behavior modification*. New York: Holt, Rinehart & Winston.

Banus, B. (Ed.). (1979). *The developmental therapist*. Thorofare, NJ: Charles B. Slack.

Bruner, J. (1966). *Studies in cognitive growth*. New York: Wiley.

Carlson, M., & Dunlea, A. (1995). Further thoughts on the pitfalls of partition: A response to Mosey. *American Journal of Occupational Therapy, 49*, 73–81.

Clark, F., Zemke, R., Frank, G., Parham, D., Neville-Jan, A., Hedricks, C., Carlson, M., Fazio, L., & Abreu, B. (1993). The issue is—Dangers inherent in the partition of OTand occupational science. *American Journal of Occupational Therapy, 47*, 184–186.

Diasio, K. (1968). Psychiatric occupational therapy: A search for a conceptual framework in light of psychoanalytic, ego psychology, and learning theory. *American Journal of Occupational Therapy, 22*, 400–407.

Dollard, J., & Miller, N. (1950). *Personality and psychotherapy*. New York: McGraw-Hill.

Erikson, E. (1950). *Childhood and society*. New York: Norton.

Fidler, G., & Fidler, J. (1963). *Occupational therapy: A communication process in psychiatry*. New York: Macmillan.

Fidler, G., & Fidler, J. (1978). Doing and becoming: Purposeful action and self-actualization. *American Journal of Occupational Therapy, 32*, 305–310.

Flavell, J. (1963). *The developmental psychology of Jean Piaget.* New York: D. Van Nostrand.

Ford, D., & Urban, H. (1963). *Systems of psychotherapy.* New York: Wiley.

Freud, A. (1965). *Normality and pathology in childhood.* New York: International University Press.

Freud, S. (1949). *An outline of psychoanalysis.* New York: Norton.

Hartman, H. (1958). *Ego psychology and the problems of adaptation.* New York: International University Press.

Jung, C. (1933). *Modern man in search of a soul.* New York: Harcourt, Brace and World.

Jung, C. (1964). *Man and his symbols.* New York: Doubleday.

Kielhofner, G. (1977). Temporal adaptation: A conceptual framework for occupational therapy. *American Journal of Occupational Therapy, 31*, 235–242.

Kielhofner, G. (Ed.). (1983). *Health through occupation: Theory and practice in occupational therapy.* Philadelphia: F. A. Davis.

King, L. J. (1978). Towards a science of adaptive responses. *American Journal of Occupational Therapy, 32*, 429–437.

Llorens, L. (1976). *Application of a developmental theory for health and rehabilitation.* Rockville, MD: American Occupational Therapy Association.

Llorens, L., & Beck, G. (1966, March). *Training methods for cognitive–perceptual–motor dysfunction.* Paper presented at the Therapy Seminar on Normal Growth and Development with Deviations, St. Louis.

Maslow, A. (1962). *Toward a psychology of being.* Princeton, NJ: D. Van Nostrand.

Mosey, A. (1968a). *Occupational therapy: Theory and practice.* Medford, MA: Pothier Brothers Press.

Mosey, A. (1968b). Recapitulation of ontogenesis: A theory for the practice of occupational therapy. *American Journal of Occupational Therapy, 22*, 426–432.

Mosey, A. (1969). Treatment of pathological distortion of body image. *American Journal of Occupational Therapy, 23*, 413–416.

Mosey, A. (1970a). The concept and use of developmental groups. *American Journal of Occupational Therapy, 24*, 272–275.

Mosey, A. (1970b). *Three frames of reference for mental health.* Thorofare, NJ: Charles B. Slack.

Mosey, A. (1971). Involvement in the rehabilitation movement 1942–1960. *American Journal of Occupational Therapy, 25*, 234–236.

Mosey, A. (1973a). *Activities therapy.* New York: Raven Press.

Mosey, A. (1973b). Meeting health needs. *American Journal of Occupational Therapy, 27*, 14–17.

Mosey, A. (1974). An alternative: The biopsychosocial model. *American Journal of Occupational Therapy, 28*, 137–140.

Mosey, A. (1976). The night of January twenty-seven. *American Journal of Occupational Therapy, 30*, 648–649.

Mosey, A. (1980). A model for occupational therapy. *Occupational Therapy in Mental Health, 1*, 11–32.

Mosey, A. (1981). Occupational therapy: Configuration of a profession. New York: Raven Press.

Mosey, A. (1985). A monistic or a pluralistic approach to professional identity? Eleanor Clarke Slagle lecture. *American Journal of Occupational Therapy, 39*, 504–509.

Mosey, A. (1986). *Psychosocial components of occupational therapy.* New York: Raven Press.

Mosey, A. C. (1992a). *Applied scientific inquiry in the health professions: An epistemological orientation.* Rockville, MD: American Occupational Therapy Association.

Mosey, A. C. (1992b). The issue is —Partition of occupational science and occupational therapy. *American Journal of Occupational Therapy, 46*, 851–853.

Mosey, A. C. (1993). Partition of occupational science and occupational therapy: Sorting out some issues. *American Journal of Occupational Therapy, 47*, 851–853.

Mosey, A. C. (1996). *Applied scientific inquiry in the health professions: An epistemological orientation* (2nd ed.). Rockville, MD: American Occupational Therapy Association.

Reilly, M. (1962). Occupational therapy can be one of the great ideas of 20th century medicine. *American Journal of Occupational Therapy, 16*, 1–9.

Reilly, M. (Ed.). (1974). *Play as exploratory learning.* Beverly Hills, CA: Sage.

Richert, G. Z. (1989). An interview with Anne Cronin Mosey. *Occupational Therapy in Mental Health, 9*, 1–15.

Schilder, P. (1950). *The image and appearance of the human body.* New York: Wiley.

Searles, H. (1960). *The nonhuman environment.* New York: International University Press.

Sechehaye, M. (1951a). *A new psychotherapy in schizophrenia.* New York: Grune & Stratton.

Sechehaye, M. (1951b). *Symbolic realization.* New York: International University Press.

Sieg, K. (1974). Applying the behavioral model to occupational therapy. *American Journal of Occupational Therapy, 7*, 421–428.

Smith, A., & Tempone, V. (1968). Psychiatric occupational therapy within a learning theory context. *American Journal of Occupational Therapy, 22*, 415–425.

Sullivan, H. S. (1953). *The interpersonal theory of psychiatry.* New York: Norton.

Trombly, C., & Scott, A. D. (1977). *Occupational therapy for physical dysfunction.* Baltimore: Williams & Wilkins.

Wolpe, J., & Lazarus, A. (1966). *Behavior therapy techniques.* New York: Pergamon Press.

Lela A. Llorens

4

Kay F. Walker and Susan Denegan Shortridge

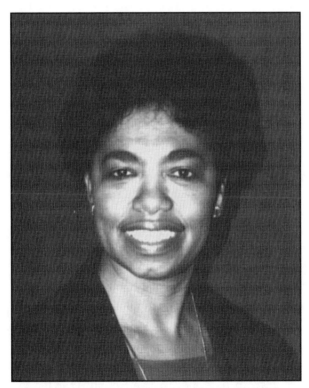

It is the task of the occupational therapist to determine at what level the individual is functioning in the various aspects along the developmental continuum and to program for facilitating growth and development in each of these areas in accordance with the needs of the individual and the demands of his age. (Llorens, 1970, p. 100)

L ela A. Llorens expressed this premise in her 1970 Eleanor Clarke Slagle Lecture, and it remained central to her deliberate and thoughtful contribution of a framework for conceptualizing and organizing the practice of occupational therapy (OT). As she stated, "This formulation does not provide a recipe for practicing occupational therapy. It simply orders some of the factors relevant to a developmental theory for practice" (1970, p. 101). Her body of work represents a consistent and coherent progression of ideas depicting the OT process, which she described simply, intricately, and comprehensively. She has shown occupational therapists how to step back and see the pieces of the therapy process in terms of an integrated whole and to apply this process in service to patients and clients, with particular sensitivity to cultural and ethnic issues.

Biographical Sketch

Lela A. Llorens (née Williams) was born in Shreveport, Louisiana, in 1933, during an era when women were not expected to have careers. In addition to the gender stereotypes of the times, she experienced the cultural limitations imposed on African American women in her Southern community. Segregation of the races in schools was the norm in the South at that time, and educational opportunities for African American children were severely limited. Recognizing these barriers, her father moved the family to Detroit, Michigan, in search of a better life and more accessible education for the children.

Perhaps the lessons of her early family history contributed to her lifelong determination and motivation for excellence. She cites her father's goal orientation—his insistence on thinking ahead and planning what you are going to do and then doing it—as a definite influence in her approach to life. When she and her sister entered school in Detroit, they were placed in a lower grade because they had come from a school in the South. Her father urged the school to give his daughters the opportunity to demonstrate their ability. Llorens noted, "We successfully passed the grade to which we advanced, and I was then advanced two grades" (personal communication, September 14, 1992).

Education

Llorens identified OT as her career choice when she read the University of Puget Sound catalog description and realized that OT matched her natural abilities in arts and crafts and her interest in medicine. She began her studies at the University of Puget Sound in 1949 and received her bachelor of science degree in occupational therapy from Western Michigan University in 1953. To support her practice goals with educational advancement, she pursued graduate work at Wayne State University, where she received a master of arts degree in vocational rehabilitation. She chose this degree program because its flexibility enabled her to elect course work that complemented her effectiveness as a therapist and as a supervisor.

Desiring to develop stronger research skills, Llorens entered a doctoral program at the University of the Pacific in Stockton, California, in 1970. She found, however, that the program's emphasis in educational psychology did not satisfy her need to learn more about research while maintaining her commitment to OT. At Walden University in both Minneapolis, Minnesota, and its campus in Naples, Florida, Llorens was able to design and complete a doctoral program that met her educational goals. She received the doctor of philosophy degree in education/occupational therapy in 1976 and completed a certificate in gerontology from San Jose State University in California in 1994.

Employment

Llorens's first position in the field was as a staff occupational therapist at the site of one of her internships, Wayne County General Hospital, where she developed programs for adult psychiatric patients. She began to identify and articulate what occupational therapy was providing to these patients. Llorens remained in this position from 1953–1957.

Despite a decrease in salary and an increase in travel time, Llorens accepted a staff position at Northville State Hospital in Michigan because it enabled her to work more with children. Although she was there for only one year, this experience confirmed her interest in pediatrics. As she stated,

> I really was fascinated with emotionally disturbed children and what occupational therapy could do for them. There was not very much in the literature regarding pediatrics . . . it was a matter of figuring out what the profession had to offer based on what was already known about adults. (L. A. Llorens, personal communication, September 2, 1983)

Llorens then worked from 1958 to 1968 at the Lafayette Clinic, beginning as supervisor of OT services in child psychiatry. She eventually became head of the OT department and supervised therapists practicing with adult psychosocial and neurological patients in addition to her practice in child psychiatry. In this job, she delineated the role of OT in a psychotherapeutic setting.

From 1968 to 1971, Llorens served as consultant to the Comprehensive Child Care Project at Mount Zion Hospital in San Francisco. This project enabled her to explore the consultant role and the expansion of OT services into community and nontraditional settings. While working on this project, she began to address cultural variables in health care delivery. She also explored the limits of OT's effectiveness in a pediatric population. This work experience confirmed for her that occupational therapy has a knowledge base that can be expanded and is viable in diverse settings such as public schools, community agencies, and outpatient clinics.

Drawing on her background as a consultant in community health practice, Llorens wrote several articles to guide other occupational therapists. She described the therapist's consulting role (1973b, 1992) and outlined a problem-solving process that consultants could use to determine how OT could best serve a new environment. In these publications, Llorens emphasized that the key to success in community health practice was the therapist's appreciation of the cultural milieu of the clients. Therapists need knowledge of clients' ethnic characteristics, socioeconomic status, and value system to communicate effectively with clients and negotiate within their community.

After about 18 years in OT, Llorens began to reflect on her original choice of profession and to explore other vocational possibilities. Her results on vocational tests were almost identical to ones from her college years that had confirmed her decision to become a health care professional. From this time of reflection, however, she decided to change her focus from clinical practice to academia.

Llorens had already acquired teaching experience throughout her employment history. For example, one of her responsibilities during the Mount Zion Hospital project was to teach growth and development to medical pediatric interns and residents. Although the hospital's Department of Pediatrics wanted her to continue with this teaching, she was faced with a career decision.

> I really felt that if I was going to teach full-time, I should teach occupational therapists. I had about 18 years experience and there were not many people around with that kind of clinical experience. . . . I felt that it should be passed on. (L. A. Llorens, personal communication, September 2, 1983)

While seeking a teaching position, Llorens investigated many OT programs. Her decision to accept an appointment as an associate professor at the University of Florida was based on several critical factors: the opportunity to be involved in the development of a graduate program, the developmental hierarchy inherent in the design of the existing curriculum, and a deep respect for the chair, Dr. Alice Jantzen, who was to become an important mentor.

This new phase of involvement in academic OT appeared to be a significant reawakening of ambition and direction for Llorens. From 1971 to 1974, she was occupied with responsibilities as an associate professor and graduate coordinator. In 1975, when Jantzen retired, Llorens assumed the role of acting department chair. In the next 2 years, she was promoted to full professor and was officially appointed chair for the OT department. She maintained this position for 6 years, during which time she contributed greatly to the department's development by facilitating the articulation of the department's frame of reference for OT education and practice and by refining the OT graduate program. In addition to promoting graduate students' interest in research, Llorens had a profound influence on the professional development of less experienced faculty.

In 1982, after 11 years at the University of Florida, Llorens became professor and coordinator of graduate studies at San Jose State University's Department of Occupational Therapy.

The following year, she was elected by the faculty to serve as chair of that department and was reelected for ensuing terms until 1993 when she was appointed as interim associate academic vice president in the Office of Faculty Affairs, a job she held for three years. She also served as codirector of the Division of Health Professions from 1990 to 1993, and as core faculty of the Geriatric Education Center at Stanford University School of Medicine. Since retiring in 1996, she has continued in emeritus roles at both San Jose State and Stanford and as adjunct associate professor in the Department of Occupational Science and Occupational Therapy at the University of Southern California.

Llorens has served as a leader in OT education throughout her academic career. Her publications in this area cover such topics as student learning and growth (Llorens, 1967c, 1982b; Llorens & Adams, 1976) and educator competency (Canfield, Williams, Llorens, & Wroe, 1973; Llorens, 1981a, 1982a). An avid supporter of graduate students in their research, she supervised some 140 projects between 1983 and 1994 (L. A. Llorens, personal communication, 2001).

Written Work

The questions "What is OT?" and "What does OT do?" have occupied most of Llorens's written work, dating to her early experiences as a student and young therapist. As a student, she was dissatisfied with not being able to explain or define occupational therapy. As a new therapist, she saw that many therapists could demonstrate the value of OT but could not articulate frames of reference or theory related to it. Not until she attended graduate school was Llorens able to explore these questions. She stated, "Term papers that I was doing for classes were essentially significant learning experiences. They were not just papers that were handed in to fulfill an assignment or requirements for a degree" (L.A. Llorens, personal communication, September 2, 1983).

Llorens's first article, "Psychological Tests in Planning Treatment Goals," was published in 1960. It revealed the impact of schooling on her professional work, as well as the influence of a mentor (Eli Rubin) and an interdisciplinary team in a work environment that promoted scholarly inquiry.

My first publication resulted from a term paper that I did for my master's degree. Although I was the single author on this paper, Eli contributed a great deal to the structure and the content. He helped me to organize which was probably the beginning of a framework or orientation to organize behaviors that we were seeing in occupational therapy. I initially used more of a psychological framework because that seemed to offer some way of beginning to look at the behaviors that we were seeing clinically. (L. A. Llorens, personal communication, September 2, 1983)

In this paper, Llorens attempted to integrate evaluation data gathered from psychological testing with behavior observations made in occupational therapy. She stated,

For occupational therapy to contribute to the therapeutic community it must be capable of contributing a specific commodity . . . [It must] participate cooperatively . . . and must be capable of a collaborative relationship. For many years, occupational therapy has maintained a dependent role to medical staff and a rivalrous, conflicting role to nursing. . . . Occupational therapy has a specific contributive function that can be realized through effective evaluation and comprehensive programming. (L. A. Llorens, personal communication, September 2, 1983)

Since her first publication, Llorens has authored or edited 8 books and authored 9 book chapters, 52 refereed journal articles, 6 newsletter articles, 13 proceedings publications, 4 book forewords, and 7 funded grants. What began as a term paper has become a written legacy of her efforts to present her answers to the first question, What is occupational therapy?

Mentors

Llorens credits several key persons who have served as mentors in her career. Mentors played an important role in her career moves, and in each new position she sought significant people within the work setting from whom to learn. As she stated, "The positions I've held have contributed to my continued growth, interest and direction in the field. This has been partly deliberate and partly opportunity" (L. A. Llorens, personal communication, September 2, 1983).

While attending Western Michigan University (1950–1953), she was a student of Marion R. Spear, chair and founder of that department, and was impressed by the high leadership expectations for graduates of that department. She also cites her supervisor in her first job, Mae McGiverin at Wayne County General Hospital, as a significant person in encouraging her interest in mental health occupational therapy.

When asked to identify persons who provided long-term guidance, she named four: Eli Rubin, Wilma West, Alice Jantzen, and Richard Whitlock (Robertson, 1992). While at the Lafayette Clinic, Llorens worked with a research team, an experience that added a new dimension to her writing and treatment capabilities. She developed a strong collaborative relationship with Eli Rubin, clinical psychologist and then coordinator of children's services at the Lafayette Clinic. Rubin encouraged her to write, conduct research, and present at conferences. He endorsed her as a part-time faculty member in her first academic teaching appointment.

Throughout her career, Llorens has been inspired by Wilma West. West was long active in the AOTA and worked in administration, education, research, and consultation. According to Llorens, "Wilma West's vision, her ability to articulate the promise of occupational therapy, and her belief in my ability to make a significant contribution to the profession were inspirational to me" (L. A. Llorens, personal communication, September 2, 1983). On West's recommendation, Llorens became consultant to the Mount Zion Project. West continued to serve as long-distance adviser to Llorens in the consultant role at Mount Zion and in subsequent appointments throughout her career.

Llorens's relationship with Alice Jantzen proved to be a significant factor in guiding her academic career toward success. As she described,

> I would also have to name Dr. Jantzen as one of my mentors. I learned a great deal from her as a strong leader within the profession, as well as in the college and department at the University of Florida. It was important to me that she was planning to remain for a number of years after I arrived. My goals, while they included a future academic administrative position, also included some other things that I thought I needed to learn. I

learned about academia from Dr. Jantzen. I learned how to
mentor young faculty and how to run an academic program as
contrasted to a rehabilitative program. I learned about higher
education as viewed by the academy, which has a different
value system than that held by helping professions. I learned
how to be an academician, as well as a therapist, teacher, and
writer. (L. A. Llorens, personal communication, September 2,
1983)

Finally, Llorens names Richard Whitlock at San Jose State
University. He assisted her in learning the system at San Jose
State. She noted that

He extended the education that I began at the University of
Florida with Alice Jantzen. The environment of a comprehensive university with a liberal arts and sciences focus and no
medical school was considerably different from that which I
had previously known. Dick Whitlock was instrumental in
helping me avoid the land mines while moving positively
ahead toward my career goals. (Robertson, 1992, p. 27)

Honors

For her leadership in theory, education, and research, Llorens
has been awarded many honors, including the highest accolades
that are bestowed in the profession of occupational therapy. Recognition of her outstanding performance began as early as her undergraduate work at Western Michigan University when she received the Marion R. Spear Scholastic Award in 1953. Llorens was
awarded the AOTA Eleanor Clarke Slagle Lectureship in 1969.
Her preparation for this lectureship initiated the evolution of her
own developmental theory.

Llorens's influence in the area of OT education was recognized at university and state levels. One of her more noteworthy
responsibilities was as chair for the Research Advisory Committee of the American Occupational Therapy Foundation (AOTF).
Her abilities as a researcher and leader in the field were apparent in her repeated appointment to this position (1978–1989).
Awards granted by the AOTA, in addition to the Eleanor Clarke
Slagle Lectureship, include the Roster of Fellows in 1973, the
Award of Merit in 1986, and a Service Award in 1989. Awards

granted by the AOTF include the Certificate of Appreciation in 1981, the A. Jean Ayres Award for research in 1988, and a Meritorious Service Award in 1989.

Llorens is also an invited keynote speaker and presenter at conferences and meetings. She has been honored as a visiting scholar at Wayne State University (1991), Texas Woman's University (1991), University of Wisconsin–Madison (1991), Medical University of South Carolina (1990), and Western Michigan University (1987). The Michigan State Senate awarded her the Certificate of Merit in 1991. Also in 1991, she was invited to submit her written works for preservation in the Blagg–Huey Library Woman's Collection at Texas Woman's University.

Theoretical Concepts

Developmental Theory for the Practice of Occupational Therapy

Llorens's first conceptualization of a developmental theory was based on 15 years of experience in OT practice and research in the OT and human development literature. As a new therapist and then in her subsequent positions, Llorens was challenged by the need for a clear description of occupational therapy that would lend credibility to the profession and to the role of occupational therapy. The task of writing for the Eleanor Clarke Slagle Lectureship presented her with the opportunity to provide that description. As she stated,

> The theory . . . has been an outgrowth of my experiences and research in the field of psychiatry, both pediatric and adult . . . in pediatric general medicine and community health. . . . These experiences have stimulated my desire to think through the function and purpose of occupational therapy as I have experienced it. (1970, p. 93)

Ten Premises

Llorens's theory was developed from the following thesis:

> That occupational therapy is a facilitation process which assists the individual in achieving mastery of life tasks and the

ability to cope as efficiently as possible with the life expectations made of him through the mechanisms of selected input stimuli, and availability of practice in a suitable environment. (1970, p. 93)

This thesis is based on the following 10 premises:

1. That the human organism develops horizontally (simultaneously) in the areas of neurophysiological, physical, psychosocial, and psychodynamic growth and in the development of social language, daily living, and sociocultural skills at specific periods of time.

2. That the human organism develops longitudinally (chronologically) in each of these areas in a continuous process as one ages.

3. That mastery of particular skills, abilities, and relationships in each of the areas of neurophysiological, physical, psychosocial, and psychodynamic development, social language, daily living, and sociocultural skills, both horizontally and longitudinally, is necessary to the successful achievement of satisfactory coping behavior and adaptive relationships.

4. That such mastery is usually achieved naturally in the course of development.

5. That the fundamental endowment of the individual and the stimulation of experiences received within the environment of the family come together to interact in such a way as to promote positive early growth and development in both the horizontal (simultaneous) and longitudinal (chronological) planes.

6. That later influences of extended family, community, social, and civic groups assist in the growth process.

7. That physical or psychological trauma related to disease, injury, environmental insufficiencies, or intrapersonal vulnerability can interrupt the growth and development process.

8. That such growth interruption will cause a gap in the developmental cycle, resulting in a disparity between

expected coping behavior and adaptive facility and the necessary skills and abilities to achieve the same.

9. That occupational therapy, through the skilled application of activities and relationships, can provide growth and development links to assist in closing the gap between expectation and ability by increasing skills, abilities, and relationships in the neurophysiological, physical, psychosocial, psychodynamic, social language, daily living, and sociocultural spheres of development as indicated both horizontally and longitudinally.

10. That occupational therapy, through the skilled application of activities and relationships, can provide growth experiences to prevent the development of potential maladaptation related to insufficient nurturing in neurophysiological, physical, psychosocial, psychodynamic, social language, daily living, and sociocultural spheres of development both horizontally (simultaneously) and longitudinally (chronologically). (Llorens, 1970, pp. 93–94)

Schematic Representation of Facilitating Growth and Development

Llorens's Schematic Representation of Facilitating Growth and Development expands the 10 premises by portraying both developmental and behavioral expectations and the activities and relationships that facilitate these expectations (Llorens, 1970, 1976). The schematic is organized into three sections (see Table 4.1).

Section I depicts developmental expectations, behaviors, and needs and their simultaneous (horizontal) and chronological (longitudinal) progression. Stage-specific development categories of human growth include those of Ayres (neurophysiological development); Gesell (physical–motor, sociocultural, social–language, and daily living development); Erikson (psychosocial development); and Hall, Grant, and Freud (psychodynamic development). Although each theorist is recognized for a particular area of expertise, Llorens stressed that these areas of growth overlap and interweave and should not be viewed in a segmental fashion. For example, although Piaget was recognized primarily for his work in cognitive development, he linked such development closely to the acquisition of sensorimotor and sociocultural skills.

In Section III, Llorens lists behavior expectations and adaptive skills that help the individual deal effectively with life and life roles. The behavior expectations and adaptive skills presented are derived from the works of Havighurst (developmental tasks); Mosey, Pearce, and Newton (ego-adaptive skills); and Piaget (intellectual development). Although behavior expectations in Section III are separated from developmental expectations in Section I of the chart, Llorens feels that they occur simultaneously. Growth in developmental tasks is facilitated by the family, environment, extended family, community, and social and civic groups.

Using the chart, one can view development as a tapestry, with each area of development overlapping and interwoven horizontally and vertically, creating a stable base for the human organism to mature. If any one area is interrupted, a thread becomes weakened, and the growth and development process is no longer stable. Physical or psychological trauma in any one of the horizontal or longitudinal parameters can disrupt the development cycle. This creates disparity between developmental expectations (Section I) and behavior expectations and adaptive skills (Section III).

Section II depicts the role of OT in providing facilitating activities and relationships to bridge this developmental gap. The first step in the intervention process is evaluation, which includes testing, interviews, record review, and systematic clinical observation.

> From these evaluation procedures the therapist determines at what level the individual is functioning in the various aspects along the developmental continuum and . . . program[s] for facilitating growth and development . . . in accordance with the needs of the individual and the demands of his age. (Llorens, 1970, p. 100)

The therapist then chooses tasks from sensorimotor activities, developmental play activities, symbolic activities, daily life tasks, and interpersonal relationships to facilitate the growth process and narrow any developmental discrepancy (Llorens, 1970). Llorens emphasized that although special attention may be placed on facilitating the process of growth in any one particular parameter, all parameters of development must be acknowledged for an integrating growth experience to occur.

Table 4.1

Schematic Representation of Facilitating Growth and Development

SECTION I

Developmental Expectations, Behaviors, and Needs (Selected for Illustrative Purposes)

Neurophysiological–Sensorimotor Ayres	Physical–Motor Gesell	Psychosocial Erikson
0–2 Sensorimotor Tactile functions Vestibular functions Visual, auditory, olfactory, gustatory functions	0–2 Head sags Fisting Gross motion Walking Climbing	Basic Trust vs. Mistrust/Oral Sensory Ease of feeding Depth of sleep Relaxation of bowels
6 mo.–4 Integration of Body Sides Gross motor planning Form and space perception Equilibrium response Postural and bilateral integration Body scheme development	2–3 Runs Balances Hand preference established Coordination	Autonomy vs. Shame and Doubt/Muscular–Anal Conflict between holding on and letting go
3–7 Discrimination Refined tactile Kinesthetic, visual, auditory, olfactory, gustatory functions	3–6 Coordination more graceful Muscles develop Skills develop	Initiative vs. Guilt/Locomotor–Genital Aggressiveness Manipulation Coercion
3– Abstract Thinking Conceptualization Complex relationships Read, write, numbers	6–11 Energy development Skill practice to attain proficiency	Industry vs. Inferiority/Latency Wins recognition through productivity Learns skills and tools
Continue development Conceptualization Complex relationships Read, write, numbers	11–13 Rapid growth Poor posture Awkwardness	Identity vs. Role Confusion/Puberty and Adolescence Identification Social Roles
Development presumably maintained	Growth established and maintained	Intimacy vs. Isolation/Young Adulthood Commitments Body and ego mastery
Alterations begin to occur in sensory functions, conceptualization, and memory	Alterations begin to occur in motor behavior, strength, and endurance	Generativity vs. Stagnation/Adulthood Guiding next generation Creative, productive
Alterations in sensory functios, conceptualizaton, and memory	Alterations in motor behavior, strength, and endurance	Ego Integrity vs. Despair/Maturity Acceptance of own life cycle

(continues)

Table 4.1 *Continued.*

SECTION I

Developmental Expectations, Behaviors, and Needs (Selected for Illustrative Purposes)

Psychodynamic Hall Grant, Freud	Socio-Cultural Gesell	Social–Language Gesell	Activity of Daily Living Gesell
0–4 Oral Dependency Initially aggressive Oral erotic activity	Individual mothering person most important Immedite family group important	Small sounds Coos Vocalizes Listens Speaks	Recognizes bottle Holds spoon Holds glass Controls bowel
0–4 Anal Independence Resistiveness Self-assertiveness Narcissism Ambivalence	Parallel play Often alone Recognizes extendeed family	Identifies objects verbally Asks "why?" Short sentences	Feeds self Helps undress Recognizes simple tunes No longer wets at night
3–6 Genital Oedipal Genital interest Possessiveness of opposite sex parent Antagonistic to same sex parent Castration fears	Seeks companionship Makes decisions Plays with other children Takes turns	Combines talking and eating Complete sentences Imaginative Dramatic	Laces shoes Cuts with scissors Toilets independently Helps set the table
6–11 Latency Primitive struggles quiescent Initiative in mastery of skills Strong defenses	Group play and team activities Independence of adults Gang interests	Language major form of communication	Enjoys dressing up Learns value of money Responsible for grooming
11– Adolescence Emancipation from parents Occupational decisions Role experiment Re-examine values	Team games Organization important Interest in opposite sex	Verbal language predominates	Interest in earning money
Outgrow need for parent validation Identify with others	Group affiliation Family, social, civic interest	Non-verbal behavior also used to communicate	Concern for personal grooming, mate, family
Emotional responsibilities may lessen Physical and economic independence accepted Shift from survival to enjoyment			Accepting and adjusting to changes of middle age
Continued growth after middle age Inner trend toward survival	↓	↓	Adjusting to changes after middle age

(continues)

Table 4.1 *Continued.*

Section II
Facilitating Activities and Relationships (Selected)

	Sensorimotor Activities	Developmental Activities	Symbolic Activities	Daily Life Tasks	Interpersonal Relationships
E **V**	Tactile stimulation Visual, auditory, olfactory, gustatory stimulation	Dolls Animals Sand Water Excursions	Biting Chewing Eating Blowing Cuddling	Recognize food Hold feeding equipment Use feeding equipment	Individual interaction
A	Physical exercise Balancing Motor planning	Pull toys Playground Clay Crayons Chalk	Throwing Dropping Messing Collecting Destroying	Feeding Dressing Toileting	Individual interaction Parallel play
L	Listening Learning Skilled tasks and games	Being read to Coloring Drawing Painting	Destroying Exhibiting	Feeding Dressing Toileting Simple chores	Individual interaction Play small groups
U **A**	Reading Writing Numbers	Scooters Wagons Collections Puppets Building	Controlling Mastery	Feeding Dressing Grooming Spending	Individual interaction Groups Teams Clubs
T	All of the above available to be recycled	Weaving Machinery tasks Carving Modeling	All of the above to be recycled	Feeding Dressing Grooming Prevocational skills	Individual interaction Groups Teams
I **O** **N**	↓	Arts Crafts Sports Clubs and interest groups Education Work ↓	↓	Feeding Dressing Grooming Life role, skills ↓	Individual interaction Groups ↓

(continues)

Table 4.1 *Continued.*

Section III

Behavior Expectations and Adaptive Skills

Developmental Tasks Havighurst	Ego-Adaptive Skills Mosey, Pearce, and Newton	Intellectual Development Piaget
Learning to: Walk Talk Take solids Elimination	Ability to respond to mothering Mastering of gross motor responses	Motor skills Integrated
Sex difference To form concepts of social and physical realit To relate emotionally to others Right	Ability to respond to routines of daily living Mastery of three-dimensional space Sense of body image	Investigative Imitative Egocentric
Wrong To develop a conscience	Ability to Follow directions Tolerate frustrations Sit still Delay gratification	Egocentricism reduced, social participation increases Language replaces motor behavior
Learn physical skills Getting along Reading, writing Values Social attitudes	Ability to perceive, sort, organize, and utilize stimuli Work in groups Mastery of inanimate objects	Orders experiences Relates parts to wholes Deductive reasoning
More mature relationships Social roles Selecting occupation Achieving emotional independence	Ability to accept and discharge responsibility Capacity for love	Systematic approach to problems Sense of equality supersedes submission to adults
Selecting a mate Starting a family Marriage, home Congenial social group	Ability to function independently Control drives Plan and execute Purposeful motion	Development established and maintained
Civic and social responsibility Economic standard of living Develop adult leisure activities Adjust to aging parents	Obtain, organize, and use knowledge Participate in primary group Participate in variety of relationships Experience self as acceptable	Alterations in other areas may effect
Adjust to decreasing physical health, retirement, death Age group affiliation Meeting social obligations	Participate in mutually satisfactory heterosexual relations	

Note. From *Application of a Developmental Theory for Health and Rehabilitation* (pp. 32–33), by L. A. Llorens, 1976, Rockville, MD: American Occupational Therapy Association. Copyright 1976 by American Occupational Therapy Association, Inc. Reprinted with permission.

An appropriate facilitation program should meet the client's needs and the demands of the client's age and life roles. The intervention process for prevention of health problems is different from that for conditions of acute illness or temporary or permanent disability. Llorens (1970) wrote that "intervention at a stage that can be identified before trauma becomes overwhelming will allow the individual to continue his growth process with a minimum of interruption and continue toward the achievement of ego-adaptive skills" (p. 100). In treatment geared toward identifiable acute illness or temporary or permanent disability, facilitation of development tasks and ego-adaptive skills must be viewed in relation to the client's needs and limitations and geared to a realistic level of attainment.

Application to Occupational Therapy

Developmental Theory and Occupational Therapy Practice Areas

Llorens's developmental theory was both derived from and applied to her research in such fields as child psychiatry, community health, and gerontology.

Child Psychiatry

Although Llorens has published in a variety of areas, including vocational rehabilitation (Llorens, 1961, 1966a, 1981e; Llorens, Levy, & Rubin, 1964), sensory integration (Hames-Hahn & Llorens, 1989; Llorens, 1968b, 1983; Llorens & Burris, 1981; Llorens & Sieg, 1975), activities of daily living and self-esteem (Bolding & Llorens, 1991), community health practice (Llorens, 1969, 1971b, 1973b, 1974), and practice with the elderly (Llorens 1988; Llorens, Hikoyeda, and Yeo, 1992; McCormack, Llorens, and Glogoski, 1991; Shiotsuka, Burton, Pedretti, & Llorens, 1992), she is best known for her work in child psychiatry. Her early works focused on emotional disturbance in children (Llorens, 1967a, 1968b; Llorens & Rubin, 1962, 1967) and OT treatment for psychosocial dysfunction (Llorens, 1960, 1968a; Llorens & Johnson, 1966; Llorens & Rubin, 1961, 1962). With her colleagues in the interdisciplinary treatment and research team at the Lafayette Clinic, Llorens also described cognitive–perceptual–motor (CPM) dysfunction in children and made recommendations about its treatment (Beck et al., 1965; Braun, Rubin, Llorens, & Beck, 1967; Braun et al., 1965; Llorens, 1966b, 1967a; Llorens & Beck, 1966; Llorens, Rubin, Braun, Beck, & Beall, 1969; Llorens, Rubin, Braun, Mottley, & Beall, 1964; Rubin, Braun, Beck, & Llorens, 1972).

To demonstrate that OT for children with emotional disturbances was therapeutic, Llorens had to establish a baseline delineating the effects of emotional disturbance on children's development (Llorens & Rubin, 1961). Thus, even very early in her career, Llorens began to address what would become a central theme in her developmental theory (Premises 7 and 8): the influence of physical or psychological trauma on the developmental process. In her work on CPM dysfunction, she would similarly explore the adverse effect of this condition on growth and development (Beck et al., 1965) and hypothesize that CPM deficits could create an inability to cope with environmental demands (Llorens, Levy, & Rubin, 1964).

In her early writings on emotional disturbance, Llorens recognized that the absence of emotional problems resulted in the acquisition of skills through practice and mastery. She hypothesized that these skills later became problem-solving methods that directly affected the child's self-confidence, self-concept, and self-esteem (Llorens & Rubin, 1961). As a stronger relationship between emotional disturbance and CPM deficits emerged in the Lafayette team's research, it became apparent that mastery must be an integral part of the treatment protocol for CPM dysfunction:

> Many of the activities are those that children usually master through maturation and environmental stimulation. However, since some children do not, for a variety of reasons, such as inadequate experiences, master them successfully, the retraining process provides a sequence through which the child can progress artificially, thus enabling him to correct his deficit in primary adaptive functions. (Beck et al., 1965, pp. 236–237)

The importance of mastery would later be elaborated on in Premises 3 and 4 of Llorens's developmental theory.

Llorens's involvement with CPM research also led her to address the relationship of environmental factors to the child's CPM dysfunction. Such factors included parental attitude, early schooling, and environmental feedback (Braun et al., 1967). A definitive move from the medical model can be seen in Llorens's involvement with the Lafayette research team's effort to clarify environmental causes of deficits and put aside classification according to diagnostic category. This recognition of the effects of the environment on developmental process would be incorporated into Premises 5 and 6 of the developmental theory.

Community Health

Llorens's appointment as consultant to the Comprehensive Child Care Project at Mount Zion Hospital led her to explore in even more depth the role of environmental factors in child development. She asserted, for example, that child rearing and health care practices in the African American community, which were themselves influenced by larger social factors, had a profound impact on the psychological development of African American children:

> All children must master specific developmental tasks and ego adaptive skills between infancy and adolescence. . . . Some of these skills will be learned in school. In this society, the combination of financial means, the lifestyle of the family, and its aspirations, along with knowledge of and availability of resources, play a large part in influencing the extent to which African American children are able to develop in these areas. (Llorens 1971a, p. 148)

Llorens's research concerns produced a book on community-based health care, *Consultation in the Community: Occupational Therapy in Child Health* (1973b), as well as articles on community child health (Llorens, 1971b, 1974, 1975), the effect of sociological and cultural variables in health care delivery for children (Llorens, 1971a, 1971b, 1973b) and elders (Llorens, 1988; Llorens et al., 1992; McCormack et al., 1991; Ross, Washington, & Llorens, 1990; Llorens, Umphred, Burton, & Glogoski-Williams,

1993), ecology of environment and individual (Llorens, 1984), and accommodations for students with disabilities (Llorens, Burton, & Still, 1999).

Gerontology

Although Llorens is usually identified with pediatric practice, her developmental theory is a lifespan theory and, as such, includes aging. She described the expected decline in certain functions, especially physical, with age and the ways in which OT intervention can foster continued growth and adaptation (Llorens, 1970, 1977, 1991). In 1990 and 1991, she served as presenter and facilitator at conferences and meetings that addressed elder and ethnic issues. Topics included ethnogeriatrics, cultural diversity and the aging workforce, and intergenerational issues and minority aging. Llorens's publications in the area of aging include articles on the culturally diverse elderly (McCormack et al., 1991), activities of daily living and elders with right versus left cerebrovascular accident (Shiotsuka et al., 1992), independence in self-feeding (Hames-Hahn & Llorens, 1989), and health care for ethnic elders (Llorens, 1988; Llorens, Umphred, et al., 1993).

Developmental Theory and Occupational Therapy Practice Process

Occupational Therapy Process

Llorens (1981b) described the OT process, shown in Table 4.2 (Killingsworth, Llorens, Southam, Down, & Schwartz, 1992), as beginning with the client who has a condition: wellness, illness, disability, or dysfunction. Through the evaluation process, the occupational therapist determines how the client is functioning and whether intervention is indicated. Evaluations include observation, interview, history, and testing. The therapist then initiates one or more types of intervention: prevention, health education, modification of maladaptive behavior, adaptive change, health maintenance, or rehabilitation. Intervention includes purposeful activity and interpersonal relationships on an individual, group, or indirect service basis. A dynamic process and developmentally based intervention is begun at the level at

Table 4.2
A Schematic Outline of the Occupational Therapy Process

Patient/Client with a Condition

Wellness (preventative needs)
Illness (due to disease, stress, etc.)
Disability (secondary to a chronic condition, trauma, etc.)
Dysfunction (occupational role performance)

Patient/Client Occupational Roles

Worker, student, volunteer, homemaker, parent, son, daughter, mate, sibling, peer, and best friend/chum.

Evaluation

From the evaluation results of the areas listed below and a consideration of the age and gender of the patient/client, the need or lack of need for occupational therapy services is determined based on occupational dysfunction indicated by problems in the occupational performance skill areas or in occupational performance subskills.

A. Occupational performance skill areas

Determined by:

Skill areas	Determined by
Self-care/self-mainanance	Observation of performance
Work/education	Interview/questionnaire
Play/leisure	History taking/review
Rest/relaxation	Testing (standardized and non-standardized) or self-care, time utilization, job/work, other

B. Occupational performance subskills

Determined by:

Subskills	Determined by
Neurosensory function	Observation of performance
Physical/motor performance	Interview/questionnaire
Psychological state/skills	History taking/review
Social/interpersonal skills/adaptation	Testing specific to performance, subskills, functions for specific age groups

C. Environmental Factors

Determined by:

Environmental Factors	Determined by
Physical setting (home, job)	Results from above assessments and community/home survey
Support system (family, friends, agencies, etc.)	
Culture	
Religion/spiritual system	
Socioeconomic status	
General community aspects (mores, values, etc.)	

(continues)

Table 4.2 *Continued.*

Goal Setting

If treatment is needed, whether for prevention, modification of behavior, maintenance, habilitation, or rehabilitation, then *intervention should begin at the level(s) at which the patient/client can succeed and/or benefit.* The patient/client should be actively involved in the selection and establishment of goals. These goals should then be *monitored, graded, continuously re-evaluated, and changed,* as necessary.

Intervention/Treatment

Treatment/intervention includes enabling purposeful and functional activity and enhancement of sensory, motor, psychological, social/interpersonal, and cognitive abilities. It also includes a variety of activities to facilitate self-care, pre-work and work, education, and play/recreation/leisure performance. Intervention occurs on a one-on-one basis, in small and large groups, and through indirect learning experiences to facilitate change in the desired direction(s). Multiple options are given for selection and choice to involve the person actively in the treatment/intervention process. Rehabilitation may include the use of adaptive equipment, splinting, and other compensatory techniques to assist the patient/client to achieve his/her highest level of function in all possible areas.

Outcome(s)

Learning of new function/activities (habilitation)
Maintenance of present function (maintanance)
Restoration of function (rehabilitation)
Improvement of function (rehabilitation)
Loss of function (with adaptation as loss occurs)

Research

Research is needed in all phases of this process for validation.

Note. Adapted from *Course Reader, OCTH 113: Human Adaptation,* by A. Killingsworth, L. A. Llorens, M. Southam, J. Down, and K. Schwartz, 1992, San Jose, CA: San Jose State University Department of Occupational Therapy. Reproduced with permission of Lela A. Llorens.

which the client can succeed or benefit and is monitored, graded, continuously evaluated, and changed accordingly. Outcomes of intervention are observed as improvement of function, restoration of function, maintenance of function, or retrogression of function.

Activity and Activity Analysis

Llorens (1970) described the OT process as the skilled application of activities and relationships (p. 94). She explained why occupational therapists use activities, tasks, and occupations, and how these activities make a difference in a client's functioning (Llorens, 1981b, 1981c). She described activity programs for children with emotion disturbances (Llorens & Bernstein, 1963; Llorens & Rubin, 1962, 1965; Llorens & Young, 1960) and adolescent girls (Hardison & Llorens, 1988), as well as the use of activities in evaluation in child psychiatry (Llorens, 1967b, 1967d).

In the application of activity, Llorens emphasized the need for gradation, the presentation of activity at the client's level, and the use of specific activities for specific goals (Llorens, 1967a; Llorens & Beck, 1966; Llorens & Johnson, 1966; Llorens & Rubin, 1962). She recommended treatment procedures as activities that begin at a level commensurate with the child's ability, allow for successful accomplishment and mastery, and present opportunities to raise the child's level of skill (Llorens & Rubin, 1962, p. 287).

Activity analysis is used to guide the decision making in activity selection. By analyzing what is required to perform a task, activity, or occupation, the therapist can decide how a given task will meet certain therapeutic goals. Activity analysis provides the therapist with a rationale for what the activity does in the therapeutic process (Llorens, 1981b). Llorens tested her idea that there are inherent aspects to an activity by asking 80 occupational therapy students to experience five activities and report the presence or absence of 29 features of the activity (Llorens, 1986). She reported agreement at 80% for 10 of the 29 features. When she asked 47 occupational therapists to view tapes of these students and report their observations of the 29 features, she found that inherent, recognizable aspects to a task were reliably observable (Llorens, 1993).

Llorens provided a framework (Figure 4.1) for analyzing activities (Llorens, 1973a, 1981b, 1986; Llorens & Burris, 1981) and for explaining the influence of activity on adaptation. (Llorens, 1991). Activities, tasks, occupations, and personal interactions provide stimuli to the central nervous system (CNS) and influence integration for adaptive responses. These activities and interactions have input to the CNS via the sensory systems:

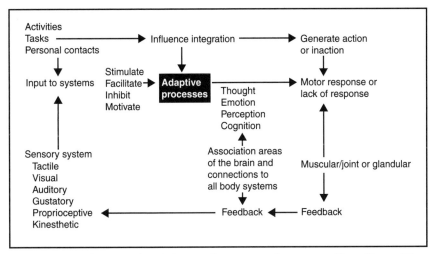

Figure 4.1. Influence of activity on human performance. *Note.* From "Performance Tasks and Roles Throughout the Life Span," by L. A. Llorens in *Occupational Therapy: Overcoming Human Performance Deficits* (p. 50), by C. Christiansen and C. Baum (Eds.), 1991, Thorofare, NJ: Charles B. Slack. Copyright 1991 by SLACK, Inc. Reprinted with permission.

tactile, visual, auditory, gustatory, proprioceptive, and kinesthetic. This input can stimulate, facilitate, inhibit, or motivate thoughts, emotions, perceptions, or cognition in the CNS. The internal action of the CNS (especially association areas of the brain and connections to body systems) is observable through motor responses (or lack of responses) that are generated through muscular, joint, or glandular activity in the organism. Motor responses generate feedback to the organism, which is conveyed to the CNS as new input. Llorens's activity analysis emphasized the need for therapists to be aware of this impact on the organism when they introduce activities and interactions, and to be able to explain the rationale for using activity.

Occupational Performance and Occupational Performance Components

Llorens described occupational performance areas and occupational performance components as the focus of OT evaluation and intervention (Llorens, 1976, 1982a). These terms had been defined earlier by the AOTA Task Force on Target Populations and published in the *Project to Delineate the Roles and Functions of*

Occupational Therapy Personnel (AOTA, 1972) in an attempt to define the parameters of OT and to establish a uniform terminology for the profession. Llorens completed a comprehensive literature review on occupational performance and occupational performance components, and developed and refined these concepts (Llorens, 1982c, 1991).

In her descriptions of normal development, Llorens often referred to the concept of "mastery" as the means to achieve and to measure human development. Through mastery of developmental tasks, one achieves behavior expectations and gains adaptive skills. Although different phases of development gain primacy at specific periods of time during the developmental lifespan, Llorens (1970) explained that for one to "achieve in the adaptive areas of functioning, it is necessary . . . to experience satisfaction and mastery" in all areas of development (p. 95). She views health and wellness in terms of the individual's ability to master developmental tasks successfully and thus to achieve appropriate adaptive skills. She considers achievement a healthy state, although normal deviations may occur. Moreover, the "achievement of competence, mastery and adaptation is central to occupational performance" (Llorens, 1991, p. 46).

Llorens defined occupational performance as the "accomplishment of tasks related to self-care/self-maintenance; work/education; play/leisure; and rest/relaxation" (1991, p. 46). Occupational performance components or subskills, such as sensory perception, sensory integration, motor coordination, psychosocial and psychodynamic responses, sociocultural development, and social language responses, enable one to achieve competence, mastery, and adaptation in the tasks of occupational performance. These, in turn, enable one to function in one's occupational roles, such as worker, parent, sibling, or mate. (See Table 4.3.) Llorens used the concepts of occupational roles, occupational performance, and occupational performance enablers in her Developmental Analysis Evaluation and Intervention Schedule (DAEIS; 1976) and her Occupational Therapy Sequential Client Care Record (SCCR; 1982c).

Developmental Analysis Evaluation and Intervention Schedule

In her book *Application of a Developmental Theory for Health and Rehabilitation*, Llorens (1976) restated her developmental theory

Table 4.3
Levels of Mastery for Successful Adaptation

Level 3: Occupational Roles

Worker	Daughter
Student	Mate
Volunteer	Sibling
Homemaker	Peer
Parent	Best friend/Chum
Son	

Level 2: Activities and Tasks of Occupational Performance

Skill Areas:

Self-care/Self-maintanance	Work/Education
Play/Leisure	Rest/Relaxation

Level 1: Occupational Performance Enablers

Subskills:

Sensory perception	Psychosocial and psychodynamic responses
Sensory integration	Sociocultural development
Motor coordination	Social language responses

Note. From "Performance Tasks and Roles Throughout the Life Span," by L. A. Llorens, 1991, in *Occupational Therapy: Overcoming Human Performance Deficits* (p. 47), by C. Christiansen and C. Baum (Eds.), Thorofare, NJ: Charles B. Slack. Copyright 1991 by SLACK Inc. Reprinted with permission.

and described its application to clients ranging from children to elders. She presented the DAEIS for use in developmental case analysis. The DAEIS provides therapists with a framework for applying the developmental theory. It guides the therapist through the OT process and brings to conscious awareness the thinking processes that the therapist uses in evaluation and treatment planning. Using the DAEIS, the therapist considers the "client as a biological, psychological and social being" (Llorens, 1982c, p. 3); the OT goals; the areas of human development that are affected by the client's condition; and the OT evaluation and intervention approaches.

Llorens (1976) applied the DAEIS to 15 clients whose growth and development had been adversely affected. Her case analyses described clients of all ages and with varied areas of disruption. Occupational therapy tools used in the treatment or facilitation process were described, and standardized and nonstandardized assessment procedures were differentiated. Activity analysis provided the theoretical rationale for the use of sensorimotor activities, developmental activities, and interpersonal relationships.

OT Sequential Client Care Record

To improve the usefulness of the DAEIS as a data collection tool for OT, Llorens incorporated the Problem-Oriented Medical Record (POMR; Weed, 1971) into the DAEIS to produce a client care record with a stronger scientific base. This became the SCCR (Llorens, 1982c) (see the outline of the SCCR in Table 4.4). Subsequent research on the SCCR's usefulness found that the variables of completeness, organizational sequence, and understandability for research and education were statistically significant features in its usability (Llorens & Schuster, 1977). The SCCR documents the OT process systematically while providing a viable communication tool to be used with colleagues, clients, and clients' families. It can be used to monitor quality care and accountability of OT services. The SCCR has served as an educational tool for OT students. Llorens proposed the use of the SCCR as a record-keeping system for clients served in OT that could potentially provide a large national database for research (Llorens, 1982c).

Theory Validation and Research

Llorens has promoted OT research in her academic career, her work with the AOTF, and her publications. She coauthored a research guide for the health science professional (Oyster, Hanten, & Llorens, 1987). She identified areas of research that need to be initiated by occupational therapists (Llorens, 1981d, 1984; Llorens & Gillette, 1985; Llorens & Snyder, 1987) and encouraged professional responsibility in the area of research (Llorens, 1979, 1990; Llorens & Donaldson, 1983). Her SCCR (Llorens, 1982c) provides a framework for collecting data for OT research. Aside from promoting research in the profession, she conducted studies of activity analysis (Llorens, 1986; 1993), pediatrics (Bolding & Llorens, 1991; Llorens, 1968b; Llorens & Rubin, 1961; Llorens, Rubin, et al., 1969), elders (Hames-Hahn & Llorens,

Table 4.4
Outline of Llorens's *Occupational Therapy Sequential Client Care Record* (SCCR)

Overview

The SCCR is a method to record and report the occupational therapy (OT) process in a comprehensive, sequential recording system that produces a complete record of the client, spanning the total time the client is served. The SCCR is designed to:

- Document therapy process
- Communicate information regarding therapy to colleagues
- Conduct research
- Contribute to the education of OT students

Sections of SCCR

Section 1: Database

- Demographics
- Areas of occupational performance to be considered
- Occupational performance components to be considered
- Evaluation techniques and procedures indicated
- Evaluation data from procedures used
- Areas of occupational performance affected
- Occupational performance components affected

Section 2: Problem Identification

- Problems list

Section 3: Initial Plan

- Occupational therapy plan
- Therapy procedures indicated
- Location of therapy

Section 4: Progress Notes

- Narrative notes
- Flow sheets: therapy procedures/dates/comments

Section 5

- Results of therapy
- Reevaluation of data from procedures used
- Occupational performance status
- Occupational performance component status
- Disposition

Note. Adapted from *Occupational Therapy Sequential Client Care Record,* by L. A. Llorens, 1982, Laurel, MD: Ramsco.

1989; Shiotsuka, et al., 1992), and education (Llorens & Adams, 1976). These studies were consistent with the models of activity analysis, the occupational therapy process, and the impact of occupational therapy on development.

Llorens has been a long-term advocate for the development of OT as an academic discipline, the science of "occupationology" (Llorens & Gillette, 1985). She has emphasized the need to define the existing body of OT knowledge and to validate and expand this knowledge through research. As she stated,

> Within the practice of our profession, there are predictable aspects relative to cause and effect in the use of activities and the application of relationships which must be identified, applied repeatedly in a systematic manner, analyzed and documented in order to establish their validity. (Lorens 1970, p. 101)

Three-Dimensional Model for Organizing OT Knowledge and the Study of OT

Llorens (1981b) proposed a three-dimensional model for organizing the knowledge and study of OT by client age or developmental stage, by practice phase, and by therapy techniques and outcomes (see Figure 4.2). Occupational therapy client groups are organized into seven age or developmental stages: infants, children, adolescents, young adults, middle adults, mature adults, and aged adults. Practice phases include prevention, treatment or therapy, and rehabilitation and health maintenance. Occupational therapy techniques can be organized into screening or evaluation techniques, intervention modalities, and outcomes. Llorens contends that "occupational therapy has a rich body of knowledge that needs to be organized for study. Through categorization and classification, the body of knowledge becomes accessible for collective appraisal" (1981b, p. 10).

An example of how this three-dimensional model can be used for selecting and designing a study of an area of OT is included in Figure 4.3. First, the infant client group and the prevention phase of OT practice are selected as the areas for study from the first two dimensions of the model. Then a study is designed to investigate a question regarding screening and evaluation, intervention modalities, or therapy outcomes from the third dimension of the

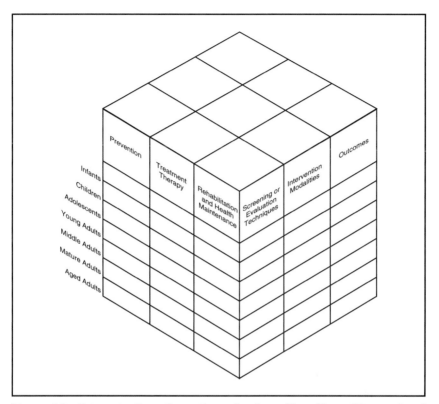

Figure 4.2. Categorization of practice technology. *Note.* From "Occupational Therapy: State of the Art, Potential for Development," by L. A. Llorens, 1981, in *Proceedings of the New Zealand Association of Occupational Therapists Annual Conference* (p. 13), Auckland, New Zealand: Auckland Metro. Reprinted with permission.

model. Thus, a given study would address one unit of the model—for example, therapy outcomes of OT prevention with infants.

Critique

A critical analysis of Llorens's developmental theory reveals several identifiable strengths. The theory has made an enduring and significant contribution to the field of occupational therapy. It provides a frame of reference that is applicable to all clients along the developmental continuum and a framework that the occupational therapist can use to conceptualize his or her practice.

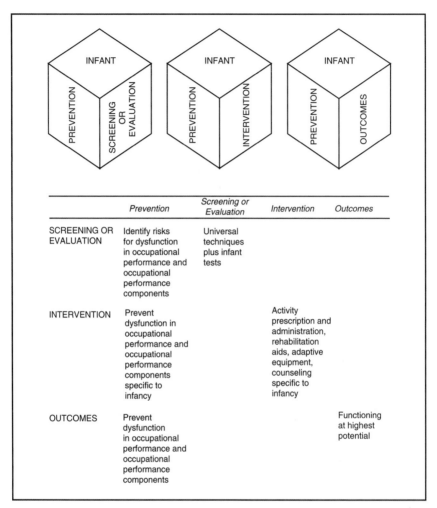

Figure 4.3. Example of Llorens's "Three-Dimensional Schemata for Knowledge Organization" in which knowledge in the area of prevention and the age group of infancy can be addressed in terms of screening/evaluation, intervention, or outcomes.

A review of Llorens's publications reveals her consistency, her common sense, and a distinct progression and refinement of her theoretical constructs. Llorens organizes material in a logical, clear, simple, and orderly fashion and presents schematic representations that lend visual clarity to her concepts.

Llorens's commitment to writing, research, and education has enhanced her theory's credibility by making it accessible to the profession. She circulated her information to new audiences by selecting a variety of communication methods, such as workshops, journals, newsletters, and lectureships, to convey her concepts. Through these modes, Llorens has contributed to making theory development an integral aspect of OT knowledge generation and practice.

Her theory purports to be applicable to clients of all ages, although, at the time of its inception, it was more easily applied to the younger client due to the lack of human growth and development research that was available on the adult when the theory was first developed. Llorens (1970) alluded to this age issue in the theory's initial presentation in her Eleanor Clarke Slagle Lecture.

Many of the concepts in Llorens's theory have long been accepted by the OT profession, but these concepts have not yet been clearly substantiated or refuted through systematic study. However, the usefulness of her facilitating growth and development model is reflected in its inclusion in major textbooks in the profession, including *Occupational Therapy for Children* (Case-Smith, 2001; Case-Smith, Allen, & Pratt, 1996; Pratt & Allen, 1985, 1989), *Willard and Spackman's Occupational Therapy* (Hopkins & Smith, 1978, 1983, 1988, 1993; Neistadt & Crepeau, 1998), and others (Christiansen & Baum, 1997; Llorens, 1991). In addition, Llorens served as one of three advisers at the inception of the OT doctoral program at Texas Woman's University (L. A. Llorens, personal communication, November 6, 2000); the program was founded upon the "occupational adaptation" model (Schkade & Schultz, 1992), which included Llorens's facilitating growth and development model.

Therapists seeking techniques for evaluation and treatment may find Llorens's theory lacking because she has not created new modalities. Instead, she has provided a way to describe and conceptualize the OT process, a way "to think through the function and purpose of occupational therapy as [she has] experienced it" (Llorens, 1970, p. 93). As she stated, "The theory has served me well as a way to conceptualize occupational therapy and to approach patients, both as practitioner and in attempting to teach the practice discipline to undergraduate and graduate students" (L. A. Llorens, personal communication, September 2, 1983).

Future of Occupational Therapy

In speculating on the future direction of OT, Llorens hypothesized that OT will "identify a common core from the numerous formulations that have been advanced . . . synthesized and analyzed . . . [and] will emerge with a universal theory of occupational therapy" (L. A. Llorens, personal communication, September 2, 1983). More than one frame of reference will be applied to different populations. Through this organizational process, the profession will be able to identify and organize evaluation and intervention techniques that are congruent with the theoretical base and frames that are established (L. A. Llorens, personal communication, September 2, 1983). As to the future of her own facilitating growth and development theory, she commented that in her work with graduate students, she

> made a conscious decision to assist students with their research and try to facilitate their growth and development, if you will, at the point in my career when I believed that the next steps in development would come from its incorporation with other frames of reference as at [Texas Woman's University] and as a way of understanding the relationship of development to occupational therapy practice and it would come through generations to follow as my professional life was coming to a close. (L. A. Llorens, personal communication, November 6, 2000)

Llorens has contributed greatly to the OT profession. She has advanced the philosophical idea of a universal theory for the profession, and she has contributed to this theory herself by organizing the principles and concepts of a developmental theory. When asked, "What advice would you give to therapists struggling to identify their professional frame of reference?" she replied,

> Try to be in touch with what you have been doing right as a practicing therapist . . . recognize the history of occupational therapy and theory development, there is more of that available to look at now, than there was. . . . It is important to struggle with the analysis and synthesis of one's own practice, values, and belief systems and to try to know what those are in relationship to the prevailing theoretical frames of reference,

and theory of occupational therapy. What you will find is that the ideas that you have and the values you have shared are common with many who have written or with whom you are working. You will begin to be able to identify with the community of occupational therapy, rather than seeing yourself as an isolated therapist in a practice setting. (L. A. Llorens, personal communication, September 2, 1983)

Bibliography

1960

Llorens, L. A. (1960). Psychological tests in planning treatment goals. *American Journal of Occupational Therapy, 14*, 243–246.

Llorens, L. A., & Young, G. G. (1960). Fingerpainting for the hostile child. *American Journal of Occupational Therapy, 14*, 306–307.

1961

Llorens, L. A. (1961). Bridging the gap: Vocational rehabilitation counseling in a psychiatric setting. *Michigan Rehabilitation Association Digest, 2*, 24–26.

Llorens, L. A., & Rubin, E. Z. (1961). Occupational therapy is therapeutic: A research study with emotionally disturbed children. In *Proceedings of 1961 AOTA National Conference*. Detroit, MI: American Occupational Therapy Association.

1962

Llorens, L. A., & Rubin, E. Z. (1962). A directed activity program for disturbed children. *American Journal of Occupational Therapy, 16*, 287–290.

1963

Llorens, L. A., & Bernstein, S. P. (1963). Fingerpainting for the compulsive child. *American Journal of Occupational Therapy, 17*, 120–121.

1964

Llorens, L. A., Levy, R., & Rubin, E. Z. (1964). The work adjustment program: A prevocational experience. *American Journal of Occupational Therapy, 18*, 15–19.

Llorens, L. A., Rubin, E. Z., Braun, J. S., Mottley, N., & Beall, D. (1964). Training in cognitive–perceptual–motor functions: A preliminary report. *American Journal of Occupational Therapy, 18*, 202–209.

1965

Beck, G. R., Rubin, E. Z., Braun, J. S., Llorens, L. A., Beall, D., & Mottley, N. (1965). Educational aspects of cognitive–perceptual motor functions in children: A suggested change in approach. *Psychology in Schools, 2* (3), 233–238.

Braun, J. S., Rubin, E. Z., Llorens, L. A., Beck, G. R., Beall, D., & Mottley, N. (1965). Cognitive perceptual motor function in school children: A suggested change in approach. *Journal of School Psychology, 3*, 1–5.

Llorens, L. A., & Rubin, E. Z. (1965). A directed activity program for emotionally disturbed children. In J. C. Gowan & G. D. Demos (Eds.), *The guidance of exceptional children* (pp. 168–174). New York: David McKay.

1966

Llorens, L. A. (1966). Aspects of pre-vocational evaluation with psychiatric patients. *Canadian Journal of Occupational Therapy, 33*, 5–12.

Llorens, L. A. (1966). Cognitive–perceptual–motor dysfunction: Evaluation and training. In J. M. Kiernat (Ed.), *Perceptual motor dysfunction evaluation and training* (pp. 271–292). Madison: University of Wisconsin.

Llorens, L. A., & Beck, G. R. (1966). Treatment methods for cognitive–perceptual motor dysfunction. In M. J. Fehr (Ed.), *Normal growth and development with deviations in the perceptual motor and emotional areas* (pp. 155–177). St. Louis, MO: Washington University.

Llorens, L. A., & Johnson, P. A. (1966). Occupational therapy in ego-oriented milieu. *American Journal of Occupational Therapy, 20*, 178–181.

1967

Braun, J. S., Rubin, E. Z., Llorens, L. A., & Beck, G. R. (1967). Cognitive motor deficits: Definition and intervention. In *Proceedings of the International Convocation on Learning Disabilities*. Pittsburgh: Crippled Children's Home.

Llorens, L. A. (1967). Cognitive–perceptual–motor dysfunction and training. In *Selected papers from professional program segments of the United Cerebral Palsy's Annual Conference*. New Orleans: United Cerebral Palsy Association.

Llorens, L. A. (1967). An evaluation procedure for children 6 to 10 years of age. *American Journal of Occupational Therapy, 21*, 64–69.

Llorens, L. A. (1967). Gauging emotional, intellectual and professional growth in students. *Educational Newsletter, 2*(2), 2.

Llorens, L. A. (1967). Projective technique in occupational therapy. *American Journal of Occupational Therapy, 21*, 226–229.

Llorens, L. A., & Rubin, E. Z. (1967). *Developing ego functions in disturbed children: Occupational therapy on milieu*. Detroit, MI: Wayne State University Press.

1968

Llorens, L. A. (1968). Changing methods in treatment of psychosocial dysfunction. *American Journal of Occupational Therapy, 22*, 26–29.

Llorens, L. A. (1968). Identification of the Ayres' syndrome in children with behavior maladjustment. *American Journal of Occupational Therapy, 22*, 286–288.

1969

Llorens, L. A. (1969). The occupational therapist in a community health program. In *Proceedings of SCOTA Annual Conference*. Southern California Occupational Therapy Association.

Llorens, L. A. (1969). The role of the occupational therapist in a children and youth project. In *Proceedings of the National Conference of Children and Youth Projects*, Southern California Occupational Therapy Association.

Llorens, L. A., Rubin, E. Z., Braun, J. S., Beck, G. R., & Beall, C. D. (1969). The effects of cognitive–perceptual–motor training approach on children with behavior maladjustment. *American Journal of Occupational Therapy, 23*, 502–512.

1970

Llorens, L. A. (1970). Facilitating growth and development: The promise of occupational therapy. Eleanor Clarke Slagle lecture. *American Journal of Occupational Therapy, 24*, 93–101.

1971

Llorens, L. A. (1971). Black culture and child development. *American Journal of Occupational Therapy, 25*, 144–148.

Llorens, L. A. (1971). Occupational therapy in community child health. *American Journal of Occupational Therapy, 25*, 335–339.

1972

Llorens, L. A. (1972). Facilitating growth and development: The promise of occupational therapy. In *Eleanor Clarke Slagle Lectures 1966–1972* (pp. 191–208). Dubuque, IA: Kendall/Hunt.

Llorens, L. A. (1972). Problem-solving the role of occupational therapy in a new environment. *American Journal of Occupational Therapy, 26*, 234–238.

Rubin, E. Z., Braun, J. S., Beck, G. R., & Llorens, L. A. (1972). *Cognitive–perceptual motor dysfunction: From research to practice.* Detroit, MI: Wayne State University Press.

1973

Canfield, A. A., Williams, M. R., Llorens, L. A., & Wroe, M. C. (1973). Competencies for allied health educators. *Journal of Allied Health, 2*(4), 180–186.

Llorens, L. A. (1973). Activity analysis for cognitive–perceptual–motor dysfunction. *American Journal of Occupational Therapy, 27*, 453–456.

Llorens, L. A. (1973). A case presentation: Billy. In E. K. Oremland & J. D. Oremland (Eds.), *Effects of hospitalization on children.* Springfield, IL: Charles C Thomas.

Llorens, L. A. (Ed.). (1973). *Consultation in the community: Occupational therapy in child health.* Dubuque, IA: Kendall/Hunt.

Llorens, L. A. (1973). What journal editors want. In M. K. Morgan, D. M. Filson, & A. A. Canfield (Eds.), *Publishing in the health professions.* Gainesville: University of Florida.

1974

Henderson, A., Llorens, L., Gilfoyle, E., Myers, C., & Prevel, S. (Eds.). (1974). *The development of sensory integrative theory and practice.* Dubuque, IA: Kendall/Hunt.

Llorens, L. A. (1974). The effects of stress on growth and development. *American Journal of Occupational Therapy, 28*, 82–86.

Llorens, L. A. (1974). Learning disability, occupational therapy and community programming. In *Proceedings of the Sixth International Congress World Federation of Occupational Therapists.* World Federation of Occupational Therapists.

1975

Llorens, L. A. (1975). Consultation in occupational therapy programs for children. *Canadian Journal of Occupational Therapy, 41*, 114–116.

Llorens, L. A. (1975). Occupational therapy consultation in community programs for children. In *Proceedings from Consultation in the Community: A Conference for Occupational Therapists.* Gainesville: University of Florida.

Llorens, L. A., & Sieg, K. W. (1975). A profile for managing sensory integrative test data. *American Journal of Occupational Therapy, 29*, 205–208.

1976

Llorens, L. A. (1976). *Application of a developmental theory for health and rehabilitation.* Rockville, MD: American Occupational Therapy Association.

Llorens, L. A., & Adams, S. P. (1976). Entering behavior: Student learning styles. In C. W. Ford & M. K. Morgan (Eds.), *Teaching in the allied health profession* (pp. 86–93). St. Louis, MO: Mosby.

1977

Llorens, L. A. (1977). A developmental theory revisited. *American Journal of Occupational Therapy, 31*, 656–657.

Llorens, L. A., & Schuster, J. J. (1977). Occupational therapy client care recording system: A comparative study. *American Journal of Occupational Therapy, 31*, 367–371.

1978

Llorens, L. A., & Adams, S. P. (1978). Learning style preferences of occupational therapy students. *American Journal of Occupational Therapy, 32*, 161–164.

1979

Llorens, L. A. (1979). Thinking research in occupational therapy. *Development Disabilities SIS Newsletter, 2*, 1.

1981

Llorens, L. A. (1981). Maintaining credibility: The academic occupational therapist. *OT Education Bulletin*, pp. 10–11.

Llorens, L. A. (1981). Occupational therapy: State of the art, potential for development. In *Proceedings of the New Zealand Association of Occupational Therapists Annual Conference* (pp. 9–17). Auckland, New Zealand: Aukland Metro.

Llorens, L. A. (1981). On the meaning of activity in occupational therapy. *Journal of the New Zealand Association of Occupational Therapists, 32*, 3–6.

Llorens L. A. (1981). Research in occupational therapy: The need, the response. *Occupational Therapy Journal of Research, 1*, 3–6.

Llorens, L. A. (1981). The role of occupational therapy in vocational rehabilitation. *Mental Health Special Interest Section Newsletter, 4*(3).

Llorens, L. A., & Burris, B. (1981). Development of sensory integration in learning disabled children. In J. Gottlieb & S. Strichart (Eds.), *Development theories and research in learning disabilities* (pp. 57–79). Baltimore: University Park Press.

1982

Llorens, L. A. (1982, Summer). Continuing clinical competency for the occupational therapy educator. *Journal of the New Zealand Association of Occupational Therapists*.

Llorens, L. A. (1982). Facilitating achievement of higher level behaviors. In J. H. Henry (Ed.), *Readings in clinical education: A resource manual for clinical instructors*. Augusta: Medical College of Georgia.

Llorens, L. A. (1982). *Occupational Therapy Sequential Client Care Record*. Laurel, MD: Ramsco.

1983

Llorens, L. A. (1983). The DSM III. Sensory integration and child psychiatry: Implications for treatment and research. *Sensory Integration Special Interest Section Newsletter, 6*(1), 2.

Llorens, L. A. (1983, Winter). Educating for professional competence: Accountability theory in practice. *Journal of the New Zealand Association of Occupational Therapists*.

Llorens, L. A., & Donaldson, K. (1983). Documentation of occupational therapy: A process model. *Canadian Journal of Occupational Therapy, 50*, 171–175.

1984

Llorens, L. A. (1984). Changing balance: Environment and individual. *American Journal of Occupational Therapy, 38*, 29–34.

Llorens, L. A. (1984). Semantic uses of sensory integration questioned. *Occupational Therapy Journal of Research, 4*(3), 244–245.

Llorens, L. A. (1984). Theoretical conceptualizations of occupational therapy: 1960–1982. *Occupational Therapy in Mental Health, 4*, 1–13.

Llorens, L. A., Ward, J. M., Still, J. R, & Eyler, R. K. (1984, Spring). The role of professional education for occupational therapy. *Occupational Therapy Education Bulletin*, pp. 6–9.

1985

Llorens, L. A., & Gillette, N. P. (1985). Nationally speaking: The challenge for research in a practice profession. *American Journal of Occupational Therapy, 39*, 143–146.

1986

Llorens, L. A. (1986). Activity analysis: Agreement among factors in a sensory processing model. *American Journal of Occupational Therapy, 40*, 103–110.

Llorens, L. A. (1986). An analysis of occupational therapy theoretical approaches for mental health: Are the profession's major treatment approaches truly occupational therapy? A response. *American Journal of Occupational Therapy, 40*, 103–110.

1987

Llorens, L. A., & Snyder, N. V. (1987). Nationally speaking: Research initiatives for occupational therapy. *American Journal of Occupational Therapy, 41*, 491–493.

Oyster, C. K., Hanten, W. P., & Llorens, L. A. (1987). *Introduction to research: A guide for the health science professional*. Philadelphia: Lippincott.

1988

Hardison, J., & Llorens, L. A. (1988). Structured craft group activities for adolescent girls. *Occupational Therapy in Mental Health, 8*(3), 101–118.

Llorens, L. A. (Ed.). (1988). Health care for ethnic elders: The cultural context. In *Proceedings of Stanford Geriatric Education Center Conference*. Palo Alto, CA: Stanford Geriatric Education Center.

1989

Hames-Hahn, C. S., & Llorens, L. A. (1989). Impact of a multisensory occupational therapy program on components of self-feeding behavior in the elderly. *Physical and Occupational Therapy in Geriatrics, 6*(3/4), 63–86.

Kibele, A., & Llorens, L. A. (1989). Going to the source: The use of qualitative methodology in a study of the needs of adults with cerebral palsy. *Occupational therapy in health care. Developmental disabilities: A handbook for occupational therapists*. New York: Haworth Press.

Llorens, L. A. (1989). Health care system models and occupational therapy. *Occupational Therapy in Health Care, 5*(4).

1990

Llorens, L. A. (1990). Research utilization: A personal/professional responsibility. *Occupational Therapy Journal of Research, 10*(1), 3–6.

Ross, H. S., Washington, W. N., & Llorens, L. A. (1990, March/April). Health promotion in a multicultural community. *Health Education*.

1991

Bolding, D. J., & Llorens, L. A. (1991). The effects of habilitative hospital admission on self-care, self-esteem and frequency of physical care. *American Journal of Occupational Therapy, 45*, 796–800.

Llorens, L. A. (1991). Performance tasks and roles throughout the life span. In C. Christiansen & C. Baum (Eds.), *Occupational therapy: Overcoming human performance deficits* (pp. 45–66). Thorofare, NJ: Charles B. Slack.

McCormack, G., Llorens, L., & Glogoski, C. (1991). The culturally diverse elderly. In J. Kiernat (Ed.), *Occupational therapy for the older adult: A clinical manual* (pp. 11–24). Gaithersburg, MD: Aspen.

1992

Killingsworth, A., Llorens, L. A., Southam, M., Down, J., & Schwartz, K. (1992). *Course reader, OCTH 1131: Human adaptation*. San Jose, CA: Department of Occupational Therapy, San Jose State University.

Llorens, L. A. (1992). Program consultation for children and adults. In E. Jaffe & C. F. Epstein (Eds.), *Occupational therapy consultation: Theory, principles and practice* (pp. 356–363). St. Louis, MO: Mosby.

Llorens, L. A. (1992). Roles for occupational therapist consultation in higher education. In E. Jaffe & C. F. Epstein (Eds.), *Occupational therapy consultation: Theory, principles and practice* (pp. 496–500). St Louis, MO: Mosby.

Llorens, L. A., Hikoyeda, N., & Yeo, G. (Eds.). (1992). Diabetes among elders: Ethnic considerations. In *Proceedings of Stanford Geriatric Education Center Conference*. Palo Alto, CA: Stanford Geriatric Education Center.

Shiotsuka, W., Burton, G., Pedretti, L., & Llorens, L. A. (1992). An examination of performance scores on activities of daily living between elders with right and left cerebrovascular accident. *Physical and Occupational Therapy in Geriatrics, 10*(4), 47–57.

1993

Llorens, L. A., (1993). Activity analysis: Agreement between participant and observers on perceived factors in occupation components. *Occupational Therapy Journal of Research, 13*(3), 198–211.

Llorens, L. A., Umphred, D. B., Burton, G. U. & Glogoski-Williams, C. (1993). Ethnogeriatrics: Implications for occupational therapy and physical therapy. *Physical and Occupational Therapy in Geriatrics, 11*(3), 59–69.

1999

Llorens, L. A., Burton, G., & Still, J. R. (1999). Achieving occupational role: accommodations for students with disabilities, *Occupational Therapy in Health Care, 11*(4), 1–7.

References

American Occupational Therapy Association. (1972). *Project to delineate the roles and functions of occupational therapy personnel*. Rockville, MD: Author.

Beck, G. R., Rubin, E. Z., Braun, J. S., Llorens, L. A., Beall, D., & Mottley, N. (1965). Educational aspects of cognitive–perceptual motor functions in children: A suggested change in approach. *Psychology in Schools, 2*(3), 233–238.

Bolding, D. J., & Llorens, L. A. (1991). The effects of habilitative hospital admission on self-care, self-esteem and frequency of physical care. *American Journal of Occupational Therapy, 45,* 796–800.

Braun, J. S., Rubin, E.Z., Llorens, L. A., & Beck, G. R. (1967). Cognitive motor deficits: Definition and intervention. In *Proceedings of the International Convention on Learning Disabilities.* Pittsburgh: Crippled Children's Home.

Braun, J. S., Rubin, E. Z., Llorens, L. A., Beck, G. R., Beall, D., & Mottley, N. (1965). Cognitive perceptual motor function in school children: A suggested change in approach. *Journal of School Psychology, 3,* 1–5.

Canfield, A. A., Williams, M. R., Llorens L. A., & Wroe, M. C. (1973). Competencies for allied health educators. *Journal of Allied Health, 2*(4), 180–186.

Case-Smith, J. (2001). *Occupational therapy for children* (4th ed.). St. Louis, MO: Mosby.

Case-Smith, J., Allen, A.S., & Pratt, P.N., (1996). (3rd ed.). *Occupational therapy for children* St. Louis, MO: Mosby.

Christiansen, C., & Baum, C. (1997). *Occupational therapy: Enabling function and well-being.* Thoroughfare, NJ: SLACK.

Hames-Hahn, C. S., & Llorens, L. A. (1989). Impact of a multisensory occupational therapy program on components of self-feeding behavior in the elderly. *Physical and Occupational Therapy in Geriatrics, 6*(3/4), 63–86.

Hardison, J., & Llorens, L. A. (1988). Structured craft group activities for adolescent girls. *Occupational Therapy in Mental Health, 8*(3), 101–118.

Hopkins, H. L., & Smith, H. D., (1978). *Willard and Spackman's Occupational Therapy* (5th ed). Philadelphia: Lippincott.

Hopkins, H. L., & Smith, H. D., (1983). *Willard and Spackman's Occupational Therapy* (6th ed.). Philadelphia: Lippincott.

Hopkins, H. L., & Smith, H. D., (1988). *Willard and Spackman's Occupational Therapy* (7th ed.). Philadelphia: Lippincott.

Hopkins, H. L., & Smith, H. D., (1993). *Willard and Spackman's Occupational Therapy* (8th ed.). Philadelphia: Lippincott.

Killingsworth, A., Llorens, L. A., Southam, M., Down, J., & Schwartz, K. (1992). *Course reader, OCTH 113: Human adaptation.* San Jose, CA: Department of Occupational Therapy, San Jose State University.

Llorens, L. A. (1960). Psychological tests in planning treatment goals. *American Journal of Occupational Therapy, 14,* 243–246.

Llorens, L. A. (1961). Bridging the gap: Vocational rehabilitation counseling in a psychiatric setting. *Michigan Rehabilitation Association Digest, 2,* 24–26.

Llorens, L. A. (1966a). Aspects of pre-vocational evaluation with psychiatric patients. *Canadian Journal of Occupational Therapy, 33,* 5–12.

Llorens, L. A. (1966b). Cognitive–perceptual–motor dysfunction: Evaluation and training. In J. M. Kiernat (Ed.), *Perceptual motor dysfunction evaluation and training* (pp. 271–292). Madison: University of Wisconsin.

Llorens, L. A. (1967a). Cognitive–perceptual–motor dysfunction and training. In *Selected papers from professional program segments of the United Cerebral Palsy's Annual Conference.* New Orleans: United Cerebral Palsy Association.

Llorens, L. A. (1967b). An evaluation procedure for children 6 to 10 years of age. *American Journal of Occupational Therapy, 21,* 64–69.

Llorens, L. A. (1967c). Gauging emotional, intellectual and professional growth in students. *Educational Newsletter, 2*(2), 2.

Llorens, L. A. (1967d). Projective technique in occupational therapy. *American Journal of Occupational Therapy, 21*, 226–229.

Llorens, L. A. (1968a). Changing methods in treatment of psychosocial dysfunction. *American Journal of Occupational Therapy, 22*, 26–29.

Llorens, L. A. (1968b). Identification of the Ayres' syndrome in children with behavior maladjustment. *American Journal of Occupational Therapy, 22*, 286–288.

Llorens, L. A. (1969). The occupational therapist in a community health program. In *Proceedings of Southern California Occupational Therapy Association Annual Conference.*

Llorens, L. A. (1970). Facilitating growth and development: The promise of occupational therapy. Eleanor Clarke Slagle lecture. *American Journal of Occupational Therapy, 24*, 93–101.

Llorens, L. A. (1971a). Black culture and child development. *American Journal of Occupational Therapy, 25*, 144–148.

Llorens, L. A. (1971b). Occupational therapy in community child health. *American Journal of Occupational Therapy, 25*, 335–339.

Llorens, L. A. (1972). Problem-solving the role of occupational therapy in a new environment. *American Journal of Occupational Therapy, 26*, 234–238.

Llorens, L. A. (1973a). Activity analysis for cognitive–perceptual–motor dysfunction. *American Journal of Occupational Therapy, 27*, 453–456.

Llorens, L. A. (Ed.). (1973b). *Consultation in the community: Occupational therapy in child health.* Dubuque, IA: Kendall/Hunt.

Llorens, L. A. (1974). Learning disability, occupational therapy and community programming. In *Proceedings of the Sixth International Congress World Federation of Occupational Therapists.* World Federation of Occupational Therapy.

Llorens, L. A. (1975). Consultation in occupational therapy programs for children. *Canadian Journal of Occupational Therapy, 41*, 114–116.

Llorens, L. A. (1976). *Application of a developmental theory for health and rehabilitation.* Rockville, MD: American Occupational Therapy Association.

Llorens, L. A. (1977). A developmental theory revisited. *American Journal of Occupational Therapy, 31*, 656–657.

Llorens, L. A. (1979). Thinking research in occupational therapy. *Development Disabilities SIS Newsletter, 2*, 1.

Llorens, L. A. (1981a). Maintaining credibility: The academic occupational therapist. *OT Education Bulletin*, pp. 10–11.

Llorens, L. A. (1981b). Occupational therapy: State of the art, potential for development. In *Proceedings of the New Zealand Association of Occupational Therapists Annual Conference* (pp. 9–17). Auckland, New Zealand: Aukland Metro.

Llorens, L. A. (1981c). On the meaning of activity in occupational therapy. *Journal of the New Zealand Association of Occupational Therapists, 32*, 3–6.

Llorens, L. A. (1981d). Research in occupational therapy: The need, the response. *Occupational Therapy Journal of Research, 1*, 3–6.

Llorens, L. A. (1981e). The role of occupational therapy in vocational rehabilitation. *Mental Health Special Interest Section Newsletter, 4*(3).

Llorens, L. A. (1982a, Summer). Continuing clinical competency for the occupational therapy educator. *Journal of the New Zealand Association of Occupational Therapists.*

Llorens, L. A. (1982b). Facilitating achievement of higher level behaviors. In J.H. Henry (Ed.), *Readings in clinical education: A resource manual for clinical instructors.* Augusta: Medical College of Georgia.

Llorens, L. A. (1982c). *Occupational Therapy Sequential Client Care Record.* Laurel, MD: Ramsco.

Llorens, L. A. (1983). The DSM III, sensory integration and child psychiatry: Implications for treatment and research. *Sensory Integration Special Interest Section Newsletter, 6*(1), 2.

Llorens, L. A. (1984). Changing balance: Environment and individual. *American Journal of Occupational Therapy, 38,* 29–34.

Llorens, L. A. (1986). Activity analysis: Agreement among factors in a sensory processing model. *American Journal of Occupational Therapy, 40,* 103–110.

Llorens, L. A. (Ed.). (1988). Health care for ethnic elders: The cultural context. In *Proceedings of Stanford Geriatric Education Center Conference.* Palo Alto, CA: Stanford Geriatric Education Center.

Llorens, L. A. (1990). Research utilization: A personal/professional responsibility. *Occupational Therapy Journal of Research, 10*(1), 3–6.

Llorens, L. A. (1991). Performance tasks and roles throughout the life span. In C. Christiansen & C. Baum (Eds.), *Occupational therapy: Overcoming human performance deficits* (pp. 45–66). Thorofare, NJ: Charles B. Slack.

Llorens, L. A. (1992). Program consultation for children and adults. In E. Jaffe & C. F. Epstein (Eds.), *Occupational therapy consultation: Theory, principles and practice* (pp. 356–363). St. Louis, MO: Mosby.

Llorens, L. A. (1993). Activity analysis: Agreement between participant and observers on perceived factors in occupation components. *Occupational Therapy Journal of Research, 13*(3), 198–211.

Llorens, L. A., & Adams, S. P. (1976). Entering behavior: Student learning styles. In C. W. Ford & M. K. Morgan (Eds.), *Teaching in the allied health professions* (pp. 86–93). St. Louis, MO: Mosby.

Llorens, L. A., & Beck, G. R. (1966). Treatment methods for cognitive–perceptual motor dysfunction. In M. J. Fehr (Ed.), *Normal growth and development with deviations in the perceptual motor and emotional areas* (pp. 155–177). St. Louis, MO: Washington University.

Llorens, L. A., & Bernstein, S. P. (1963). Fingerpainting for the compulsive child. *American Journal of Occupational Therapy, 17,* 120–121.

Llorens, L. A., & Burris, B. (1981). Development of sensory integration in learning disabled children. In J. Gottlieb & S. Strichart (Eds.), *Development theories and research in learning disabilities.* (pp. 57–79). Baltimore: University Park Press.

Llorens, L. A., Burton, G., & Still, J. R. (1999). Achieving occupational role: Accommodations for students with disabilities. *Occupational Therapy in Health Care, 11*(4), 1–7.

Llorens, L. A., & Donaldson, K. (1983). Documentation of occupational therapy: A process model. *Canadian Journal of Occupational Therapy, 50,* 171–175.

Llorens, L. A., & Gillette, N. P. (1985). Nationally speaking: The challenge for research in a practice profession. *American Journal of Occupational Therapy, 39,* 143–146.

Llorens, L. A., Hikoyeda, N., & Yeo, G. (Eds.). (1992). Diabetes among elders: Ethnic considerations. In *Proceedings of Stanford Geriatric Education Center Conference*. Palo Alto, CA: Stanford Geriatric Education Center.

Llorens, L. A., & Johnson, P. A. (1966). Occupational therapy in ego-oriented milieu. *American Journal of Occupational Therapy, 20*, 178–181.

Llorens, L. A., Levy, R., & Rubin, E. Z. (1964). The work adjustment program: A prevocational experience. *American Journal of Occupational Therapy, 18*, 15–19.

Llorens, L. A., & Rubin, E. Z. (1961). Occupational therapy is therapeutic: A research study with emotionally disturbed children. In *Proceedings of 1961 AOTA National Conference*. Detroit, MI: American Occupational Therapy Association.

Llorens, L. A., & Rubin, E. Z. (1962). A directed activity program for disturbed children. *American Journal of Occupational Therapy, 16*, 287–290.

Llorens, L. A., & Rubin, E. Z. (1965). A directed activity program for emotionally disturbed children. In J. C. Gowan & G. D. Demos (Eds.), *The guidance of exceptional children* (pp. 168–174). New York: David McKay.

Llorens, L. A., & Rubin, E. Z. (1967). *Developing ego functions in disturbed children: Occupational therapy milieu*. Detroit, MI: Wayne State University Press.

Llorens, L. A., Rubin, E. Z., Braun, J. S., Beck, G. R., & Beall, C. D. (1969). The effects of cognitive–perceptual–motor training approach on children with behavior maladjustment. *American Journal of Occupational Therapy, 23*, 502–512.

Llorens, L. A., Rubin, E. Z., Braun, J. S., Mottley, N., & Beall, D. (1964). Training in cognitive–perceptual–motor functions: A preliminary report. *American Journal of Occupational Therapy, 18*, 202–209.

Llorens, L. A., & Schuster, J. J. (1977). Occupational therapy client care recording system: A comparative study. *American Journal of Occupational Therapy, 31*, 367–371.

Llorens, L. A., & Sieg, K. W. (1975). A profile for managing sensory integrative test data. *American Journal of Occupational Therapy, 29*, 205–208.

Llorens, L. A., & Snyder, N. V. (1987). Nationally speaking: Research initiatives for occupational therapy. *American Journal of Occupational Therapy, 41*, 491–493.

Llorens, L. A., Umphred, D. B., Burton, G. U., & Glogoski-Williams, C. (1993). Ethnogeriatrics: Implications for occupational therapy and physical therapy. *Physical and Occupational Therapy in Geriatrics, 11*(3), 59–69.

Llorens, L. A., & Young, G. G. (1960). Fingerpainting for the hostile child. *American Journal of Occupational Therapy, 14*, 306–307.

McCormack, G., Llorens, L., & Glogoski, C. (1991). The culturally diverse elderly. In J. Kiernat (Ed.), *Occupational therapy for the older adult: A clinical manual* (pp. 11–24). Gaithersburg, MD: Aspen.

Neistadt, M. E., & Crepeau, E. B. (1998). *Willard and Spackman's occupational therapy*, Philadelphia: Lippincott.

Oyster, C. K., Hanten, W. P., & Llorens, L. A. (1987). *Introduction to research: A guide for the health science professional*. Philadelphia: Lippincott.

Pratt, P. N., & Allen, A. S. (1985). *Occupational therapy for children*. St. Louis, MO: Mosby.

Pratt, P. N., & Allen, A. S. (1989). *Occupational therapy for children* (2nd ed.). St. Louis, MO: Mosby.

Robertson, S. C. (1992). *Find a mentor or be one*. Rockville, MD: American Occupational Therapy Association.

Ross, H. S., Washington, W. N., & Llorens, L. A. (1990, March/April). Health promotion in a multicultural community. *Health Education.*

Rubin, E. Z., Braun, J. S., Beck, G. R., & Llorens, L. A. (1972). *Cognitive–perceptual motor dysfunction: From research to practice*. Detroit, MI: Wayne State University Press.

Schkade, J. K., & Schultz, S. (1992). Occupational adaptation: Toward a holistic approach for contemporary practice, part 1. *American Journal of Occupational Therapy, 46*, 829–837.

Shiotsuka, W., Burton, G., Pedretti, L., & Llorens, L. A. (1992). An examination of performance scores on activities of daily living between elders with right and left cerebrovascular accident. *Physical and Occupational Therapy in Geriatrics, 10*(4), 47–57.

Weed, L. L. (1971). *Medical records, medical education and patient care*. Chicago: Year Book Medical Publishers.

A. Jean Ayres

5

Kay F. Walker

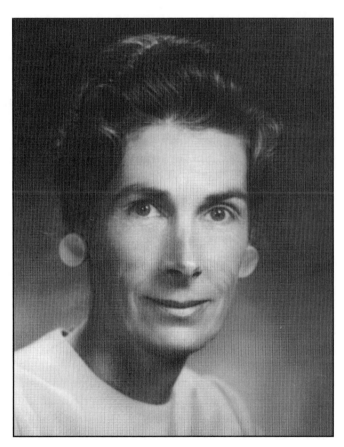

Learning is a function of the brain; learning disorders are assumed to reflect some deviation in neural functioning. (Ayres, 1972d, p. 1)

T hose first words in Ayres's book, *Sensory Integration and Learning Disorders,* reflect the central concern of her neurobehavioral theory that addressed the relationships of sensory and motor processing to learning and behavior. In this chapter, I seek to review the body of work, on sensory integration theory, testing and treatment that Ayres produced in her impressive 42-year career as an occupational therapy (OT) clinician and researcher. Before turning to her theory and research, I chronicle the life of Jean Ayres, the individual.

Biographical Sketch

Childhood

Anna Jean Ayres was born 1923 in California and lived there until her death in 1988. She grew up on a farm in Vasalia where she was friends with the trees and the earth. With her brother and younger sister, she created games and enjoyable activities from whatever was available in their rural surroundings (A. J. Ayres, personal communication, June 29, 1981; June 3, 1987). Playtimes with her brother and younger sister afforded Jean comfort from the tensions of an unhappy relationship with her mother and older sister.

Throughout childhood, she had health problems and suffered from what she termed "constitutional inadequacy." She thought of herself as a bad, difficult, and shameful child who deserved her mother's complaints about her "ugly disposition." Her father was stern and distant, but loving. He embodied a strong work ethic and instilled in his children the principles of efficiency, economy, hard work, and responsibility for self and others. An educator until he could afford to farm, he placed a high value on education and made many sacrifices to be able to send his children to college (A. J. Ayres, personal communication, June 29, 1981; June 3, 1987).

The happiness and love relationships that Ayres lacked in childhood she found in her marriage. She dedicated her first book, *Sensory Integration and Learning Disorders* (1972d), to her husband, Franklin Baker. "I will say that I have a nearly perfect, just nearly perfect marriage. Just a real love relationship. A complete pair bond. That's where the love is" (A. J. Ayres, personal communication, June 29, 1981).

Schooling

Ayres attended a country school that was a mile-and-a-half walk from home and had no electric lights or running water. School offered little reprieve from her unhappy home life, and she did not perform well during the first years of school. She found it hard to express herself and to understand what others were saying, especially if they had an accent. Learning to read gave Ayers her first true understanding of how some words sounded. As an adult, she cited her "damaged left hemisphere" as the cause of her problems, and although she disseminated her life's work through numerous publications and presentations, writing and speaking remained difficult for her (A. J. Ayres, personal communication, June 29, 1981).

She obtained her bachelor's degree in OT in 1945, her master's degree in OT in 1954, and her doctoral degree in educational psychology in 1961, all from the University of Southern California (USC). From 1964 to 1966, she engaged in postdoctoral work at the Brain Research Institute at the University of California, Los Angeles (UCLA). This, she says, "was the most fortunate experience I ever had." Although her ideas were not popular at UCLA and she was "low man on the totem pole among all of the scientists" during her years there, her work at the institute enabled her to study with neuroscientists and to gain knowledge of the brain (A. J. Ayres, personal communication, June 29, 1981).

Work

Ayres took her first OT job in a Veteran's Administration Hospital in 1946. Next she established an OT program at a private psychiatric hospital, where she drafted her first journal article (Ayres, 1949). From there she went to the Kabat Kaiser Institute, where she served as head occupational therapist from 1948 to 1953. While working toward her master's degree, she gained experience in the areas of cerebral palsy and vocational training. From 1955 throughout the remainder of her career, she held academic appointments at USC in special education or occupational therapy.

In the years after receiving her doctoral degree, she felt that her OT colleagues at USC did not support her work because her focus on brain function was not synchronous with the prevailing social science perspective in the department. She spoke frankly of her experiences:

> It isn't so much to what group I give that which I develop, but what group will accept me. Initially, occupational therapy would not accept me. I could not cope with the resistance and hostility and other negative attitudes. I became so disgusted with occupational therapy in general because I kept wanting to push the field and the field pushed back. I finally became so disgusted and had such a hard time relating to occupational therapists, I said to hell with OT, I'm going to go my way and they can go their way. That's when I left the OT department [at USC] because I just couldn't tolerate the negativism toward me. (A. J. Ayres, personal communication, June 29, 1981)

Ayres saw the rejection of new ideas as not unusual in a university, which she described as potentially a "teeth and claws" place, and stated, "I don't cope well with teeth and claws." She resolved these conflicts by taking the attitude, "I'd just have to be satisfied within myself. I cannot satisfy anyone else. I just wanted to satisfy myself and the committees that grant research funds in Washington, D.C." (A. J. Ayres, personal communication, June 29, 1981).

For eight years after her postdoctoral work, Ayres held a faculty appointment in the special education department of USC. She stated that she found acceptance there because she brought in research funds: "If you bring in research funds and you produce enough, you can keep your desk. If you have a desk and you have an appointment and you have an account number, you can make it at a university" (A. J. Ayres, personal communication, June 29, 1981).

After 1971, Ayers's federal grants were not renewed and there was no funding of any type from the OT profession. Just when it seemed as though Ayres's work would go unsupported, an event of great significance occurred. Two occupational therapists, Lorraine Kovalenko and Patricia Wilbarger, recognized the importance of Ayres's line of inquiry and established a nonprofit foundation (now Sensory Integration International) to serve as a receiving agency for donated funds. Ayres raised research funds, primarily though lecturing, and with this funding base she was qualified to submit proposals for private foundation grants. Lecturing widely throughout the United States and abroad for 2½ years, she brought gradual grassroots acceptance and financial support for the theory of sensory integration (SI). Explaining sensory integration to parents and others in her book, *Sensory Integration and the Child* (Ayres, 1979), she says:

> Sensory integration is the organization of sensory input for use. The "use" may be a perception of the body or the world, or an adaptive response, or a learning process, or the development of some neural function. Through sensory integration, the many parts of the nervous system work together so that a person can interact with the environment effectively and experience appropriate satisfaction. (p. 184)

Ayres did not perceive her initial lack of financial and professional support as the greatest obstacle she had to overcome. Rather,

> The major obstacle is my own brain—my left cerebral hemisphere, in particular. Sensory integrative dysfunction is so complex, so great, that I don't really have the neuronal capacity to handle it as well as I'd like to. That's the biggest obstacle. That, and the problems presented as sensory integrative dysfunction. (A. J. Ayres, personal communication, June 29, 1981; June 3, 1987)

Ayres consistently disseminated her thinking through publications. After her first professional journal article (Ayres, 1949), which was published when she was 26 years old, she wrote 55 more professional publications, including two books. In addition, she prepared four films and numerous test manuals. Throughout her life, she continued to pose questions, report research findings, and offer theories, thus allowing her work to be utilized and examined.

In 1977, she opened the Ayres Clinic, a private facility in Torrance, California. In this carefully designed environment for sensory integrative therapy, she provided therapy for children, conducted research, and developed test instruments and theory. Through her affiliation with USC as an adjunct faculty member, she offered postbaccalaureate clinical residencies and trained numerous master's students and therapists from throughout the nation and abroad. In 1984, she retired from the Ayres Clinic and turned her energies to the Sensory Integration and Praxis Tests (SIPT; Ayers, 1989) standardization project (American Occupational Therapy Association [AOTA], 1985). Until her death in 1988, she continued her affiliation with USC in an emeritus status and served in an advisory capacity at the Ayres Clinic and for Sensory Integration International.

Recognition

Ayres received some of the highest accolades in the profession from AOTA: the Eleanor Clarke Slagle Lectureship in 1963, the Award of Merit in 1965, the Roster of Fellows in 1973, and appointment as a charter member of the Academy of Research in 1983. In 1987, the American Occupational Therapy Foundation established the A. Jean Ayres Award for outstanding achievement in occupational therapy research, theory, or practice (AOTA, 1987). Despite the controversy surrounding her work, Ayres nonetheless made a great impact on OT theory.

On December 16, 1988, Ayres succumbed to a lengthy struggle with cancer. Finding "orthodox treatment of cancer not working well," she engaged in "some nonorthodox approaches" and concentrated her attention on her work with the SIPT (A. J. Ayres, personal communication, June 3, 1987). Before her death, she was able to see their completion.

In a special tribute to Ayres at the 1989 AOTA conference, President Elnora Gilfoyle stated,

> For all her genius and complexity, she had an acute appreciation of the commonplace rhythms of life. The intricacies of the nervous system, the change of seasons, the instinctive capabilities of animals, the human drive to accomplish. These were the forces that caught her fascination and inspired inquiry. The fact that she dedicated her life to the study of the most basic, yet poorly understood, aspects of human function reflects her essence. (AOTA, 1989b, p. 4)

As Florence Clark remembers Ayres's influence, "Jean taught me to search for authenticity, strive to achieve the highest academic standards, be vigilantly responsive to the needs of others and to stay on the right course despite resistance in order to help the world" (AOTA, 1989a, p. 15). In a tribute to Ayres's scholarship, Charlotte Royeen (1998) remarked that SI theory "in its complexity, scope, and depth is equal to the more commonly known theories of Freud, Piaget and Jung. As with the passing of any truly innovative leader, a vacuum follows in her wake" (p. 240).

Theory Overview and Development

Theory Synopsis

The central concept in SI theory is that neural integration of sensation is essential to movement and learning and, in addition to the visual and auditory sensory systems, the tactile, kinesthetic, proprioceptive, and vestibular sensory systems are important for these functions. In addition, subcortical neural structures that mediate postural responses and intersensory integration are highlighted for their contribution to cognitive functions. Children who have learning, movement, or behavioral problems, despite no known neurological problems, presented the clinical puzzlement that drove Ayers to this theory development. Ayres's questioning of how to help these children led her to develop test instruments, conduct factor analytic studies to hypothesize constructs of SI, build a therapy clinic with sensory integrative procedures and equipment, promote examiner competency in test administration, disseminate her work through publications and presentations, and carry out therapy efficacy studies. Supporters of Ayres's work developed a certification process for test administration and continuing education courses in SI theory, test administration, interpretation, and therapy. SI therapy has also been applied to a variety of patient problems. Ayres's original constructs have been further developed and subjected to examination in research, mostly by occupational therapists, and have remained somewhat controversial within OT and without wide acceptance outside the profession.

Contemporary Theoretical Context

The first words in the preface to Ayres's book, *Sensory Integration and Learning Disorders* (1972d), were, "This book presents a neurobehavioral theory" (Ayres, 1972d, p. ix). Ayres developed her theories at a time when learning disabilities and developmental dyslexia (Critchley, 1964) were just beginning to be described (Mercer, 1983) and the condition "minimal brain dysfunction" was being proposed (Clements & Peters, 1962). The brain researchers of the 1950s and 1960s are cited in textbooks today for their frontier work in areas such as visual perception (Benton, 1964), brain function (Brodal, 1964; Eccles, 1966; Luria, 1966; Penfield & Roberts, 1959), motor mechanisms (Evarts & Thach, 1969), language (Geschwind, 1965), pain mechanisms (Melzack & Wall, 1965), limbic functions (Pribram, 1961), neuropsychiatry (Schilder, 1964), and hemisphere functions (Sperry & Gazzaniga, 1967), as well as in more specific studies such as Harlow's (1958) work on the tactile system and attachment, and Kluver and Bucy's (1939) work on temporal lobe functions. Groundwork developmental theories had been put in place by Piaget (1952) in the area of cognitive development and Gesell (1940) in the area of motor milestones. In rehabilitation, various neural-based therapy approaches were proposed: Bobath and Bobath's (1964) neurodevelopmental treatment, Fay's (1954) motor patterns, Kabat and Knott's (1948) neuromuscular reeducation, and Rood's (1954) neurophysiology-based treatment. (Incidentally, Ayres credits Margaret Rood, who was not a prolific writer, as having a contribution "far greater than appears from citations alone" [Ayres, 1972d, p. ix].) Ayres's contemporaries in education were Frostig (Maslow, Frostig, Lefever, & Whittlesey, 1964), Kephart (1960), and Cratty (1964), all of whom invited educators to consider perceptual and motor relationships in learning and learning disorders. In short, Ayres developed her ideas in the context of an era of explosion of knowledge about the neural basis for behavior and learning.

Ayres sought to apply the animal and cellular neural studies of her contemporaries in neuroscience to the questions and explanations of clinical problems she observed in children with learning disabilities. Her work was unique from her colleagues in education; she emphasized the discovery of underlying sensorineural processes of learning problems instead of developing curricula to address the problem. In OT, Ayres led the way in work with children with subtle central nervous system (CNS) dysfunction and in demonstrating a scholarly approach to clinical problems through the processes of theory, research, practice, and standardized testing. Followers of SI theory looked to Ayres to distill the literature and to provoke thinking beyond the obvious clinical observations to search for the neural underpinnings and to challenge understandings in light of the neuroscience literature. The lack of knowledge about SI, she asserted,

> must be faced and dealt with in as adequate manner as possible with full recognition of the limitations involved and with the realization that any conceptual framework is in some respects erroneous and will require constant modification as new knowledge unfolds. (Ayres, 1968b, p. 43)

Theory Development

Ayres developed and tested her theories through clinical practice, literature review, and research studies. She used factor analyses and cluster analyses in theory development and test construction. She used clinical studies to investigate the effectiveness of SI therapy for children with learning disabilities and for other patient groups.

Clinical Practice

Ayres cited the problems of her clients as the central inspiration for her work: "They have certain conditions, responsibility for modification of which I assume; therefore, I must learn what I need to know to ameliorate their condition" (A. J. Ayres, personal communication, June 24, 1981). Throughout her career, Ayres was actively involved in clinical practice. In the therapy setting, she identified problems, formulated questions, and applied her theoretical approaches. The real world of clinical practice consistently guided her research and theory development efforts. In her clinical research, she investigated patterns of perceptual-motor and then SI dysfunction, primarily in children with learning disabilities, but also in participants with autism, aphasia, and hearing and visual impairments. She explored the effects of SI therapy on a variety of behavior problems, perceptual-motor problems, and skill deficits in children with learning disabilities, neurological disorders, autism, and schizophrenia.

Literature Review

Ayres consistently used literature in the fields of neuroscience, neuropsychology, neurobehavior, and neurophysiology to support her assumptions, pose questions, extrapolate findings, and interpret clinical problems. The neuroscience body of knowledge is a continuing resource for the development of new theory. SI theory is a neurologically based theory that seeks to bridge the gap between basic science research and its application to human clinical problems. For example, while contemporaries focused on visual-perceptual deficits, Ayres sought alternative answers. "You get that [contribution of vestibular and proprioceptive systems to visual perception] more from studying neurology, and even then you have to make a lot of inferences. You have to go well beyond the printed word to come up with that interpretation" (A. J. Ayres, personal communication, June 29, 1981). Rather than waiting for someone else to extract clinical applications from the literature, Ayres did so, explaining,

> Therapists dash in where scientists fear to tread. It's a dangerous thing to do, but it's what builds theory. Theory is not the facts. Theory is putting the facts together so you can use them and in our case to enhance the development of children. This is always my end objective. (A. J. Ayres, personal communication, June 29, 1981)

Although references to neuroscience literature are found in nearly all of Ayres's writings, her book *Sensory Integration and Learning Disorders* (1972d) provided the most complete discussion of the conceptual bases of her theory. It included a comprehensive review of principles of brain function, integrative processes, CNS levels, sensory modalities and factors, syndromes, and neural systems as they related to SI theory. Chapters on specific disorders included sections on neurological, neuroanatomical, and neuro-physiological considerations (Ayres, 1972d).

Research

Factorial designs are useful for summarizing interrelationships among variables concisely and accurately. Ayres used the R-technique and Q-technique, the most frequently used types of two- and three-mode factor analysis at the time. The R-technique was used to factor variables from each subject, thus preserving information about the test but obscuring information about the individual (when pairs of a subject's scores are summed, information about the subject is lost). The Q-technique was used to factor an individual's data collected at the same time from a number of variables (test scores). Computation of Q involves correlations among various subjects' scores on a given test, preserving information about subjects but obscuring information about tests. Thus, the R-technique is useful when one wishes to know how test scores are grouped but is not concerned with the subjects' characteristics. Conversely, the Q-technique is useful when one wishes to group subjects and identify types of individuals but is not concerned with test characteristics (Gorsuch, 1983).

Cluster analysis is useful for discovering groupings of subjects (Knox, Mack, & Mailloux, 1988). Cluster techniques seek to group subjects into meaningful clusters so that subjects within the group are similar and subjects from different clusters are not alike. Although Ayres used factor analysis for most of her work, she also used cluster analysis for diagnostic groupings on the SIPT (Ayers, 1989).

Having established five syndromes of SI dysfunction in children with learning disabilities that were not observed in normal children, Ayres proceeded to sharpen the definitions of and provide specific guidelines for diagnosing types of SI dysfunction and to revise the Southern California Sensory Integration Tests (SC-SIT; Ayres, 1972e). Implicating left hemisphere dysfunction in the auditory language factor and right-hemisphere dysfunction with the factor "poorer coordination on the left than right side of the body," Ayres (1969) began to differentiate SI dysfunction from hemisphere dysfunction. This and subsequent studies of academic, language, and SI measures of children with learning problems (Ayres, 1971, 1972f, 1977a) helped Ayres to differentiate the role of SI dysfunction in auditory-language and learning problems and to provide guidelines for test interpretation.

Theoretical Concepts

Sensory Integration—The Term

For many years, writers and researchers have used the term *sensory integration* in the general sense to refer to the use of sensory information for neural processing. In recent years, persons in OT and other fields have used this term synonymously with *sensory stimulation*, *sensory processing*, and, sometimes, *sensory modulation*. Lack of precision in the use of these terms presents confusion in evaluating research findings and therapy approaches and in differentiating what is being observed about an individual versus what is inferred about what is going on inside the individual's nervous system (Miller & Lane, 2000).

Ayres described the term *sensory integration* as the brain's ability to "filter, organize and integrate the masses of sensory information" for learning (Ayres, 1968b, p. 43). Although she used the terms *sensation* and *integration* frequently in her early writings (Ayres, 1958, 1960, 1961b, 1963b), it was not until 1968 that she combined these terms into sensory integration (SI) (Ayres 1968a, 1968b). Learning, she asserted, was a function of this neuropsychological ability, and reading could be described as "the end product of a long evolutionary course in which the increased capacity of SI, accompanied by the ability to emit an adaptive motor response, has furnished a critical foundation" (Ayres, 1968a, p. 170). "Certain types of learning disability," therefore, could "be interpreted partially in terms of dysfunction within the brain's integrative functions" (Ayres, 1968b, p. 43). Although Ayres acknowledged that "exactly how sensory integration occurs in the brain remains elusive," she insisted that that lack of knowledge should "not be an excuse for avoiding an issue basic to all learning" (Ayres, 1968b, p. 43). She considered auditory language functions to be part of the total SI process but stated that they were not the focus of her investigations (Ayres,

1968a, 1968b). The term *SI* took on special meanings and new terminology emerged as the theory of SI evolved. In developing the theory of SI, Ayres drew from developmental and neurological foundations.

Developmental Foundations

In her early writings, Ayres discussed phylogenetic and ontogenetic principles related to hand function (1954), visual-motor function (1958, 1961a), treatment (1966a), and reading (1968a), as well as neuromuscular, neurodevelopmental, and motor theories (Ayres, 1963b). She applied two phylogenetic principles to SI theory: (a) the importance of sensation and (b) the interdependence of higher and lower CNS structures and functions. According to the first principle, vertebrate organisms survived over millions of years because they evolved increasingly complex neural systems that enabled them to interact successfully with their environment. These neural changes resulted either by chance from genetic mutations or through the modification of the CNS via sensory input. SI theory emphasized the latter cause, claiming that "sensory input from the environment actually modified the nervous system because it called for new types of responses" (Ayres, 1963b, p. 364). The evolution of vertebrates coincided with their increase in numbers of sensory nerve fibers and their development of complex systems for processing sensory information. "Enlarging the scope of information supplied to the brain enabled it, in turn, to develop increasingly complex adaptive response" (Ayres, 1972d, p. 23). The second phylogenetic principle states that as vertebrates evolved, their earlier, simple neural structures were retained and new structures were added. The functions ascribed to the earlier systems remained and were not replaced, but instead were modified and integrated as each new neural level evolved.

> Each structure remained capable of receiving information, integrating it, and organizing an appropriate motor response. While the highest or youngest structure present at any one time in evolution or in any one species today (in humans it is the cerebral cortex) exerted critical influence over all lower structures, the higher centers still maintained a dependence upon lower structures. (Ayres, 1972d, p. 23)

According to an ontogenetic developmental principle, the development of the individual organism recapitulates the development of the species. For example, the motor development of human infants replays the evolutionary progression of vertebrates, which were first capable of swimming movements, then quadrapedal ambulation, and finally bipedal ambulation and dexterous upper extremities. Similarly, the development of motor control progresses from cephalad to caudal, proximal to distal, gross to fine, flexion to extension, adduction to abduction, ulnar to radial, movement in straight planes to rotational movement, and reflexive contraction to voluntary contraction (Ayres, 1963b).

Hypothesized Development of Sensory Integrative Processes

Ayres (1964a) hypothesized a sequence of perceptual-motor development (see Figure 5.1), in which academic skills and an ability to conceptualize (Level IV) are based on visual-spatial perception and motor skills (Level III), which, in turn, evolved from body scheme and motor planning (Level II) that were founded on tactile and visual perception and proprioception (Level I). The integration of tactile, proprioceptive, and visual sensations provide a body scheme and the ability to plan movements. Body scheme provides a postural model (Ayres, 1961a) or postural frame of reference (Ayres, 1964a) for movement and is also a result of the processing of sensory impulses that are generated through movement. "Motor planning and body scheme are two

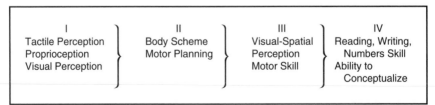

Figure 5.1. Hypothesized sequences in perceptual motor development. *Note.* From "Perceptual-Motor Training for Children," by A. J. Ayres, 1964, in *Approaches to the Treatment of Patients with Neuomuscular Dysfunction* (p. 18), by C. Satterly (Ed.), Dubuque, IA: William C. Brown, Publishers. Copyright 1964 by William C. Brown, Publishers.

sides of the same coin. The development of each is dependent upon the other" (Ayres, 1964a, p. 19). Body scheme is

> the knowledge we have of the construction and spatial relationships of the different anatomical elements, such as fingers, legs, arms, that make up our body. It involves being able to visualize these elements in movement and in different positional relationships. (Ayres, 1960, p. 308)

Visual-spatial perception guides movement and is derived from the integration of vision, proprioception (including vestibular), and cutaneous sensations as movement occurs. Visual-spatial perception develops in concert with manual manipulation and body scheme, and includes the perception of form, direction, or position in space and space visualization. As the child handles, explores, and experiments with objects and moves through and experiences space, he or she formulates perceptions and concepts of form and space. The role of vision is to verify what is experienced tactiley and kinesthetically. "Visual impressions reinforce and become associated with the manual impressions so that later visual cues can recall the cutaneous and proprioceptive, and the latter can recall the visual" (Ayres, 1958, p. 132). Likewise, the visual stimuli are essential for interpretation of the stimuli arising from manual manipulation. Thus "the same activities which enhance efficiency of motor planning also provided the basis of visual space perception" (Ayres, 1964a, p. 20). According to this model, body scheme, motor planning, and visual-spatial perception are the foundations for academic abilities.

By 1979, Ayres had refined this model (see Figure 5.2) to tie what can be observed about human behavior—that is, the "end products"—to what may be inferred about the sensory system processing that contributes to those end products. This model serves as an organizing framework for illustrating the role of sensory systems in human behavior, for interpreting SI tests (Ayres, 1976b, 1989), and for explaining test results to parents, teachers, and team members. She hypothesized four stages of SI development, which were roughly equivalent to the first year of life, the toddler stage, the preschool stage, and the school-age stage. The end products (concentration, organization, self-esteem, self-control, self-confidence, academic learning, abstract thinking, and specialization of the brain and body sides) of the fourth stage were thought

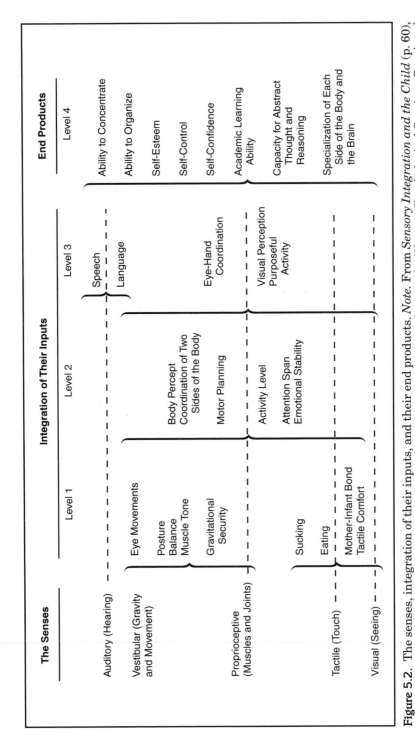

Figure 5.2. The senses, integration of their inputs, and their end products. *Note.* From *Sensory Integration and the Child* (p. 60), by A. J. Ayres, 1979, Los Angeles: Western Psychological Services. Copyright 1979 by Western Psychological Services. Reprinted with permission.

to develop as the result of many years of integration of the sensory systems (auditory, vestibular, propioceptive, tactile, and visual).

Consistent with SI theory, Ayres emphasized the roles of the tactile, proprioceptive, and vestibular systems in development. In the early months of life (Level 1), the tactile system contributes to the survival functions of sucking and eating, and the psychological functions of mother-infant bonding and tactile comfort. Vestibular and proprioceptive sensations provide a basis for eye movements, posture, balance, muscle tone, and gravitational security. In toddlerhood (Level 2), vestibular, proprioceptive, and tactile systems converge to contribute to the formation of a body percept and to the coordination of the two sides of the body, motor planning, activity level, attention span, and emotional stability. By about age 3 (Level 3), the child works to refine skills in eye-hand coordination, visual perception, and speech and language, and to engage in purposeful activity. At this level, audition and vision join the three basic senses to bring about skill development. Although vision and audition are obviously very important senses, Ayres deemphasized their role in development and dramatized the contribution of the less obvious senses: vestibular, tactile, and proprioceptive (Ayres, 1979).

Level 4 includes the end products of the integration of sensation that occurs during the first six years of life. For formal schooling, the child needs a foundation on which to develop the ability to concentrate, organize, and reason abstractly. Self-control, self-esteem, and self-confidence are important for human relationships in the classroom and at home. To provide a neurological basis for academic learning, the specialized functions of the cerebral hemispheres and right and left body sides must be well lateralized. Ayres proposed that these Level 4 abilities develop through the brain's ability to integrate sensory processes, beginning at birth (Ayres, 1979).

Neurological Bases

Ayres emphasized four concepts of neural functioning in her theory of SI: sensory integrative processes for concept formation; sensory integrative processes for movement; tactile, proprioceptive, and vestibular bases for auditory and visual functions; and subcortical functions.

Integrative Processes for Concept Formation

To function effectively, the brain must be able to organize sensory input from many sources into a meaningful pattern that can be used for movement and learning. It must be able to take information received from an isolated sensory source and compare it to another sensory source for clarification and validation. Because the brain has many more afferents than efferents, it must be able to structure the massive sensory input it receives if it is to perform effectively. The brain's ability to organize, compare, and structure sensory information is referred to as its integrative function.

Intersensory or intermodality integration is the capacity of the CNS to associate information from two or more different sensory modalities (Ayres, 1968a). Convergent, multisensory neurons that are activated by input from several sensory modalities provide a neuroanatomical basis for intersensory integration. These neurons are found throughout the neuroaxis, providing intersensory integration at the spinal cord, brain stem, cerebellum, and cerebrum levels (Ayres, 1972d). The brain gives meaning to the combined input from several sources, and one sensory modality can "predict" what the information would be from another sensory system. This interplay among the sensory systems allows one to develop concepts and to learn (see Figure 5.3). For example, in the case of concept formation, through sensory experiences with oranges, one develops the concept of "orangeness" and can identify an orange simply by its scent. Future sensory encounters with an orange through one sense—for example, its scent—will produce associations with its appearance, texture, and taste.

Integrative Processes for Movement

Sensation is one of the first components of a motor act. According to Ayres (1963b),

> Motor acts are initiated either directly or indirectly by some environmental factor that became known to the individual through sensory stimulation. One sees a pencil before one grasps it; one feels too warm and throws off the covers; one hears a horn at the side and changes the direction of the car; one feels the bag of groceries slipping and gives it a firmer hold. (p. 365)

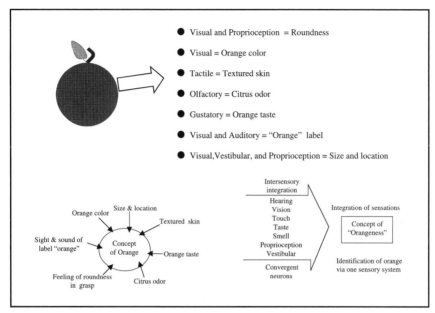

Figure 5.3. Integrative process for concept formation.

To produce movement, the CNS must integrate sensation. It must organize incoming sensations, combine them with past sensory processes, and use them to formulate an anticipated motor response. Once the movement is under way, the CNS must monitor, evaluate, and alter it as needed for future reference. Although movement is a product of CNS organization, the process of integrating sensation for movement can also be said to have an organizing effect on the CNS.

Movement, as it occurs, generates sensations that provide additional data for CNS processing. These include tactile, kinesthetic, proprioceptive, and vestibular sensations that arise from the body as it moves. These sensations inform the CNS about the movement as it is being produced: the stretch of the skin as it moves over a joint; joint motion and position; the relative position of body parts; the position of the head in relation to the body and to the earth's gravitational force; and the speed, duration, and strength of muscle contraction. The CNS must integrate this sensory information from the body with that from visual, auditory, and other senses to determine whether the intended movement was executed. The analysis of sensory information enables the CNS to adjust the formulation of subsequent motor responses. The integration of the sensations that are generated through movement enables the development and refinement of sensorimotor abilities.

The integration of sensation for movement not only is important for sensorimotor functions, but, also contributes to learning and cognition. Humans became intelligent creatures through the evolution of a motor system that afforded them the opportunity to explore and learn about their environment. Ayres suggested that the sensory integrative aspects that enable one to become a competent sensorimotor being are related to competence in early academic skills and that the brain's ability to integrate sensations for movement underlies the brain's ability to organize sensations for learning. In short, she proposed that "sensory integrative processes [for movement] subserve some aspects of cognition" (Ayres, 1975a, p. 304).

Tactile, Proprioceptive, and Vestibular Bases for Visual and Auditory Functions

The contribution of vision and audition to neural organization for academic performance is readily apparent and has been widely studied by numerous researchers and theorists. In contrast, Ayres theorized that the tactile, proprioceptive, and vestibular systems also had an impact on sensory processing for learning. Drawing on neuroscience literature from the 1960s and 1970s, Ayres reported that the tactile, proprioceptive, and vestibular systems mature in utero earlier than the visual and auditory systems. "There is quite general agreement that the phyletically older systems (tactile, olfactory, gustatory, vestibular, and proprioceptive) mature before the younger auditory and visual systems" (Ayres, 1975a, p. 314). During fetal life the stimulation of these older systems results first in reflex movements of the neck and mouth and then in reflex movements of the arms, legs, and trunk (tactile); eye movements (vestibular); and muscle contraction (proprioceptive). The functioning of these systems early in life makes possible the life-sustaining abilities to suck, swallow, breathe, and move.

If the sensory systems develop in concert with one another and not independently of each other and if, through SI, each sensory system influences and is influenced by other sensory systems, it follows that sensory systems that develop earlier have an impact on those that develop later. Thus, the functioning of the earlier systems influences the functioning of the later developing systems: "The normal development of visual perception requires intersensory integration from other sources, especially somatosensory and vestibular" (Ayres, 1968b, p. 46). Ayres hypothesized that auditory processing is probably enhanced through the stimulation of other senses (e.g., vestibular), and that visual perception and auditory processing are to a certain extent dependent on the processing of stimuli from the tactile and vestibular systems (Ayres, 1972c, p. 83).

Following this line of reasoning further, if early developing systems influence later developing systems, then dysfunction in the development of the early systems may affect the development of the later systems. Ayres surmised that dysfunction involving tactile, proprioceptive, or vestibular systems might contribute to learning problems observed in the performance of auditory or visual tasks. The child's learning difficulties may be due not only to problems in auditory or visual processes, but also to the SI deficits caused by problems in tactile, proprioceptive, and vestibular processes. Applying these principles to therapy, Ayres proposed that the goal of SI therapy is to enhance the brain's ability to learn through auditory and visual modes by ameliorating SI dysfunction involving the tactile, proprioceptive, and vestibular systems (Ayres, 1958, 1968b, 1972a, 1972c, 1972d, 1975a).

Subcortical Functions

SI theory explains how the CNS integrates sensation for human learning and movement. Unlike theories and research that focus on cortical processes for learning and movement, this theory emphasizes the functions of subcortical structures for human performance. Subcortical structures include the thalamus, basal ganglia, cerebellum, and brain stem. Of these structures, Ayres emphasized the role of the brain stem, including the thalamus. Although Ayres modified SI theory to address cortical functions in her later formulations regarding praxis, a review of hierarchical neural processes, as described by Ayres, remains useful for understanding SI theory.

The cerebral cortex, also called the neo- (or new) cortex, developed last phylogenetically and is responsible for the complex cognitive abilities and skilled manipulation capabilities that characterize humans. However, in keeping with phylogenetic principles, the earlier developing neural structures were not replaced and the functioning of these structures was not eliminated. Instead, the neocortex developed additively upon these older structures by integrating and refining the functions of earlier systems. Functions became replicated with increasing complexity as the neuroaxis evolved from spinal cord to brainstem to cerebrum. "Cortical functions, then, are in some respects still dependent upon brainstem functions" (Ayres, 1975a, p. 318).

The brain stem is one of the major structures in which SI occurs (Ayres, 1975a).

> At one time in the evolutionary process, the brainstem, as the highest neural structure, provided sufficient organization and direction to enable the organism to interact adaptively with its environment, albeit at a primitive level. Those functions, although greatly modified, still operate in man today. (Ayres, 1972d, p. 40)

The major nuclei of the brain stem, including the thalamus, are (a) sensory nuclei for the vestibular, tactile, proprioceptive, auditory, visual, and gustatory systems; (b) motor nuclei for eye, facial, and throat movements; eye and postural reflexes; and muscle tone; (c) limbic nuclei for mood and for stereotypical motions associated with survival functions; (d) autonomic nuclei for cardiovascular, gastrointestinal, and pulmonary functions; and (e) reticular nuclei for arousal, alerting, and attending functions. The brain stem is in a position to perform major integrative functions and to influence the functioning of the neocortex. Ayres argued,

> Any major neural structure receiving sensory input from many sources is apt to have widespread influence over the rest of the brain. Multiplicity of input usually means convergence of input, and where there is convergence of input there is integration of input. (1972c, p. 82)

The brain stem and thalamus are "good examples of structures to which the principle is applicable" (Ayres, 1972d, p. 53). Ayres emphasized the role of the reticular formation in the brain stem and the thalamus in receiving and integrating "sensory input from every sensory modality" (Ayres, 1972c, p. 40) and in serving as a master control mechanism in the CNS. The reticular formation has both descending pathways to the spinal cord to influence postural responses and ascending pathways for alertness and attention. She concluded, "The majority of children with disordered learning show some dysfunction that can be linked to the brain stem, especially the reticular formation" (Ayres, 1972d, p. 45).

In addition to the brain stem, other subcortical structures have important intersensory integration functions. The cerebellum

> receives input from all sensory sources over the afferent neurons and from much but not all of the cerebral cortex, processes it, and then uses it to influence ongoing neuronal activity, especially down the spinal cord, to brainstem nuclei, the thalamus, basal ganglia and cortex. (Ayres, 1972d, p. 47)

The cerebellum plays a role in the smoothness and timing of movements, muscle tone, vestibular functions, and limbic functions. The basal ganglia regulate posture and movements of the body in space and are involved in the production of complex motor acts. They appear to be "involved in a type of sensory integration that allows one type of sensory input to influence the integration of another type and to utilize that input for moderately complex postural and other bodily movements" (Ayres, 1972d, p. 49). The limbic system

> is concerned with primitive patterns of behavior necessary for individual and species survival, including vegetative functions, defending the body against attack, and the simple perceptual motor functions needed to fulfill these survival functions. Its function is clarified when it is considered the primary cortical structure in a large proportion of vertebrates. Fish have no neocortex; amphibians, reptiles, and birds have little, yet all of these animals show basic but well integrated behavior including perceptual, motor, and simple learning and memory. (Ayres, 1972d, p. 49)

In summary, Ayres proposed that SI for sensorimotor functions occurs in all subcortical levels and provides a foundation for cortical functions. Furthermore, SI dysfunction at the subcortical level may contribute to difficulties in cognitive processes. SI therapy aims to enhance cognitive processing by improving SI functions mediated in subcortical structures (Ayres, 1967, 1968b, 1972b, 1972c, 1972d, 1975a). Evaluation and assessment of SI dysfunction is the first step in addressing these problems in the clinic.

Evaluation and Assessment

Test construction occupied much of Ayres's efforts throughout her career. She developed, revised, and reformulated tests for identifying what were termed perceptual–motor problems in the 1960s and, later, SI dysfunction. She said, "I needed to develop tests to really get at the problem, and in learning situations, problems are not easily measured, determined, even recognized. When I started out, there weren't any really good tests for looking at dysfunction in children" (A. J. Ayres, personal communication, June 29, 1981). She developed the Motor Accuracy Test before her doctoral work but did not standardize it until after she received her degree. In her doctoral program, she "wanted to have the kind of instruction, guidance and supervision of test construction that I could see I was going to need later in research" (A. J. Ayres, personal communication, June 29, 1981).

Initially, Ayres focused on developing visual–perceptual tests. She reported, "I spent a lot of time and a lot of money developing visual perception tests that never reached the market" (A. J. Ayres, personal communication, June 29, 1981). Like several of her contemporaries, she wanted to pursue the obvious role of visual perception in reading and other academic tasks.

> When Marianne Frostig (who developed the Frostig Developmental Test of Visual Perception) found out I was developing a test of visual perception, she called me on the telephone and asked me not to develop it because she was developing one and I told her I didn't think there would be much conflict. (A. J. Ayres, personal communication, June 29, 1981)

Eventually, however, Ayres began to look beyond visual perception.

It wasn't a good area to pursue, but it took me a long time to figure [that] out. We could see that visual processing problems were central to learning disorders, but we needed to look beyond vision. If you just look at children from a behavioral standpoint and do behavioral-type research and modeling, you'll never really discover that a main foundation to visual perception is the vestibular system, with proprioception and other senses also contributing. (A. J. Ayres, personal communication, June 29, 1981)

Ayres published her first test, the Ayres Space Test, in 1962 and continued throughout her career to develop and revise tests (see Table 5.1). At the time of her death in 1988, the national restandardization of the SIPT was completed. This fulfilled her goals of remedying some of the psychometric properties of the SCSIT) Ayres, 1972e, 1980b), expanding the normative samples beyond Southern California (Ayres, Mailloux, & McAtee, 1985), and improving test–retest reliability (Kinnealey & Wilbarger, 1993). A list of the tests included in the SIPT is shown in Table 5.2.

Sensory Integrative Dysfunction

Ayres described SI dysfunction in children with learning or behavior problems who had no known peripheral nervous system or CNS deficits. Like her contemporaries in the 1960s, she was intrigued by the question "Why can't Johnny learn?" when Johnny has normal intelligence, hearing, vision, speech, and results on a neurological exam. Psychologists, special educators, and language pathologists explained learning problems as "processing deficits," although CNS structures and the peripheral nerves conveying information to and from the CNS were intact. Whereas other researchers focused on specific problems with visual perception, speech and language, and reading, Ayres investigated somatosensory, motor, and vestibular processing deficits as indicators of SI dysfunction.

Much of Ayres's work focused on constructing and refining typologies of SI dysfunction. Her first typology was based on a factor analytic study of 100 children with learning disabilities and 50 normal children. She identified five discrete patterns of dysfunction: developmental apraxia, perceptual dysfunction of

Table 5.1
Tests Developed by Ayres

Test	Date	Properties/Revisions
Ayres Space Test	1962	Sixty-item test of form perception and visual manipulation in space of egg and diamond shapes. Normative data on children in Southern California.
Southern California Motor Accuracy Test	1964b	Test of manual speed and dexterity in tracing with pencil by each hand. Normative data on children in Southern California.
Southern California Figure Ground Visual Perception Tests	1966d	Test of visual selection of stimulus from competing background. Normative data on children in Southern California.
Southern California Kinesthesia and Tactile Perception Tests	1966e	Tests of arm movement kinesthesia, finger identification, tactile discrimination, and tactile localization. Normative data on children in Southern California.
Southern California Perceptual–Motor Tests	1968c	Combined prior tests and added imitation of postures, bilateral motor coordination, crossing the body midline, standing balance, and right–left discrimination. Normative data on children in Southern California.
Southern California Sensory Integration Tests (SCSIT)	1972e	Compiled 17 tests into one kit, renamed Ayres Space Test to Space Visualization Test and reduced its number of items, Extended norms for the Figure–Ground Visual Perception Test and Motor Accuracy Test, and normed two new tests: the Position in Space Test and the Design Copying Test.
Southern California Postrotary Nystagmus Test	1975b	Test of vestibulo–ocular reflex function. Normative data on children in Southern California.
Southern California Motor Accuracy Test— Revised 1980	1980a	Southern California Motor Accuracy Test norms for three speeds of right- and left-hand performance.
Southern California Sensory Integration Tests (SCSIT) Revised	1980b	Revised to include post rotary nystagmus and new norms of motor accuracy.
Sensory Integration and Praxis Tests (SIPT)	1989	Seventeen subtests normed on 2,000 children in the United States and Canada. Omission of several tests from SCSIT. Addition of four new praxis tests. Computer scoring and interpretation of test results.

Table 5.2
Brief Descriptions of the 17 Subtests of Ayres's
Sensory Integration Praxis Tests

1. Space Visualization (SV). In this puzzle-like test, the child indicates which of two forms will fit a formboard. This test measures visual perception and mental rotation of objects.

2. Figure–Ground Perception (FG). The child points to pictures that are hidden among other pictures. This test measures how well the child visually perceives a figure against a confusing background.

3. Manual Form Perception (MFP). The child identifies unusual shapes held in the hand. This test measures tactile perception and visual perception.

4. Kinesthesia (KIN). The child attempts to put his or her finger back to where the therapist had previously placed it. This test assesses the sense of arm position and movement.

5. Finger Identification (FI). The child points to his or her finger that the therapist touched. This test measures tactile perception.

6. Graphesthesia (GRA). The child draws with a finger the same simple design the therapist drew on the back of the child's hand. This test measures tactile perception and motor planning.

7. Localization of Tactile Stimuli (LTS). The child points to the spot where the therapist has lightly touched the child's arm or hand with a pen. This test measures tactile perception.

8. Praxis on Verbal Command (PrVC). The child executes a series of coordinated movements that have been described verbally. This test assesses ability to translate verbal description into various postures.

9. Design copying (DC). The child copies a series of increasingly complex line drawings, following detailed instructions. This test measures two-dimensional constructional praxis and visuomotor coordination.

10. Constructional Praxis (CPr). The child builds with blocks, using structures built by the therapist as models. This test measures three-dimensional constructional praxis.

11. Postural Praxis (PPr). In this test, the child imitates unusual body postures demonstrated by the therapist. The ability to conceptualize, plan, and execute movements is assessed.

12. Oral Praxis (OPr). The child imitates movements of the tongue, lips, and jaw. The ability to plan and execute facial movements is assessed.

13. Sequencing Praxis (SPr). The child imitates a series of simple arm and hand movements. This test measures bilateral coordination and the ability to plan and execute sequential movements.

(continues)

Table 5.2 *Continued.*

14. Bilateral Motor Coordination (BMC). The child imitates a series of arm and foot movements. This test evaluates the ability to coordinate the two sides of the body.

15. Standing and Walking Balance (SWB). The child holds various standing and walking postures, with eyes open and eyes closed. This test reflects the integration of sensations from gravity and proprioceptors.

16. Motor Accuracy (MAc). In this test, the child draws a line on top of a long, curving printed line. Visuomotor coordination and motor planning are measured.

17. Postrotatry Nystagmus (PRN). The child is rotated clockwise and counterclockwise on a rotation board. This test measures processing of vestibular sensory input.

Note. From *Sensory Integration and Praxis Tests,* by A. J. Ayres (1989), Los Angeles: Western Psychological Services. Copyright 1988 by Western Psychological Services. Reprinted by permission of the publisher.

form and position in two-dimensional space, tactile defensiveness, the deficit of integration of function of the two sides of the body, and perceptual dysfunction of visual figure-ground discrimination. This classification scheme, presented in her Eleanor Clarke Slagle lecture (Ayres, 1963a), provided the framework for test development and theory building in SI (Ayres, 1963a, 1965). The absence of these five syndromes in the normal subjects supported areas of dysfunction that were not characteristic of normal development (Ayres, 1965, 1966b, 1966c). Although the specific characteristics of these areas of dysfunction shifted somewhat in the progression of studies, four areas of dysfunction were described:

- Visual form and space dysfunction
- Developmental dyspraxia
- Deficits in vestibular and bilateral integration
- Tactile defensiveness

Visual Form and Space Dysfunction

Ayres (1958) described perception as "a function of afferent neural interaction for the purpose of interpreting and organizing afferent neural interaction for insight and use" (p. 130) and, along with Maslow et al. (1964), described aspects of visual perception and potential areas of visual form and space dysfunction as visual figure-ground, form constancy, spatial orientation, and spatial relationships. She found a relationship between form and space perception deficits and learning problems in several factor analytic studies of the SCSIT (Ayres, 1965, 1969, 1972f, 1977a). Tests that loaded on the form and space perception factor included those that were purely visual (space visualization), those that tapped visual and motor functions (design copying), and those that involved visual, motor, tactile, and proprioceptive functions (graphesthesia, kinesthesia, and manual form perception).

In contrast to the prevailing viewpoint that visual form and space dysfunction could be identified and treated in isolation, Ayres found that it often accompanied praxis, postural, ocular, and somatosensory dysfunction in children with learning and behavior problems. Elaborating on Trevarthen's (1968) hypothesized dual modes of vision, Ayres (1972d) contrasted ambient vision, or perception of the surrounding environment, with focal vision, or perception of near visual stimuli. Ambient vision relies on a spatial map of the environment that the organism develops through subcortically mediated, postural–ocular experiences with gravity and space as locomotion progresses through prone, sitting, quadraped, and bipedal postures. Focal vision, in contrast, requires precise attention to details of orientation and form in central vision and is a function of the cerebral cortex. According to Ayres, the ability to discriminate the orientation of a letter on a page is derived from cortical, focal visual functions and also from the environmental spatial map provided by subcortical structures. Although the ambient-focal vision and cortical–subcortical dichotomies are not as separate as Ayres suggested, these concepts were useful for bringing attention to the possible linkage of somatosensory, proprioceptive, and motor functions to visual perception.

The association of visual form and space functions with praxis was further supported by the factor analytic studies and cluster analyses of the SIPT (Ayres, 1989). Because of the "common conceptual link between praxis and visual perception" (Ayres & Marr, 1991, p. 210), a factor composed of three overlapping components—form and space perception, visuomotor coordination, and visual construction—was named "visuopraxis" (Ayres & Marr, 1991; Fisher & Murray, 1991). Cluster

analysis of the SIPT identified children in a visuo- and somatodyspraxia cluster group (Ayres & Marr, 1991). Although Ayres
identified visual form and space problems in many studies, she
consistently viewed these problems in the context of somatosensory, proprioceptive, and praxis functions rather than
primarily as problems in processing by the visual system. She
considered visual form and space perception to be an end product of sensory integration. Consequently, she did not emphasize
visual–perceptual training as part of SI therapy.

Developmental Dyspraxia

Developmental dyspraxia is "a disorder of sensory integration in-
terfering with praxis, e.g., the ability to plan and execute skilled
or nonhabitual motor tasks" (Ayres, 1972d, p. 165). The ability to
sequence movements to produce a coordinated series of actions is
faulty. Although the child can learn new tasks, doing so takes
longer and is more difficult than for children with normal SI development. The child may find everyday activities such as fas-
tening buttons and riding a bicycle to be laborious and frustrating. Such skills may be late to develop. Praxis problems in
planning and executing movements occur, according to the classical definition, in the absence of identified muscle weakness,
tremors, spasticity, or sensory loss, and similarly, developmental
dyspraxis is not associated with identified neurological problems
(unlike adult-onset apraxia which is often associated with a left,
language-dominant hemisphere lesion or with a right hemisphere lesion.

Having consistently found a relationship between low scores
on praxis tests and low scores on tactile tests (Ayres, 1965, 1969,
1971, 1972f, 1977a), Ayres theorized that the development of
praxis was related to tactile (skin) and proprioceptive (muscle,
tendon, and joint) somatosensory processing. Cutaneous, muscle, joint, tendon, and deep tissue receptors are constantly activated as muscles contract, joints move, and the skin slides over
moving muscles and joints. The resultant flow of sensory input
to the CNS sustains and provides the basis for development of a
body scheme, which in turn provides a dynamic map that the
brain uses for organizing, ordering, and timing movements. If
the information, which the body receives from its somatosensory
receptors, is not precise due to faulty sensory integration, "the

brain has a poor basis on which to build its scheme of the body; consequently, the capacity to motor plan cannot develop normally" (Ayres, 1972d, p. 170).

Ayres differentiated the sensory basis for praxis and postural and bilateral integration:

> While postural and bilateral integration appear to be especially and directly dependent upon vestibular input, praxis is especially and directly dependent upon discriminative tactile functions with the vestibular system providing more of a substrate. Both systems are dependent upon proprioceptors, with posture more related to the muscle spindle and praxis to joint receptors. . . . The major substrate of praxis is believed to be diencephalic and cortical while the brain stem is the major integrating site for postural and bilateral integration. (Ayres, 1972d, p. 171)

In the 1980s, Ayres elaborated upon conceptual and cognitive processes mediated by the cerebral cortex, especially the left hemisphere, in developmental dyspraxia. Drawing on others' investigations of clumsy children and research in adult dyspraxia, as well as on her own insights from her clinical practice and research, she proposed three processes in developmental dyspraxia: "ideation or conceptualization; planning a scheme of action; and motor execution" (Ayres, 1985, p. 19).

In a study of 182 children with learning or behavior problems, Ayres, Mailloux, and Wendler (1987) sought to determine the existence of a unitary dyspraxia function or to differentiate types of developmental dyspraxia associated with sensory (i.e., visual, tactile, kinesthetic, proprioceptive, and vestibular) or auditory language functions. Neither a single dyspraxia function nor a type of dyspraxia was supported, and there was insufficient evidence of differential associations with sensory systems. However, the "data supported the idea of a general practice function with different practice skills defined by behavioral tasks" (Ayres & Marr, 1991, p. 210). Linkages between tactile functions and praxis and between visual processes and praxis were again shown. The authors concluded that there was evidence for a somatopractic function and that "two basic elements of the general practic function appear to be tactile processing and ideation or concept formation" (Ayres et al., 1987, p. 105). They related visual perception to ideational processes for praxis because the visual tests that had the strongest associations with praxis were those that required considerable concept formation.

Subsequent factor and cluster analyses of the SIPT (Ayres, 1989; Ayres & Marr, 1991) revealed three factors related to praxis: somatopraxis, visuopraxis, and praxis on verbal command associated with prolonged postrotary nystagmus. The somatopraxis factor included low scores on tests of praxis and somatosensory/proprioceptive processing. Ayres labeled the somatosensory tests in a separate factor (Ayres & Marr, 1991); however, the coexistence of low praxis scores with low somatosensory scores remains a requisite for diagnosing somatodyspraxia (Cermak, 1991).

The visuopraxis factor was described in the previous section on visual form and space dysfunction. Low scores on visuopraxis tests in the absence of tactile or somatosensory dysfunction were considered to indicate hemisphere dysfunction rather than a sensory integration disorder (Fisher & Murray, 1991). Children identified in the visuosomatodyspraxia cluster may have low praxis scores and low scores on tests of somatosensory processing, visual processing, or both. However, Ayres notes that the "visuopraxis scores should be delineated instead as form and space perception, visuomotor coordination, or visual construction deficits" (Ayres & Marr, 1991, p. 227).

The Praxis on Verbal Command Subtest of the SIPT assesses the individual's ability to assume postures in response to verbal instructions. Low scores on this subtest loaded with high scores on the Postrotary Nystagmus Subtest (prolonged postrotary nystagmus presumably indicates faulty central inhibition of vestibular input). The praxis on verbal command pattern of SIPT scores was found in a study of children with language disorders, and Ayres interpreted this pattern as suggestive of left hemisphere rather than sensory integrative dysfunction (Ayres & Marr, 1991). Finally, praxis components comprise three of the six clusters (Table 5.3) used in the computer-scored Western Psychological Services (WPS) SIPT Test Report (Figure 5.4): visuo- and somatodyspraxia, dyspraxia on verbal command, and low-average sensory integration and praxis.

In summary, Ayres's theory of praxis emphasized conceptual processes that are dependent on somatosensory integration. In her later work, Ayres continued to emphasize the importance of tactile, kinesthetic, proprioceptive, and vestibular system functioning as a basis for cortical processes of ideation, planning,

Table 5.3

Six Comparison Groups on the Western Psychological
Services (WPS) Sensory Integration and Praxis Test Report

Group	Definition
Generalized sensory integration dysfunction	Tends to have below-average integration scores on all SIPT subtests and both practice and somatosensory deficits.
Visuo- and somatodyspraxia	Low scores on design copying, finger identification, graphesthesia, postural praxis, bilateral motor coordination, standing and walking balance, motor accuracy, and kinesthesia. Has the lowest postrotary nystagmus score of the six groups.
Dyspraxia on verbal command	Severe difficulties with praxis on verbal command and the highest postrotary nystagmus score of the six groups.
Deficit in bilateral integration and sequencing	Low-average scores on standing and walking balance, bilateral motor coordination, oral praxis, sequencing praxis, and graphesthesia.
Low-average sensory integration and praxis	Tends to have low-average scores on all areas of the SIPT.
High-average sensory integration and praxis	Above-average functioning in all areas of the SIPT.

and sequencing (Ayres, 1985). She also continued to view dyspraxia as a sensory integrative disorder when it was associated with disorders in the somatosensory system. She claimed that in the absence of other signs of SI disorders, problems related to visuopraxis and praxis on verbal command were not sensory integrative disorders but rather possible *outcomes* of poor praxis or related to hemisphere dysfunction.

Bilateral Integration and Vestibular Dysfunction

As Ayres's factor analytic studies (1965, 1969) demonstrate, bilateral integration deficits are linked to postural problems, and both disorders show an association with low academic achievement. As early as 1963, in her Eleanor Clarke Slagle lecture, Ayres speculated that the association between diminished body

178 👪 Kay F. Walker

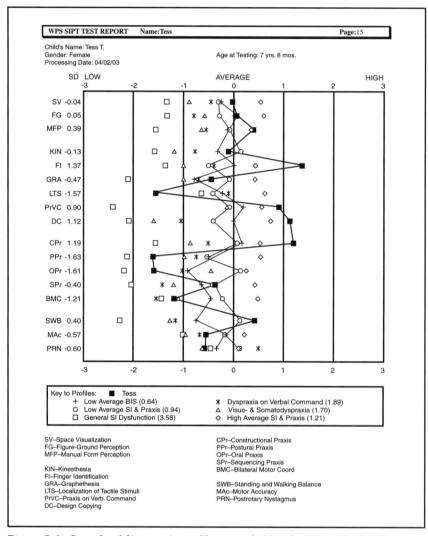

Figure 5.4. Sample of diagnostic profiles revealed by cluster analysis of Sensory Integration and Praxis Tests. From *Sensory Integration and Praxis Test.* Copyright 1988–1996 by Western Psychological Services. Reprinted by permission of the publisher, Western Psychological Services, 12031 Wilshire Boulevard, Los Angeles, CA 90025; www.wpspublish.com. *Note.* In this sample, the examinee's profile is most like low-average BIS (+) and low-average SI and Praxis (O).

balance and poor integration of sides of the body might be due to a neurophysiological deficit that was basic to both (Ayres, 1963a). In 1972, Ayres proposed a syndrome of postural and bilateral integration (PBI), with major symptoms, including poorly integrated postural and ocular mechanisms, poor bilateral integration, and poor visual perception (Ayres, 1972d). Later research led her to implicate the vestibular system in this syndrome, and eventually to propose that vestibular system dysfunction played a significant role in problems of interhemispheral communication and hemispheric specialization. Ayres (1975a) wrote,

> the postulate that the brainstem interhemispheral integrating mechanism is functionally associated with the brain stem postural reflexes and reactions and, furthermore, that inadequate maturation of the brainstem-mediated postural reactions interferes with maturation of the brainstem interhemispheral integrative mechanisms. The resultant dysfunction interferes with the development of specialization of function of the cerebral cortex. (p. 342)

In 1976, Ayres redefined the PBI as a syndrome of vestibular and bilateral integration (VBI) dysfunction that involved poor interhemispheral communication, inadequate cerebral specialization, and deficits in the vestibular system (Ayres, 1976a). Symptoms of VBI include inadequate integration of the two body sides, hyporesponsive nystagmus, and deficient postural responses. The diagnosis of VBI depended on the Postrotary Nystagmus and Bilateral Motor Coordination subtests of the SIPT and a variety of clinical observations (i.e., poor eye pursuits across the midline, lack of agreement of eye–hand preference, lack of agreement of ear–hand preference); a lack of definite right ear superiority on the dichotic listening test; a lower preferred hand score on the Motor Accuracy subtest; a low score on contralateral use of the hands on the subtest, Space Visualization; immature righting and equilibrium responses; poorly integrated primitive postural reflexes; lack of flexibility in rotation around the longitudinal axis of the body; reduced postural background movements to orient and adjust the body posturing to a task; muscle hypotonicity; poor cocontraction; and poor discrimination of right and left body sides (Ayres, 1976b).

Ayres's theory of vestibular dysfunction evolved over a period of several years and was based on several studies of the effectiveness of SI therapy, which stimulates the vestibular system and encourages the maturation of postural responses in treating learning disabilities. In one such study, Ayres (1972b) evaluated the success of SI therapy in improving the academic performance of children in whom auditory language problems were identified as the cause of their academic difficulties. Five months after the termination of therapy, greater gains in academic scores were made by the experimental group that received SI therapy than by the control group. To explain how this nonacademic therapy could improve academic performance, Ayres proposed that the vestibular and somatosensory input provided by SI therapy enhanced the brain's capacity for intersensory integration of visual, auditory, vestibular, and somatosensory processing, thereby enhancing the brain's capacity for learning. She also hypothesized that "normalization of postural mechanisms organized in the midbrain enable[s] better cortical interhemispheral communication upon which reading must be quite dependent" (Ayres, 1972b, p. 342).

Once Ayres had developed the Southern California Postrotary Nystagmus Test (PRN test; Ayres, 1975b), she could assess an ocular reflex related to vestibular functioning. A subsequent study (Ayres, 1976a) using PRN test results as a variable enabled her to make significant additions to a theory implicating vestibular-based dysfunction in learning disabilities of children. Ayres compared academic gains made by matched groups of children with hyporesponsive, normal, or prolonged (hyperreactive) postrotary nystagmus who did or did not receive SI therapy in addition to special education. Among the three groups that received only special education, those in the hyporesponsive nystagmus group profited less from this regimen than those in the hyperreactive nystagmus or normal nystagmus group. She found that children with hyporesponsive nystagmus who received SI therapy in addition to special education made academic gains, whereas children with hyporesponsive nystagmus who received only special education showed no change in achievement level. Ayres concluded that hyporesponsive nystagmus identifies a type of vestibular disorder that interferes with academic learning.

The children with learning disabilities who had hyporesponsive nystagmus accounted for nearly one half of the sample and appeared less dysfunctional and more capable than the children with normal or prolonged nystagmus. Children in the hyporesponsive nystagmus group had higher intelligence scores, were in better physical condition, had better auditory language functions, and showed a higher baseline of academic achievement than children in the normal or prolonged nystagmus groups. The fact that children with hyporesponsive nystagmus made up nearly half of the sample, whereas the normal incidence is 14%, indicates that the more capable children with learning disabilities likely had a vestibular disorder. Children with prolonged duration nystagmus seemed to have more neurological involvement, and some of them had signs of left cerebral hemisphere dysfunction; this group was less responsive to SI therapy.

As part of the same study, Ayres investigated the predictability of the Dichotic Listening Test for SI dysfunction in children with learning disabilities. (The dichotic listening test presents competing stimuli simultaneously to each ear, and the child reports the stimulus heard, enabling the tester to determine which ear and thus which hemisphere is attending to the stimulus.) Patterns of associated scores were identified, but were not statistically significant. Children with infrequent use of the left hemisphere scored poorly on tests of auditory language function (Ayres, 1977b). Two explanations were offered: (a) poor interhemispheral communication leading to poor hemispheric specialization and (b) poor left hemisphere functioning. Because nearly half of the sample population had hyporeactive nystagmus, the involvement of the vestibular system was implicated in interhemispheric communication and specialization (Ayres, 1976a).

In short, this important 1976 study yielded many useful theoretical, diagnostic, and clinical results. It showed that children with learning disabilities who had vestibular SI dysfunction could make academic as well as sensory integrative gains when SI therapy was provided in addition to special education. It also laid the groundwork for delineation of the syndrome of vestibular and bilateral integration (Ayres, 1976a). Vestibular disorder, as characterized by hyporesponsive nystagmus, was linked to academic deficits, including auditory language dysfunction (Ayres, 1978).

The association between the vestibular system and auditory language functions was again demonstrated in a 1981 study (Ayres & Mailloux, 1981) of four aphasic children. Using a single-case method, Ayres found that the rate of growth in language comprehension increased in all four children and expressive language improved in two of the children after they received SI therapy. Hyporesponsive postrotary nystagmus, indicative of vestibular disorder, was found in the pretesting of the two children who made the greatest gains in expressive language. The therapy emphasized, and all the children sought, experiences in vestibular stimulation.

These results led to the hypothesis that SI therapy promotes auditory processing in those neural systems that are dependent on vestibular and somatosensory processing. Further, Ayres concluded that SI therapy was effective in facilitating language development in children with aphasia and somatosensory and vestibular processing disorders, and suggested that the vestibular system was one of a complex of contributing mechanisms underlying expressive language.

The development of additional subtests in the SIPT and subsequent factor and cluster analyses of the SIPT led to further refinement of a disorder of bilateral integration (Ayres, 1989; Ayres & Marr, 1991). A bilateral integration and sequencing (BIS) factor and cluster were identified. In addition, low scores on postural praxis were observed in the cluster analysis, but BIS disorder is often seen without low postural praxis scores (Knox et al., 1988). The BIS label is used in the absence of somatopraxis or other explanations of the low scores. When low somatosensory and praxis scores are seen, the bilateral integration and sequencing scores may be more appropriately considered as part of the praxis picture. In addition, when there is evidence of higher-level dysfunction, such as with high postrotary nystagmus and low praxis on verbal command scores, the bilateral integration and sequencing problem is not considered a sensory integration problem.

Tactile Defensiveness, Sensory Defensiveness, Sensory Registration, and Sensory Modulation

The disinhibition syndrome of hyperactivity and distractibility has long been recognized as a major problem in many children with learning deficits. Ayres identified what she termed *tactile defensiveness* as part of this syndrome in 1964. Others have described the role of sensory functioning in contexts of sensory defensiveness, sensory registration, and sensory modulation.

Tactile Defensiveness Tactile defensiveness is characterized by expressions of "feelings of discomfort and a desire to escape the situation when certain types of tactile stimuli are experienced" (Ayres, 1964c, p. 8). Ayres did not develop tests for tactile defensiveness. Instead, she suggested that the examiner observe the child's negative reactions to tactile stimuli during tactile testing. Questions about when the test would end, comments about not liking the test, withdrawing the hand or moving the body away from the examiner, complaints of a painful stimulus, giggling, or angry comments were all clues that the child found tactile stimuli to be aversive (Ayres, 1964c). Other examples of tactile defensive behavior include avoiding or dislike of bathing, haircuts, being touched on the face, sand play, going barefoot, and wearing certain fabrics (Ayres, 1979). Assessments of tactile defensiveness include Larson's (1982) sensory history, Royeen and Fortune's (1990) Touch Inventory for Elementary School-Aged Children, and Dunn's (1999) Sensory Profile.

An example of the refinement of theory through research findings was seen in changes in Ayres's ideas about tactile defensiveness in regard to protective versus discriminative tactile systems. In an early work, Ayres (1964c) proposed that tactile defensiveness was a result of the predominant influence of the protective tactile system, which led to diffuse, alerting, and warning reactions in response to tactile stimuli with concomitant fright, flight, or fight responses. The protective system is older phylogenetically, develops early ontogenetically, and must be inhibited for discriminative functions to develop. The discriminative tactile system develops later and provides for the tactile discrimination of two- and three-dimensional objects and for tactile localization. Ayres thought that predominance of the protective system prevented optimal functioning of the discriminative system. According to this hierarchical tactile system, the presence of tactile defensiveness could contribute to poor performance on tactile discrimination tests that are susceptible to distractibility or that include a light tactile stimulus. However, tests of tactile discrimination were found to have stronger correlations with praxis tests, whereas somatosensory scores may or may not be depressed in the presence of tactile defensiveness. Thus, tactile defensiveness seems to be a problem of disinhibition involving the tactile system rather than a product of a disordered tactile system itself (Ayres, 1976b). Tactile defensiveness and poor tactile discrimination are two separate disorders involving the tactile system, and thus it does not follow that when tactile defensiveness is reduced, improvements in tactile discrimination should be expected (Fisher & Dunn, 1983).

Sensory Defensiveness   According to Ayres, prolonged postrotary nystagmus (Ayres, 1975b) and choreoathetosis (Ayres, 1977c) share an underlying neurological basis with tactile defensiveness, in that all three could be considered indicators of CNS disinhibition or hyperexcitability. Finding that choreoathetosis shared variance with the effect of the asymmetrical tonic neck reflex on equilibrium, Ayres suggested that choreoathetosis was a release phenomenon (1977b) and a problem of insufficient inhibition of motor responses (1977c). In a study of children with choreoathetoid movements who received SI therapy compared with those who received special education only, those receiving therapy made gains in eye–hand coordination after a year of SI therapy (although the gains were not statistically significant). Whether the SI therapy affected the SI substrates of eye–motor coordination or the motor release problem itself was not clarified in this study (Ayres, 1977c).

The term *sensory defensiveness* has been introduced to refer to several types of defensive responses to sensory stimuli (Knickerbocker, 1980; Wilbarger & Wilbarger, 1990). Tactile defensiveness has been viewed as one type of sensory defensiveness that is similar to gravitational insecurity and aversive responses to vestibular–proprioceptive stimuli (Royeen & Lane, 1991). Gravitational insecurity refers to a fearful, defensive reaction to vestibular–proprioceptive stimuli when the body is not in contact with the floor, such as when swinging on suspended equipment (Fisher, 1991). Aversive responses to vestibular–proprioceptive stimuli include autonomic nervous system responses such as nausea, sweating, and dizziness.

Sensory Registration   Ayres (1979) described three types of sensory processing problems in children with autism: registration, modulation, and motivation. She noted that the child with autism ignores stimuli to which most persons would respond. It is as if the child does not "register" or notice stimuli or may notice it sometimes but not others. If the child does register the stimulus, he or she may have difficulty moderating the response and overreact or react defensively. Children with autism seem to lack the innate drive or motivation to engage and explore their environment. In a study of 10 children with autism, Ayres and Tickle (1980) investigated the level of responsiveness to auditory, visual, tactile, vestibular, proprioceptive, olfactory, and gustatory stimuli as a predictor of response to SI therapy. Results indicated that SI therapy could be effective in treating sensory defensiveness and tactile defensiveness in particular. The children's reactions to 14 sensory stimuli were classified as hyporesponsive, normal, or hyperresponsive. After one year, the group was divided into the best and poorest respondents to therapy. Children with hyperresponsivity (e.g., tactile defensiveness, avoidance of movements, gravitational insecurity) and who exhibited an orienting response to an air puff on the skin were the best respondents. Ayres and Tickle (1980) concluded that those autistic children who were able to register sensory input but could not modulate it benefited more from the organizing effect of SI therapy than did those children who were hyporesponsive to or did not orient to sensory stimuli.

Sensory modulation A range of sensory registration and responsivity has been suggested by various authors (Cermak, 1988; Lai, Parham, & Johnson-Ecker, 1999; Knickerbocker, 1980; Miller & McIntosh, 1998; Royeen & Lane, 1991). At one end of the spectrum is sensory dormancy, characterized by hyporesponsivity and failure to orient, and at the other end is sensory defensiveness characterized by hyperresponsivity and overorientation. Presumably, the range of optimal functioning lies in the modulation of responses within these two extremes and varies with one's "sensory diet"—that is, the "optimum amount of organizing and integrating sensations being registered by one's central nervous system at all times" (Wilbarger, 1984, p. 7). Children who have difficulty with sensory modulation may have excessive variations in responses to incoming sensory stimuli and experience difficulties in information processing (Kimball, 1993). More recently, an ecological view of sensory regulatory problems considers physical environment, cultural, task, and relationship contextual variables that influence a child's ability to regulate responses to sensation (Miller, Reisman, McIntosh, & Simon, 2001).

Royeen and Lane (1991) suggested that tactile defensiveness, gravitational insecurity, and aversive responses to vestibular stimuli are examples of sensory defensiveness, a disorder of sensory modulation that results from an imbalance of descending mechanisms for modulation of sensory stimuli. They suggested that the limbic system is the neurological correlate of sensory defensiveness. Excessive excitation of the reticular formation through the diffuse thalamic projection system is the neurological correlate for the syndrome of hyperactivity, distractibility, and tactile defensiveness. For unknown reasons, in some individuals, the arousal functions of the reticular activating system predominate and interfere with cortical association and recruitment responses needed for perceptual, attention, and cognitive processes. Sensory input is inadequately modulated, resulting in heightened responsiveness to sensation and difficulty in controlling behavioral responses and focusing attention.

Regulatory Disorder

Although SI theory has been applied primarily within occupational therapy, parallels of SI theory with initiatives outside the field are evident. One example is in the regulatory disorders described in the *Diagnostic Classification of Mental Health and Developmental Disorders of Infancy and Early Childhood* (Greenspan, 1994). This classification describes conceptualizations of mental health and developmental disorders in infancy and early childhood to provide a common language for clinical diagnosis and empirical study. Regulatory disorders are described as "difficulties in regulating behavior and physiological, sensory, attentional, motor or affective processes and in organizing a calm, alert or affectively positive state" (p. 31). These disorders include four types: hypersensitive; underreactive; motorically disorganized, impulsive; and other. Some of the descriptors of sensory regulation problems are not unlike those discussed in SI theory and can serve as reminders of the importance of precision in SI terminology. As interest in sensory and motor processing continues to grow, it becomes even more important to differentiate SI terminology from neurophysiology terminology (Lane, Miller, & Hanft, 2000) and to differentiate observable behaviors from inferred CNS processes (Hanft, Miller, & Lane, 2000) so as to have a common language for knowledge exchange and research within and outside of the field of OT.

Treatment

Principles

Ayres (1979) described sensory integration therapy as follows:

> The central idea of this therapy is to provide and control sensory input, especially the input from the vestibular system, muscles and joints, and skin in such a way that the child spontaneously forms the adaptive responses that integrate those sensations. Making this idea work with a dysfunctional child requires a skilled therapist and a large room with a lot of simple yet special equipment. When the therapist is doing her job effectively and the child is organizing his nervous system, it looks as if the child is merely playing. Life is full of paradoxes; this is one of them . . . We are not trying to teach the child the activity he is doing, or any other motor skill . . . We want him to become more capable of learning any motor skill, or academic ability, or type of good behavior he needs in his life. Motor activity is valuable in that it provides the sensory input that helps to organize the learning process. (p. 140)

Sensory integrative therapy focuses on control of selected sensory input that proceeds according to developmental sequences and requires an adaptive response. Sensory integration therapy is a movement-based therapy. Movement is used for its sensation-producing effect. Movement generates vestibular, tactile, and proprioceptive sensations that are integrated with visual and auditory sensations. Movement both imposes organization on sensation and is an indicator of the status of that organization (Ayres, 1979).

The therapist carefully selects therapeutic activities for the desired somatosensory, proprioceptive, vestibular sensation, and motor responses. Through activity analysis, the therapist identifies sensations needed for and generated by the activities. The reaction being facilitated or inhibited and the SI requirements for the motor response are carefully observed as the child interacts with the activity (Ayres, 1979).

Sensory integrative therapy incorporates normal developmental sequences. Activities emphasize postural responses and intersensory integration. Generally, the treatment sequence begins with improving SI in general through broad stimulation of vestibular and tactile systems. It proceeds with enhancement of the maturation of postural responses and the body's dynamic relationship with the earth's gravitational force. Treatment then emphasizes (a) development of the capacity to organize and sequence movement (motor planning) and (b) encouragement of interaction of the two body sides. These steps provide the basis for the development of form and space perception and related behavioral, perceptual, and cognitive functions that are important for learning (Ayres, 1975a).

Adaptive responses require organized interaction between the child and the environment and are a natural outcome of accurate and precise sensory input. Thus, adaptive responding is desirable for integrating sensations for motor behavior for effective interaction with the environment. Adaptive responses may be as simple as figuring out how to get one's body in a prone position on a scooter board or as complex as writing one's name. A procedure is considered therapeutic if it helps the child make increasingly mature responses to the therapy environment (Ayres, 1979).

The child's responses are used to guide the treatment. The therapist closely observes the child's spontaneous movements, postural responses, motor patterns, and skills for the desired adaptive behavior. Responses to a given activity or piece of equipment indicate how the child's nervous system interprets the stimuli. Activities that the child enjoys and seeks are generally considered indicative of those things that are integrating to the child's nervous system. Self-initiated activity in a selected environment is thought to be more integrative than imposed activities or tasks. Such an approach offers pleasurable, playful experiences that tap into the child's innate drive toward sensory integration. This invitational approach to therapy is referred to as the "art" of therapy (Ayres, 1979).

The sensory and motor experiences involved in SI therapy have the potential to result in over- or underarousal states. Therapists should observe the child for signs of nausea, hyperexcitability, sleepiness or sleeplessness, undesirable increases or decreases in muscle tone, and defensive responses. Adherence to safety factors, such as well-padded floors, durable suspension supports, and equipment maintenance procedures, is important in ensuring a safe therapy environment (Ayres, 1975a, 1979).

Sensory integration therapy is most effective when used in conjunction with services that address other needs of the child and when the child's family is involved (Koomar & Bundy, 1991; Murray & Anzalone, 1991; Parham & Mailloux, 2001). The ultimate aim of SI therapy is to enable the child to function well in his or her occupational roles.

Equipment

Sensory integrative equipment is essential to providing SI therapy. This equipment enables movement in a variety of planes and requires innumerable combinations of muscular, balance, and coordination responses. Equipment developed in the Ayres Clinic includes the suspended hammock, scooter board ramp, platform swing, carpeted barrel, quadruped balancing board, inner-tube barrel, suspended "helicopter" apparatus, and vibrating table. Scooter boards, large therapy balls, suspended bolsters, and T-stools developed in other sensory motor therapies are used in SI therapy as well (Ayres, 1979).

Therapy Emphasis in Various Forms of SI Dysfunction

Therapy for developmental dyspraxia addresses problems with ideation or concept of the activity, planning a course of action, and executing the plan. For the child with ideational problems, the therapist selects the simplest activity that the child can perform using his or her whole body in relation to the therapeutic equipment. For severe ideational problems, the therapist helps the child through the activity manually, verbally, and through modeling. Because the typical therapy equipment may be too complicated for the child with these conceptual problems, the therapist may need to create simplified activities.

For the child with problems in planning and executing movements, the therapist selects activities that elicit strong motor responses to provide massive sensory flow from somatosensory and proprioceptive systems. These activities, which emphasize total flexion, extension, rotary, and diagonal movements, provide the postural basis for planning and executing movements. Planning and executing movements proceed from simple praxis activities, such as moving effectively from one place to another, to more complex praxis activities involving sequences of movement (Ayres, 1985). Koomar and Bundy (1991) suggested a progression of activities from isolated to combined movements, from movements of the whole body to movements that activate one part of the body and inhibit others, and from feedback-dependent to feedforward-dependent actions. Feedback-dependent activities are those that require the individual to depend upon feedback arising from movement as it occurs; feedforward-dependent activities require the individual to anticipate the sequence of movements that will be needed to perform the activity. The more complex the activity, the greater the demands for adequate processing of sensory information for feedback and feedforward to plan and execute activities in time and space.

Therapy for vestibular-based dysfunction emphasizes motion, rotation, and starting and stopping actions to activate the vestibular system. Extension postures and alternating flexion and extension for cocontraction and bilateral activities are incorporated into the treatment. Righting and equilibrium responses are facilitated in prone, supine, and upright positions. The rate of vestibular stimulation is varied to produce desired calming or excitatory effects. Because of the autonomic reactions associated with vestibular stimulation, the therapist must observe for signs of autonomic distress such as sweating, pallor, respiratory changes, flushing, nausea, seizures, or dizziness.

Problems with the modulation of sensory input (overresponsiveness, underresponsiveness, fluctuating responsiveness, or delayed responsivity) manifest as tactile defensiveness, gravitational insecurity, aversive response to vestibular stimulation, and diminished sensory registration. These conditions require the therapist to calibrate sensory input carefully and to monitor the child's responses (Koomar & Bundy, 1991).

Application to Occupational Therapy

Scope

According to Meleis (1985, p. 158), "The final test of any theory is whether or not it is adopted by others." A theory's "circle of contagiousness" indicates where the theory is used geographically; how the theory has been used for research, education, administration, and clinical practice; and whether the theory has been used cross-culturally (Meleis, 1985).

The literature on SI published by persons other than Ayres provides a means to assess the circle of contagiousness of SI theory. This theory has been applied in research and clinical practice and has influenced education in occupational therapy. SI theory is the most widely researched model for practice in OT. Through the organization Sensory Integration International (SII) and the collaboration between the University of Southern California and Western Psychological Services, courses are taught throughout the United States and in Canada, Ireland, Israel, Japan, South Africa, and other countries. A review of the literature spawned by SI theory, research, and practice is beyond the scope of this chapter. The reader is referred to other sources (Fisher, Murray, & Bundy, 1991; Kimball, 1993; Parham & Mailloux, 2001; Roley, Schaaf, & Blanche, 2001) for more specifics on clinical practice of SI theory and other reviews based on neuroscience literature.

Assessment

One of Ayres's major contributions to OT was in the area of measurement and test development. Ayres was the first occupational therapist to develop a comprehensive battery of standardized assessments, including the Southern California Motor Accuracy Test (1964b, 1980a), SCSIT (1972e, 1980b), Southern California Postrotary Nystagmus Test (1975b), and SIPT (1989). She introduced occupational therapists to standardized test administration, moving OT assessment beyond checklists, scales, and clinical observations. The development of valid and reliable measurement instruments to assess psychoneurological behaviors, especially in children, is difficult and calls for strict adherence to standards for test administration to maximize accurate and consistent use of the tests. Ayres taught occupational therapists to develop efficient psychomotor skills for handling test materials, to use consistent verbal instructions, and to develop the objectivity of the tester role. She insisted that test administration to an individual child replicate, as closely as possible, test administration used in the standardization process.

Ayres trained therapists in test administration in the Ayres Clinic and, through SII, developed a three-course test administration certification process for the nation. In the 1970s, SII convened interested and qualified therapists to become the faculty for teaching the theory-test, administration-test interpretation course series to occupational therapists and physical therapists in the United States and other countries. Participants who successfully completed the course requirements were certified to administer and interpret SI tests. In the mid-1990s, Western Psychological Services, the publisher of Ayres's tests, and the University of Southern California Department of Occupational Therapy also developed a three-course series.

Ayres's dream that this educational process become part of OT graduate education has not been realized in elective graduate courses at USC. However, specialty education in SI remains, mostly in the area of continuing education. Nevertheless, Ayres's work in assessment has provided OT with a model for the process of test development, the comprehensive assessment of selected sensory and motor functions, the integration of test development and theoretical constructs, and strict standardized test administration.

Appendix 5.A presents validity and reliability studies of the SIPT in the last decade. Some of the validity studies have implications for SI construct development (Mulligan, 2000), particularly for praxis (Lai, Fisher, Magalhaes, & Bundy, 1996; Parham, 1998). Other studies addressed discriminate validity of the SIPT for separate groups with and without SI dysfunction (Cermak, Morris, & Koomar, 1990; Cermak & Murray, 1991; Fanchiang, Snyder, Zobel-Lachiusa, Loeffler, & Thompson, 1990; Mulligan, 1996; Wincent & Engel, 1995) and concurrent validity of the SIPT to predict scores on related tests (Haack, Short-DeGraff, & Hanzlik, 1993; High, Gough, Pennington, & Wright 2000; Walker & Burris, 1991). An exhaustive review of test instruments other than the SIPT that are related to sensory integration is beyond the scope of this chapter; however, reviews of tests other than the SIPT that are related to SI are also found in other references provided for this chapter (e.g., Carrasco, 1993).

Therapy

Therapy for SI disorders was central to Ayres's work, and she educated therapists in the Ayres Clinic and through continuing education in the principles and procedures of SI therapy. Sensory integration therapy was a departure from other developmental approaches used in OT in that it focused on children with learning disorders, required the use of special equipment, and emphasized gross movement. In contrast developmental approaches were provided on the mat or at the table and emphasized fine motor activities and skill development.

Reimbursement for OT in pediatrics, including for SI testing and therapy, has been problematic. Key issues include the use of appropriate diagnostic and treatment procedure terminology (Stallings-Sahler, Anzalone, Bryze, Carrasco, & Pettit, 1993) and explanations of sensory integration (Stallings-Sahler, 1993a). The sensory integration code in the 1995 Current Procedural Terminology (CPT) supports reimbursement for SI therapy (Thomas, 1995), and serves as a major impetus for funding for SI.

Sensory integration therapy has been applied in various populations, such as cocaine-exposed infants (Stallings-Sahler, 1993b) and adults with profound mental retardation who engage in self-injurious behavior (Reisman, 1993). Sensory integration problems have been suggested in a variety of clinical populations (Cermak, 1994), and the appropriateness of SI therapy for certain client problems has been questioned (Nommensen & Maas, 1993). An exhaustive review of literature related to the application of SI in occupational therapy is beyond the scope of this chapter; however, Appendix 5.B provides a review of studies addressing the efficacy of SI from 1990 to 2000. In addition, meta-analyses and other reviews of SI efficacy are discussed in the next section of this chapter regarding the validation of SI theory.

Theory Validation and Research

Theory

Sensory integration is one of the more controversial therapies for learning disabilities. Sieben (1977) criticized this approach, citing as faulty its assumption that children with learning disabilities have something wrong with their brain stems. He also criticized the assumptions that controlled stimulation of vestibular and somatosensory systems improves brain stem integration for vision and hearing, and that mastery of postural skills can carry over to academic skills. In contrast, Lerer (1981) stated that the SI concepts are accurate and are based on 100 years of biomedical research efforts. He argued that SI theory concerning implication of the brain stem in sensory motor dysfunction is "probably valid" and that medical and other professionals recognize similar symptomatology in which the brain stem may be important.

Ottenbacher and Short (1985) identified literature supporting the assumption that subcortical brain areas contribute to complex processes of learning and cognition. They also noted that the "active management of children in meaningful, challenging activities that provide a vast array of multisensory and motor stimulation and feedback" (p. 304), which characterizes SI therapy, is well documented in the literature.

Ayres's attempts to link bilateral integration (as well as hemispheric communication and hemispheric lateralization) to vestibular functioning have remained speculative because the role of the vestibular system has not been clearly established. Fisher (1991) made several important points regarding this issue.

First, Ayres (1975b) used the Postrotary Nystagmus Test as an indicator of central vestibular processing—that is, brain stem CNS processing of vestibular information—and assumed intact peripheral structures and functions. Whether the duration of postrotary nystagmus reflects central or peripheral vestibular functioning remains controversial, and doubts on this matter have been used to discredit vestibular-related SI dysfunction. In defense of SI theory, Fisher (1991) urged readers

> to differentiate between those studies in which indicators of *peripheral* vestibular function are measured (peak slow-phase eye velocity during vestibular nystagmus) and those studies in which indicators of *central* vestibular processing are measured (circularvection, time course of vestibular nystagmus, duration of optokinetic afternystagmus, and postural control under conditions of sensory conflict). (p. 84)

Second, the PRN assesses one aspect of vestibular functioning: compensatory eye movements in relation to position and movements of the head. Other ocular and postural responses are tested through clinical observations that do not differentiate roles of the vestibular and proprioceptive systems. Ocular pursuits, tested as part of the postural-ocular deficits, are mediated by the visual system, not the vestibular system.

Third, although Ayres differentiated the roles of proprioceptive, tactile, and vestibular input in her views of praxis or bilateral integration (see Ayres, 1972d, p. 171), she often referred only to discriminative tactile functions and their role in praxis (Cermak, 1991; Fisher, 1991). This lack of clarity was due, in part, to the lack of tests of proprioception and the difficulty with separating proprioception from vestibular and tactile functions. (Also, generally, the term *proprioception* includes vestibular as well as muscle, joint, tendon, and deep pressure receptors.) The postural abilities that occupational therapists assess through clinical observations call for combined proprioceptive, vestibular, and tactile processing.

Fisher (1991) and Cermak (1991) refined Ayres's views on the relative contribution of tactile, proprioception, and vestibular systems. They hypothesized that dyspraxia is a dysfunction of somatosensory processing and that the bilateral integration and sequencing deficit is a dysfunction of vestibular and proprioceptive processing. Furthermore, bilateral integration dysfunction may be a form of dyspraxia that involves the proprioceptive and vestibular systems and is characterized by impaired bilateral, anticipatory responding in sequences of actions. Dyspraxia may be seen alone or in combination with bilateral integration and sequencing dysfunction.

Finally, Ayres's hypothesized brain stem interhemispheral mechanism has not been supported by neurological correlates. However, the importance of proprioceptive, vestibular, and tactile input to motor cortexes for body scheme, motor control, motor planning, anticipatory responding, attention, orientation, and sequencing has been demonstrated (Cermak, 1991; Fisher, 1991). In my opinion, continuing to view a brainstem–cortical hierarchy is no longer as useful as conceptualizing these structures as aspects of one interactive neural system.

Testing

The SCSIT (Ayres, 1972e, 1980b) were criticized for incomplete standardization information, sample size variations ranging from 13 to 70 subjects on the subtests, and a small sample size of fewer than 100 in each age group. Other concerns included reliability and validity. The SIPT (Ayres, 1989) were developed to replace the SCSIT with a psychometrically sound instrument.

Reliability of the 17 SIPT subtests was generally good. Interrater reliability coefficients ranged from .94 to .99 (Ayres, 1988). Test–retest reliability coefficients were .60 or better on all subtests except postrotary nystagmus (.48), kinesthesia (.50), localization of tactile stimuli (.53), and figure–ground perception (.56), and the median for all tests was .74. These reliability coefficients are a considerable improvement over those for the 17 SCSIT subtests. On the revised SCSIT, test–retest coefficients ranged from .01 to .94, with a median of .53 (Ayres, 1980b), and were below .70 on 73% of the subtests (Evan & Peham, 1981).

Ayres and Marr (1991) reported the results of construct and criterion-related validity studies for the SIPT. Construct validity was investigated through factor and cluster analyses. Factor analyses were conducted with a normative sample (n = 1,750), dysfunctional children (n = 125), and a combined group of dysfunctional children (n = 117) matched to children in the normative sample (n = 176). A cluster analysis was conducted on the latter combined group. The results of these studies further clarified theoretical constructs identified in Ayres's earlier factor analytic studies. Two types of criterion-related validity studies were conducted. First, in the absence of comparable sensory integration tests, SIPT profiles were compared across other diagnostic groups that had prior diagnosis and would be expected to conform to patterns that were in keeping with the diagnosis. Second, SIPT scores were compared to scores on the Kaufman Assessment Battery for Children; the Luria-Nebraska Neuropsychological Battery, Children's Revision; the Bruininks-Oseretsky Test of Motor Proficiency; and the Bender-Gestalt Test.

The validity studies of the SIPT were considerably more comprehensive than were the validity investigations of the SCSIT. The original versions of the SCSIT subtests provided some validity data (Ayres, 1962, 1964b, 1966d, 1966e) and included the ability of the test to discriminate between normal and dysfunctional groups and to correlate with similar published tests. Manuals for the later versions of the SCSIT did not include validity information (Ayres, 1972e, 1980b).

Research Methods

Factor analysis is a research method that can identify both theoretical constructs in a developing theory and the operational characteristics of those constructs. Thus, it can be used to examine both the construct validation of test instruments and the underlying theory (Gorsuch, 1983). Ayres's factor analytic studies established the construct validity of her testing instruments and the theorized syndromes of dysfunction. However, Ayres's earlier studies have been criticized for methodological inadequacies (Clark, Mailloux, & Parham, 1985). A closer look at Ayres's studies in terms of factor analytic criteria reveals some flaws.

Gorsuch (1983) recommended that factor analytic studies meet the following six conditions for generalizability of factor analysis:

1. The number of subjects should not be less than 100, and the absolute minimum ratio is five individuals to one variable.

2. Split sample analysis should be used, keeping those factors that match across the two samples; a large sample is also necessary.

3. Variables should have a history of good reliability estimates and good correlation with other variables in the analysis.

4. Factors should be highly significant based on the tests for this criterion, although significance tests in factor analysis are poor.

5. A minimum of five to six variable loadings should be used for each factor.

6. Data should be factored by several different analytical procedures, keeping only those factors that appear across the procedures used.

Most of Ayres's factor analytic studies meet Gorsuch's first criterion in that they have 100 or more dysfunctional subjects (Ayres, 1965, 1971, 1972f, 1977a; Ayres et al., 1987; Ayres & Marr, 1991), although one study of dysfunctional children (Ayres, 1969) and two of normal children (Ayres, 1966b, 1966c) do not meet this criterion. Ayres's 1965 study, which has 25 children in each of 4 groups, does not meet the criterion of a large split sample. The good reliability of the SIPT (Ayres & Marr, 1991) meets Criterion 3, but the poor reliability of the earlier SCSIT compromises Criterion 3 (Ayres, 1980b). Significances of factors of .01 and .05 are reported (Ayres, 1965, 1966b, 1966c, 1971, 1972f; Ayres et al., 1987); thus, Criterion 4 is met to some extent, assuming that .01 is considered highly significant. Ayres identified factors with six or more variables, thus meeting Criterion 5. Finally, Ayres uses Q- and R-technique factor analyses to identify factors. She retained those factors that consistently reappear: developmental dyspraxia, deficit in form and space, dysfunction in bilateral integration, and tactile defensiveness. Thus, Criterion 6 is met if applied to several studies together and not to individual studies.

Various arthors have criticized Ayres's factor analysis studies. Cummins (1991) criticized her factor analytic studies for their lack of cross-validation. His reappraisal of data in eight studies by Ayres from the period 1986 to 1987 failed to support the factors identified by Ayres. In a construct validity study, Lai et al. (1996) identified dyspraxia as a unidimensional construct, with bilateral integration and sequencing and somatopraxis as part of the dyspraxia. This finding was in contrast to the lack of support for dyspraxia as a unitary function in an earlier study by Ayres et al. (1987). More recently, Mulligan's (1998) confirmatory factor analysis of the patterns of dysfunction in 10,475 records of SIPT scores resulted in a four-factor model (visual perceptual deficit, bilateral integration and sequencing deficit, dyspraxia, and somatosensory deficit), with a generalized praxis dysfunction. In addition to a modified model of SI dysfunction, Mulligan recommended the shortening of the SIPT to eliminate subtests that did not contribute to the analysis (postrotary nystagmus; kinesthesia; standing and walking balance; motor accuracy; and figure ground perception). She also advised that therapists use caution when diagnosing types of SI dysfunction, and suggested that they design intervention that is holistic versus focusing on a type of dysfunction.

Therapy Efficacy

Therapy efficacy studies have focused on the question, Is SI therapy effective? (see Appendix 5.B for a review of studies from

1990 to 2000). Treatment effects have been observed in motor proficiency in children with motor problems (Allen & McDonald, 1995), engagement in preschool children with autism (Case-Smith & Bryan, 1999), emotional and behavior problems in infants with regulatory disorders (DeGangi, Sickel, Wiener, & Kaplan, 1996), sensorimotor functions in children with learning disabilities (LD) (Humphries, Wright, McDougall, & Vertes, 1990), gross motor functions in children with LD at 3-year follow-up (Wilson & Kaplan, 1994), sensory defensiveness in adults (O'Hara, 1998), feeding independence in the elderly (Hames-Hahn & Llorens, 1989), and time in restraint and the amount of self-injurious behavior in an adult with profound retardation (Reisman, 1993). In contrast, small or no effects were found on visual–motor integration at 12-month follow-up (Davidson & Williams, 2000); motor and SI problems (DeGangi et al., 1996); cognitive, language and academic performance in children with LD (Humphries et al., 1990); and memory and behavior problems and activities of daily living skills in adults with dementia (Robichaud, Hebert, & Desrosiers, 1994). Comparable treatment effects were found in studies of SI versus perceptual motor treatment on SI functions (Humphries, Snider, & McDougall, 1993) and on academic and motor measures (Polatajko, Law, Miller, Shaffer, & Macnab, 1991) in children with LD and SI dysfunction; of SI versus sensory stimulation on performance checklists in adults with severe LD (Soper & Thorley, 1996); and of SI versus tutoring on academic functioning in children with LD (Wilson, Kaplan, Fellowes, Gruchy, & Faris, 1992). Parents, teachers, and therapists perceived SI as extremely or somewhat effective in helping children with LD improve in skill areas (Stonefelt & Stein, 1998), and therapists' use and competency may affect their perception of the child's improvements (Case-Smith & Miller, 1999). Finally, SIPT-grouped data showed prostreatment gains in 6- to 8-year-old boys (Kimball, 1990)

SI efficacy research has been criticized as being poorly controlled, having too few subjects, not accounting for the Hawthorne effect, and being interpretive and anecdotal (Arendt, MacLean, & Baumeister, 1988; Bochner, 1978; Committee on Children with Disabilities, 1985; Densem, Nutall, Bushnell, & Horn, 1989; Lerer, 1981; Posthuma, 1983; Schaffer, 1984). Schaffer (1984) identified a likelihood of Type I and Type II errors in an analysis of five SI therapy efficacy studies. Polatajko,

Kaplan, and Wilson (1992) applied post hoc power analyses to variables in six studies to examine the treatment effect size and sample size needed for sufficient statistical power to avoid a Type II error. They concluded that SI therapy generally was found to have a minimal treatment effect, pointing to the possibility of a Type II error that may be due to a small sample size. They discussed the practicality of large-sample, randomized trials in SI therapy, as well as the feasibility of these studies when SI therapy seems to yield minimal clinical effects.

Meta-analyses of SI efficacy studies have yielded conflicting results. Ottenbacher (1982) reported a meta-analysis of eight studies, including three by Ayres, and concluded that the performance of subjects who received SI therapy was significantly better than that of subjects in the control groups. Eight of the 49 studies identified met the operational definition of SI therapy for inclusion in the analysis. Although Ayres's (1972b, 1978) effectiveness studies had emphasized improved academic functioning, Ottenbacher found that the dependent variables most affected by SI therapy were motor or reflex variables. In contrast, Kavale and Mattson (1983) conducted a meta-analysis of 180 studies, including one by Ayres (1972b) to assess the efficacy of perceptual–motor training for improving academic, cognitive, or perceptual–motor scores. The criterion for inclusion of a study in the analysis was the presence of a control group. The authors concluded that "perceptual motor training is not effective and should be questioned as a feasible intervention technique for exceptional children" (p. 165). They were surprised that not even perceptual-motor measures showed improvement. Similarly, Myers and Hammill's (1982) actuarial analysis of 35 studies conducted by Kephart, Barsch, Cratty, Getman, and Ayres found that results of these studies failed to support the perceptual-motor approaches. In contrast to studies that included SI therapy as a perceptual-motor treatment, Vargas and Camilli (1999) conducted a meta-analysis of 32 studies done from 1972 to 1995 in which the therapy was designed to "enhance development of basic SI processes with activities that provide vestibular, proprioceptive, tactile or other somatosensory inputs as modalities to elicit" (p. 191) active participation of the child. They found that in the 16 SI versus no-treatment studies, treatment effect sizes were significantly larger for earlier studies and larger effect sizes were found in the psychoeducational and motor variables.

In the 16 SI versus alternative treatment studies, SI therapy was just as effective as other forms of therapy. In an analysis of seven studies, few appreciable effects of SI therapy for children with LD were found in terms of postrotary nystagmus, sensori-motor, academic, and self-esteem measures (Hoehn & Baumeister, 1994).

In a careful review of the seven randomized clinical trials of SI treatment for children with learning disabilities that have been published since Ayres's study in 1972b, Polatajko et al. (1992) concluded that SI was no better than a placebo as an effective treatment for academic problems and that, insofar as sensory or motor variables were concerned, SI treatment is similar to perceptual-motor training. They also pointed out obstacles in SI therapy efficiency studies such as the "purity" of the compared treatments, the significance of individual gains from therapy that are not seen in group studies, and measurement, noting, "It may be that clinicians and researchers are trying to detect change with a yardstick while change is occurring in inches" (p. 338).

Several factors contribute to the conflicting and controversial results of SI efficacy research (Walker, 1991). First, SI therapy is difficult to administer in a precise, homogeneous fashion due to natural variability in individualized therapy, unique functional levels and responsiveness of the individual child, and expertise of the therapist.

Second, although the characteristics of SI therapy have been well delineated by Ayres and others, the actual type of therapy being rendered has often been ill defined or not defined in studies claiming to use SI therapy. Therapy claimed by authors to be SI therapy—such as balance beam work (Densem et al., 1989); passive vestibular stimulation to reduce self-injurious behaviors against the skin (Dura, Mulick, & Hammer, 1988); and flashing lights, rocking, vibration, and auditory stimulation to reduce self-injurious behaviors (Mason & Iwata, 1990)—violates these principles of SI therapy: individualized assessment, sensory–motor activities tailored to address underlying dysfunction, and adaptive responding. Furthermore, the specialized space, equipment, and training required for SI therapy in some cases has been overmodified to the extent that it no longer approximates SI therapy as Ayres designed it. In addition to the "mislabeling" of therapy as SI, there is a risk to the child-centered flow of treatment when the study dictates adherence to a standard treatment (Parham & Mailloux, 2001).

Third, SI therapy has been confused with other approaches such as neurodevelopmental intervention (Arendt et al., 1988), neurophysiological retraining regimens (Sieben, 1977), perceptual-motor training (Kavale & Mattson, 1983; Myers & Hammill, 1982), and sensory stimulation (Mason & Iwata, 1990). This point was made clear when AOTA President Robert Bing (personal communication, December 20, 1985) and a Sensory Integration International committee (personal communication, December 20, 1985) responded to a recommendation by the Committee on Children with Disabilities (1985) that pediatricians recommend OT for severe motor problems but not for the child who is dyspraxic or clumsy because these problems improve with age and the therapy programs have not been the subject of scientific research. Bing and the SII committee not only cited research that showed long-term effects of dyspraxia, but also differentiated SI therapy from passive patterning therapies and cited research to support its superior effectiveness.

Fourth, in contrast to assessing the efficacy of therapy over a course of time as measured by selected outcomes, studies that address what goes on within SI therapy sessions (Tickle-Degnan, 1988) focus on the therapy process and immediate effects during therapy. For example, a coding system for quantifying therapist-child interactions during SI therapy (Coster, Tickle-Degnan, & Armenta, 1995) has been used to describe symbolic play (Cross & Coster, 1997) and therapist management of the "just right challenge" in therapy (Tickle-Degnan & Coster, 1995; Dunkerley, Tickle-Degnan, & Coster, 1997).

Finally, Ayres's clinical research may have had empirical merit during the evolution of a body of SI research and theory (Cermak & Henderson, 1990). In response to critiques of SI research methodology (Lerer, 1981), AOTA President May Hightower-Van Damm said, "In many instances in medicine, psychology, and education, carefully documented behavioral changes are the most important data we have to evaluate a given approach to a presenting problem, i.e., drug therapies, psychotherapy, behavior modification and self-contained classroom instruction" (Personal communication, March 12, 1981). Using critical reviews of evidence-based practice, occupational therapists can continue to assess the clinical impact of SI therapy. Challenges to the study of SI must be addressed in order for collective research efforts to yield a consensual body of findings (Miller & Kinnealey, 1993).

Occupational therapists have been criticized for their overzealousness in promoting SI therapy for children and for overextension of research findings to other patient populations. Lerer (1981) suggested that SI therapy not be used outside the experimental research situation, and he criticized therapists for subjecting families, taxpayers, and third-party payers to the expense of this experimental therapy. He remarked that "Ayres, in her carefully conducted inquiries, is cautious about drawing definite conclusions from her theories, concepts and hypotheses" (p. 4). Posthuma (1983) questioned the widespread use of SI therapy by occupational therapists in adult psychiatry and cited cost ineffectiveness, a lack of standardized tests for adults, and confusion over SI versus other movement therapies as areas that needed to be addressed. She urged the development of research and specialty training to enable SI therapy to be appropriately applied to adults. In a review of SI studies, Ottenbacher (1982) found no studies in psychiatry, geriatrics, or physical disabilities that met empirical standards of traditional behavioral science research. He cautioned therapists not to apply SI therapy prematurely to populations for which the therapeutic effects have not been established. Similarly, Arendt et al. (1988) concluded that SI therapy for persons with mental retardation has not been empirically or theoretically supported and should only be used for research purposes with this population.

Summary of Critiques

In summary, the theoretical assumptions of SI theory have a basis in the neurosciences. However, highly selective interpretations of the neuroscience literature that support SI theory are subject to criticism. Frequent updating of neuroscience conceptual bases is a requisite for future SI theory development.

Psychometric inadequacies of the SCSIT (Ayres, 1972e) have been addressed in the SIPT (Ayres, 1989). The primary purpose of this standardization project was to develop a valid and reliable instrument for evaluation of SI dysfunction in children with LD. There continues to be a need to develop instruments for identifying SI dysfunction in other patient populations.

Research has shown SI dysfunction in some children with LD. There is some evidence that SI therapy enhances academic learning. Other gains include improvements in motor performance. Further well-designed research needs to be conducted to delineate the types of patient problems most benefited by SI therapy and to assess long-term effects of therapy. Variables of the therapy process itself need to be described as a basis for the study of within-session effectiveness.

Ayres's work has had a large impact on the OT field. Although developed for a specific patient group (i.e., children with learning problems), the theory is one of the most complete of existing OT theories. Its scope includes clinical problem identification, the formulation of theoretical constructs, theory validation research, test instrument development, therapy approaches and equipment, and therapy efficacy studies. SI theory has spawned more research, publications, and educational efforts in OT than any other OT theory to date, except possibly Kielhofner's (2002) model of human occupation. It has helped therapists to view patient problems in the context of sensory functioning and has provided another way of perceiving health and dysfunction.

Appendix 5.A Sensory Integration and Praxis Tests (SIPT) Validity and Reliability Studies from 1990 to 2000

Study	Participants	Dependent Variable	Independent Variable	Findings
Cermak & Murray (1991)	39 children ages 5 to 8 years	Constructional abilities as measured by the Design Copying and Constructional Praxis subtests of the SIPT compared to abilities measured by the Developmental Test of Visual–Motor Integration Block Design subtest of the Wechsler Intelligence Scale for Children—Revised, Primary Visual Motor Test, and Rey-Osterrieth Complex Figure Test.	Experimental group (EG): 21 children with learning disabilities; control group (CG): 18 children with no learning disabilities	Children in EG performed significantly more poorly than children in CG on both the Design Copying and the Constructional Praxis subtests. These two subtests showed moderately high correlations (.46 to .71) with the other tests of constructional abilities when both groups were combined. Correlations were mostly moderate for the EG alone but were generally not significant for the CG. The validity of the subtests was supported with the use of the contrast groups, as the EG performed significantly more poorly than the CG.

(continues)

Appendix 5.A Validity and Reliability *Continued.*

Study	Participants	Dependent Variable	Independent Variable	Findings
Cermak, Morris, & Koomar (1990)	45 children: 23 four-year-olds (mean age 55.6 months) and 22 six-year-olds (mean age 78.1 months)	Performance on the Praxis on Verbal Command subtest of the SIPT	The SIPT was administered under two conditions: (a) standard administration on verbal command and (b) administration of the same items on imitation.	There was a significant difference on the scores under the two different conditions and across the two age groups. A significant difference was found between the verbal command and initiation scores of the four-year-olds, with performance on the verbal command condition significantly less accurate. This was not the case for the six-year-olds, however, possibly due to a ceiling effect. The authors believe that, due to the inclusion of the Praxis on Verbal Command subtest, the SIPT will be a more discriminating tool in assessing praxis deficits in children.

(*continues*)

Study	Participants	Dependent Variable	Independent Variable	Findings
Fanchiang, Snyder, Zobel-Lachiusa, Loeffler, & Thompson (1990)	114 nondelinquent-prone adolescents ages 12 to 18 years and 12 delinquent-prone adolescents with learning problems	Performance on 10 of the 17 subtests of the SIPT, the Finger Posture Imitation Test, and the MacQuarrie Test for Mechanical Ability	Nondelinquent-prone versus delinquent-prone groups and age groups	There was a significant difference in the performance of the two groups, with the delinquent-prone group performing more poorly on the vestibular and praxis-related tests. Results also indicated an age correlation on the performance of the praxis tests, and on the Manual Form Perception, Graphesthesia, and Bilateral Motor Coordination subtests. The MacQuarrie Test was the best discriminator between the two groups and, therefore, could be used to screen for the detection of possible practice difficulty in adolescents ages 12 to 18 years.

(continues)

Appendix 5.A **Validity and Reliability** *Continued.*

Study	Participants	Dependent Variable	Independent Variable	Findings
Haack, Short-De-Graff, & Hanzlik (1993)	29 girls and 41 boys ages 3 years 2 months (3-2) to 5 years 11 months (5-11) who have not attended kindergarten	Ocular motor skills: visual pursuits and fixation	Postrotary nystagmus and clinical observations of vestibular functions	Significant positive correlation between ocular motor skills and vestibular-related clinical observations, indicating validity of the PRN as a measure of vestibular system integrity.
High, Gough, Pennington, & Wright (2000)	14 boys ages 5 to 11 years	Performance on the Movement Assessment Battery for Children (MAB)	Performance on Ayres's (1980) SCSIT	Both protocols provide similar diagnostic information except for the motor domain; the MAB does not provide information on motor planning and bilateral sequencing ability equivalent to that provided by the SCSIT.

(continues)

Study	Participants	Dependent Variable	Independent Variable	Findings
Kinnealey & Wilbarger (1993)	27 children (13 boys and 14 girls) ages 4-6 to 10-0 years who had been born at high risk and hospitalized in a neonatal intensive care unit in California (a subgroup of those used to determine the reliability of the SIPT reported in the 1989 manual)	Test–retest reliability of the SIPT	The SIPT as a whole and broken down into its 17 subtests comprising 4 domains: given by the same examiner once and again 2 weeks later to each subject	The test–retest reliability of the SIPT battery as a whole is excellent (.93); the test–retest reliability of the four domains of the SIPT ranges from .75 to .90, with praxis and bilateral integration and form and space being most reliable, with perception being least reliable. Test–retest reliability of individual scores ranged from .32 to .89. From this study, the test–retest reliability information reported in the SIPT manual should be interpreted in light of the fact that 80% of the children in the sample were not normal.

(continues)

Appendix 5.A Validity and Reliability *Continued.*

Study	Participants	Dependent Variable	Independent Variable	Findings
Lai, Fisher, Magalhaes, & Bundy (1996)	210 subjects	Rasch analysis results of SIPT raw scores	The five SIPT praxis subtests	Each of the five praxis subtests measures a single, unidimensional construct; all items together define a single practic function, indicating that a single component underlies (a) bilateral integration and sequencing deficits and (b) somatodyspraxia. An examination of the heirarchy of item difficulties resulted in recommendations for the development of a single screening test for developmental dyspraxia.
Mulligan (1996)	309 children with attention-deficit/hyperactivity disorder (ADHD) and 309 children without ADHD	Performance and score patterns on the SIPT	Experimental group (EG): children with ADHD; control group (CG): children without ADHD	Children in EG demonstrated relative strengths in nonmotor visual perception and localization of tactile input, as well as weaknesses in vestibular processing and in most areas of praxis and motor planning. Certain SIPT scores of children in EG differed significantly from those of children in CG. The test that best discriminated the two groups was space visualization.

(continues)

Study	Participants	Dependent Variable	Independent Variable	Findings
Mulligan (2000)	1,961 children ages 4 years to 8-11	Cluster analysis results of the SIPT	Three-, four-, five-, and six-cluster solutions were examined for best fit and theoretical rationale	The results of this study support the use of a five-cluster solution rather than the six-cluster solution currently used in the interpretation of the SIPT. These results should be cautiously applied only to children with known or suspected SI deficits because only children with suspected SI dysfunction were included in the sample. Also, the profile groups (clusters) are most useful for identifying the degree of dysfunction rather than the type or quality of dysfunction.

(continues)

Appendix 5.A Validity and Reliability *Continued.*

Study	Participants	Dependent Variable	Independent Variable	Findings
Parham (1998)	67 children ages 6 to 8 and followed up 4 years later	SI factors, reading, and arithmetic abilities measured on the SIPT and the Kaufman Assessment Battery for Children (K-ABC)	32 school-identified children with learning handicaps and 35 children without learning handicaps, were administered the SIPT and the K-ABC at ages 6 to 8 and again at follow-up	SI factors were strongly related to arithmetic achievement at early ages, but the strength of the relationship declined with time. The reverse pattern was found for reading. A strong relationship was also found between praxis and arithmetic achievement.
Walker & Burris (1991)	30 normal children with no identified learning, behavioral, or developmental problems; ages 6-5 to 9-9 (mean age of 8 years)	Performance on the SIPT	Performance on the Metropolitan Achievement Test (Prescott, Balow, Hogan, & Farr, 1978)	The correlations of the test scores did not indicate a predictive relationship between scores on achievement tests and on tests of SI. Results support the use of SI tests as discrete indicators of sensory and motor functions.

(continues)

Study	Participants	Dependent Variable	Independent Variable	Findings
Wincent & Engel (1995)	Children with migraine headaches	Vestibular–proprioceptive abilities measured on the SIPT	Migraine headache or mixed headache	Most subjects showed significantly high Postrotary Nystagmus subtest scores and strengths in the areas of sensory processing and praxis. SIPT may be helpful in determining cortical versus brain stem processing dysfunction in children with migraine headaches.

Appendix 5.B Sensory Integration (SI) Therapy Efficacy Studies from 1990 to 2000

Study	Participants	Dependent Variable	Independent Variable	Findings
Allen & McDonald (1995)	Five children with motor/learning problems ages 5 to 11 years (mean age of 7 years)	Bruininks-Oseretsky Test of Motor Proficiency pre- and posttest	10 sessions SI therapy	Four children improved in motor proficiency and one deteriorated.
Case-Smith & Bryan (1999)	Five preschoolers with autism	Nonengagement, mastery play, and interaction measured using videotape clips of each child's free play; this followed a 3-week baseline during which no occupational therapy (OT) services were provided	10 weeks of one-on-one daily SI-based treatment sessions by a therapist and consultations with teachers	Four children demonstrated a decreased frequency of nonengaged behavior and three demonstrated an increased frequency of mastery play. Improvements in the frequency of interaction were minimal.

(continues)

Study	Participants	Dependent Variable	Independent Variable	Findings
Davidson & Williams (2000)	37 children with developmental coordination disorder	Performance on the Movement ABC and the Beery-Buktenica Developmental Test of Visual–Motor Integration	10 weeks of combined SI and perceptual–motor training intervention; pretest and posttest (12 month follow-up)	10-week block of combined therapy relatively ineffective at the 12-month follow-up according to mean scores on the Movement ABC and Beery Test. Statistically significant improvements were seen only in the areas of fine motor skills and visual–motor integration; these improvements reflected an actual change that was relatively small. The design flaws of this study contributed to an exaggerated treatment effect.
DeGangi, Sickel, Wiener, & Kaplan (1996)	39 infants described as regulatory disordered and 11 normal children	Performance on an interdisciplinary assessment at initial visit, at 7 to 30 months, with a follow-up at 3 years	Control group (CG): 13 untreated infants and experimental group (EG): 26 infants treated with a 12-week intervention program using a child-centered approach and principles from SI therapy	At three years, children with regulatory disorders differed from their normal counterparts in SI, mood regulation, attention, motor control, sleep, and behavioral control. Children in CG had more emotional and behavioral problems than children in EG; EG children had more motor and SI problems than children in CG.

(continues)

Appendix 5.B Therapy Efficacy *Continued.*

Study	Participants	Dependent Variable	Independent Variable	Findings
Humphries, Snider, & McDougall (1993)	103 children from 58 to 107 months of age (mean age of 79 months) described as having both learning disability and SI dysfunction	SI functioning as measured by the SCSIT (Ayers, 1980b), the SCPRNT (Ayers 1975b), and clinical observations (instructions provided by Dunn, 1981)	SI group: 72 one-hour sessions three times a week of SI treatment ($n = 35$), perceptual–motor (PM) group: 72 one-hour sessions three times a week of PM training ($n = 35$), control group: no treatment ($n = 33$)	SI and PM groups improved significantly compared to the control group, but the improvements of the SI group were not superior to those of the PM group. These results could indicate the need to refine assessment methods of dysfunction subtypes in order to better detect subtle changes in functioning.
Humphries, Wright, McDougall, & Vertes (1990)	30 children with learning disability and SI dysfunction ages 72 to 99 months	Sensorimotor functioning and higher-level cognitive, language, and academic performance as measured by a battery of tests	Random assignment to one of three groups—SI group: 24 one-hour weekly OT treatment sessions ($n = 10$); PM group: 24 one-hour weekly perceptual-motor training sessions ($n = 10$), control group: received no treatment intervention ($n = 10$)	The SI group made significant gains in motor functioning. No group differences were found in higher-level cognitive, language, and academic performance. Therapeutic effects were demonstrated on the primary motor functioning of children who were not receiving any special education or other services that would contaminate the interpretation of the outcomes.

(continues)

Study	Participants	Dependent Variable	Independent Variable	Findings
Kimball (1990)	19 boys ages 6 to 8 years	Pretest and posttest performance on the SIPT (Ayers, 1984)	Six months of biweekly OT with SI intervention in a school setting	Significant improvement was seen in scores of grouped data on tests of praxis, somatovestibular functioning, and bilateral integration and sequencing. Individual improvement was visible in 17 of the 19 boys according to the Western Psychological Services SIPT chromagraphs. Results indicate that the SIPT may be used to document improvement in children who have received OT with SI techniques.
O'Hara (1998)	13 adults ages 23 to 43 years identified as having sensory defensiveness	Performance on the Adult Sensory Questionnaire, Revised Dimensions of Temperament Survey (DOTS-R)—Adult Form, and Adult Sensory Interview	Four weeks of SI "self-treatment" program; pre- and posttesting was completed	Dimensions on the DOTS-R did not change; greater significance between pre- and posttest scores may have been identified with a larger sample size or longer treatment period.

(continues)

Appendix 5.B Therapy Efficacy *Continued.*

Study	Participants	Dependent Variable	Independent Variable	Findings
Polatajko, Law, Miller, Schaffer, & Macnab (1991)	67 children with learning disabilities and SI dysfunction	Academic achievement, motor performance, and self-esteem as measured by the Woodcock–Johnson Psychoeducational Battery, Bruininks-Oseretsky Test of Motor Proficiency, Behavioral Academic Self-Esteem Rating Scale, and Personality Inventory for Children, administered before therapy, after 6 months of therapy, and 3 months after cessation of therapy	Random assignment to one of two groups—sensory integrative (SI): 1 hour of therapy per week for 6 months ($n = 35$) using sensory modalities to elicit an adaptive motor response; perceptual motor (PM): 1 hour of therapy per week for 6 months ($n = 32$) using activities to increase PM function	Both the SI and PM groups improved on academic and motor measures. No group differences were detected in any measure.
Reisman (1993)	Adult with profound retardation	Minutes per day in restraints; mean number of self-injurious behaviors (SIB) per minute	Five minutes per hour of tactile, proprioceptive, and vestibular input	Time in restraint and amount of SIB decreased.

(continues)

Study	Participants	Dependent Variable	Independent Variable	Findings
Robichaud, Hebert, & Desrosiers (1994)	40 adults with dementia (28 women and 12 men); mean age of 78.4 years	Outcomes measured by the Revised Memory and Behavior Problems Checklist and the Psychogeriatric Scale of Basic Activities of Daily Living	Random assignment to one of two groups—experimental group ($n = 22$): three 45-minute sessions of SI treatment per week for 10 weeks, control group ($n = 18$): no SI treatment	The SI program had no significant effects on the behaviors of the experimental group. The authors concluded that modifications to this study (i.e., session frequency and sample size) should be implemented before this type of program is labeled inefficacious.
Soper & Thorley (1996)	28 adults ages 23 to 50 years with severe learning disabilities	Performance on three checklists—Clinical Observations Checklist, Behavioral Checklist, and Ayers Scale of Adaptive Responses—used as assessment at pre- and posttest stages	Experimental group (EG) ($n = 14$): received a weekly SI-based treatment session; control group ($n = 14$): received weekly sensory stimulation	Statistically significant improvement occurred in both groups; greater statistically significant improvement occurred in the EG compared to the CG in some areas. There was no negative correlation between age and improvement in either group.

(continues)

Appendix 5.B Therapy Efficacy *Continued.*

Study	Participants	Dependent Variable	Independent Variable	Findings
Stonefelt & Stein (1998)	23 parents, teachers, and occupational therapists of children with learning disabilities who are receiving or have received an SI therapy form of OT	21 survey questions involved perceived efficacy of SI therapy in helping child improve in 12 skill areas; additional questions for the parents and teachers related to effects in the home or classroom and any adaptations made; additional questions for therapists involved SI techniques and their effectiveness.	Eight children diagnosed with learning disabilities who had received SI therapy from an OT for less than 1 year or longer; all children received treatment at least two times per week and also received speech therapy.	Most respondents identified that SI therapy was either extremely or somewhat effective in helping the children improve in 12 skill areas. All parents reported home activities, and all teachers reported classroom accommodations in efforts to help a child. The SI techniques most commonly used were linear activities, tactile stimulation, games, jumping, and bouncing. Seven occupational therapists reported using a treatment method in addition to SI, and all seven reported that the multimodal approach was more effective than SI alone.

(continues)

Study	Participants	Dependent Variable	Independent Variable	Findings
Wilson & Kaplan (1994)	22 children ages 5 to 9 years with learning disabilities or at risk for developing learning problems	3-year follow-up; academic, motor, and behavioral instruments	Seventy-five 50-minute individual SI therapy or individual tutoring sessions	Gross motor skills significantly improved in SI group; no difference was evident in reading, fine motor, visual–motor, or behavioral factors. No significant correlation occurred between improvement during treatment and maintenance of gains.
Wilson, Kaplan, Fellowes, Gruchy, & Faris (1992)	29 children ages 5 to 9 years with learning, motor coordination, and vestibular–proprioceptive problems	6- and 12-month assessments with the Woodcock-Johnson, Bruininks-Oseretsky Test of Motor Proficiency, Abbreviated Symptom Questionnaire, and Hyperactivity Index	Seventy-five 50-minute sessions of individual SI therapy or individual tutoring	No significant differences after 6 or 12 months of treatment between the two groups. SI may be as effective as tutoring for improving academic functioning, but tutoring was as effective as SI in improving motor functioning.

Bibliography

1949

Ayres, A. J. (1949). An analysis of crafts in the treatment of electroshock patients. *American Journal of Occupational Therapy, 3,* 195-198.

1954

Ayres, A. J. (1954). A form used to evaluate the work behavior of patients. *American Journal of Occupational Therapy, 8,* 73–74.

Ayres, A. J. (1954). Ontogenetic principles in the development of arm and hand functions. *American Journal of Occupational Therapy, 8,* 95-99.

1955

Ayres, A. J. (1955). A pilot study on the relationship between work habits and workshop production. *American Journal of Occupational Therapy, 9,* 264–276.

Ayres, A. J. (1955). Proprioceptive facilitation elicited through the upper extremities. *American Journal of Occupational Therapy, 9,* 1–9, 57–58, 121–126.

1957

Ayres, A. J. (1957). A study of the manual dexterity and workshop wages of thirty-nine cerebral palsied trainees. *American Journal of Physical Medicine, 36,* 6–10.

1958

Ayres, A. J. (1958). Basic concepts of clinical practice in physical disabilities. *American Journal of Occupational Therapy, 12,* 300–302.

Ayres, A. J. (1958). The visual-motor function. *American Journal of Occupational Therapy, 12,* 130–138.

1960

Ayres, A. J. (1960). Hemiplegia. In *Occupational therapy reference manual for physicians* (pp. 38–42). Dubuque, IA: William C. Brown.

Ayres, A. J. (1960). Occupational therapy for motor disorders resulting from impairment of the central nervous system. *Rehabilitation Literature, 21,* 302–310.

Ayres, A. J. (1960). Research for therapists. In *Proceedings of the American Occupational Therapy Association 1960 Conference* (pp. 79–82). Rockville, MD: American Occupational Therapy Association.

1961

Ayres, A. J. (1961). Development of the body scheme in children. *American Journal of Occupational Therapy, 15,* 99–102.

Ayres, A. J. (1961). The role of gross motor activities in the training of children with visual motor retardation. *Journal of the American Optometric Association, 33,* 121–125.

1962

Ayres, A. J. (1962). Perception of space of adult hemiplegic patients. *Physical Medicine and Rehabilitation, 43,* 552–555.

1963

Ayres, A. J. (1963). The development of perceptual-motor abilities. A theoretical basis for treatment of dysfunction. *American Journal of Occupational Therapy, 17,* 221–225.

Ayres, A. J. (1963). Occupational therapy directed toward neuromuscular integration. In H. S. Willard & C. S. Spackman (Eds.), *Occupational therapy* (3rd ed.; pp. 358–466). Philadelphia: J.B. Lippincott.

1964

Ayres, A. J. (1964). Integration of information. In C. Satterly (Ed.), *Approaches to the treatment of patients with neuromuscular dysfunction: Study Course VI. Third International Conference of the World Federation of Occupational Therapists, 1962* (pp. 49–57). Dubuque, IA: William C. Brown.

Ayres, A. J. (1964). *Perceptual-motor dysfunction in children.* Monograph from the Greater Cincinnati District, Ohio Occupational Therapy Association, Cincinnati.

Ayres, A. J. (1964). Perceptual-motor training for children. In C. Satterly (Ed.), *Approaches to the treatment of patients with neuromuscular dysfunction: Study Course VI, Third International Conference of the World Federation of Occupational Therapists, 1962* (pp. 17–22). Dubuque, IA: William C. Brown.

Ayres, A. J. (1964). Perspectives on neurological bases of reading. In M. P. Douglass (Ed.), *Claremont Reading Conference, 28th yearbook* (pp. 113–118). Claremont, CA: Claremont Graduate School Curriculum Laboratory.

Ayres, A. J. (1964). Tactile functions: Their relation to hyperactivity and perceptual-motor behavior. *American Journal of Occupational Therapy, 18,* 6–11.

1965

Ayres, A. J. (1965). A method of measurement of degrees of sensorimotor integration. *Archives of Physical Medicine and Rehabilitation, 46,* 433–435.

Ayres, A. J. (1965). Patterns of perceptual-motor dysfunction in children: A factor analytic study. *Perceptual and Motor Skills, 20,* 335-368.

1966

Ayres, A. J. (1966). Interrelation of perception, function, and treatment. *Journal of the American Physical Therapy Association, 46,* 741–744.

Ayres, A. J. (1966). Interrelationships among perceptual-motor abilities in a group of normal children. *American Journal of Occupational Therapy, 20,* 288–292.

Ayres, A. J. (1966). Interrelationships among perceptual-motor functions in children. *American Journal of Occupational Therapy, 20,* 68–71.

Ayres, A. J., & Reid, W. (1966). The self-drawing as an expression of perceptual-motor dysfunction. *Cortex, 2,* 254–265.

1967

Ayres, A. J. (1967). Remedial procedures based on neurobehavioral constructs. In *Proceedings of the 1967 International Convocation on Children and Young Adults with Learning Disabilities,* Pittsburgh, PA.

1968

Ayres, A. J. (1968). Reading—A product of sensory integrative process. In H. K. Smith (Ed.), *Perception and reading: Proceedings of the Twelfth Annual Convention of the International Reading Association* (Vol. 12, Part 4). Newark, DE.

Ayres, A. J. (1968). Sensory integrative processes and neuropsychological learning disability. In J. Hellmuth (Ed.) *Learning disorders* (Vol. 3, pp. 41–58). Seattle, WA: Special Child Publications.

1969

Ayres, A. J. (1969). Deficits in sensory integration in educationally handicapped children. *Journal of Learning Disabilities, 2,* 160–168.

Ayres, A. J. (1969). Relation between Gesell development quotients and later perceptual-motor performance. *American Journal of Occupational Therapy, 23,* 11–17.

1971

Ayres, A. J. (1971). *The challenge of the brain*. Paper presented at the Perceptual Motor Conference (sponsored by the Physical Education Division of the American Association for Health, Physical Education, and Recreation). Sparks, NV.

Ayres, A. J. (1971). Characteristics of types of sensory integrative dysfunction. *American Journal of Occupational Therapy, 25,* 329–334.

1972

Ayres, A. J. (1972, August-September). Basic concepts of occupational therapy for children with perceptual-motor dysfunction. In *Proceedings of the Twelfth World Congress of Rehabilitation International*. Sydney, Australia.

Ayres, A. J. (1972). Improving academic scores through sensory integration. *Journal of Learning Disabilities, 5,* 338–343.

Ayres, A. J. (1972). An interpretation of the role of the brain stem in intersensory integration. In A. Henderson & J. Coryell (Eds.), *The body senses and perceptual deficit: Proceedings of the Occupational Therapy Symposium on Somatosensory Aspects of Perceptual Deficits* (pp. 81–89). Boston: Boston University.

Ayres, A. J. (1972). *Sensory integration and learning disorders*. Los Angeles: Western Psychological Services.

Ayres, A. J. (1972). Sensory integration process: Implications of deaf-blind from learning disability children. In W. A. Blea (Ed.), *Proceedings of the National Symposium for Deaf-Blind* (pp. 81–89). Pacific Grove, CA.

Ayres, A. J., & Heskett, W. M. (1972). Sensory integrative dysfunction in a young schizophrenic girl. *Journal of Autism and Childhood Schizophrenia, 2,* 174–181.

Ayres, A. J. (1972). Types of sensory integrative dysfunction among disabled learners. *American Journal of Occupational Therapy, 26,* 13–18.

1975

Ayres, A. J. (1975). Sensorimotor foundations of academic ability. In W. M. Cruickshank & D. P. Hallahan (Eds.), *Perceptual and learning disabilities in children* (Vol. 2, pp. 301–358). Syracuse, NY: Syracuse University Press.

1976

Ayres, A. J. (1976). *The effects of sensory integration therapy on learning disabled children*. Los Angeles: University of Southern California.

Ayres, A. J. (1976). *Interpreting the Southern California Sensory Integration Tests*. Los Angeles: Western Psychological Services.

1977

Ayres, A. J. (1977). Cluster analyses of measures of sensory integration. *American Journal of Occupational Therapy, 31,* 362–366.

Ayres, A. J. (1977). Dichotic listening performance in learning-disabled children. *American Journal of Occupational Therapy, 31,* 441–446.

Ayres, A. J. (1977). Effect of sensory integrative therapy on the coordination of children with choreoathetoid movements. *American Journal of Occupational Therapy, 31,* 291–293.

Ayres, A.J. (1977). A response of defensive medicine. *Academic Therapy, 13,* 149–152.

1978

Ayres, A. J. (1978). Learning disabilities and the vestibular system. *Journal of Learning Disabilities, 11,* 18–29.

1979

Ayres, A. J. (1979). *Sensory integration and the child.* Los Angeles: Western Psychological Services.

Ayres, A. J. (1979). The sensory registration function in autistic and aphasic/apraxic children. In *Piagetian theory and its implication for the helping professions: Proceedings of the Ninth Interdisciplinary Conference.* Los Angeles University of Southern California. Co-Sponsors: Children's Hospital of Los Angeles, University of Affiliated Program and USC School of Education and USC School of Social Work.

1980

Ayres, A. J., & Tickle, L. S. (1980). Hyper-responsivity to touch and vestibular stimuli predict positive response to sensory integration procedures in autistic children. *American Journal of Occupational Therapy, 34,* 375-381.

1981

Ayres, A. J., & Mailloux, Z. (1981). Influence of sensory integration procedures on language development. *American Journal of Occupational Therapy, 35,* 383–390.

1983

Ayres, A. J., & Mailloux, Z. (1983). Possible pubertal effects on therapeutic gains in an autistic girl. *American Journal of Occupational Therapy, 37,* 535-540.

1984

Ayres, A. J., & Cermak, S. A. (1984). Crossing the body midline in learning-disabled and normal children. *American Journal of Occupational Therapy, 38,* 35-39.

Slavik, B. A., Kitsuwa-Lowe, J., Danner, P. T., Green, J., & Ayres, A. J. (1984). Vestibular stimulation and eye contact in autistic children. *Neuropediatrics, 15,* 33–36.

1985

Ayres, A. J. (1985). *Developmental dyspraxia and adult onset dyspraxia.* Torrance, CA: Sensory Integration International.

Ayres, A. J., Mailloux, Z., & McAtee, S. (1985). An update of the Sensory Integration and Praxis Tests. *Sensory Integration Special Interest Section Newsletter, 8*(3).

1987

Ayres, A. J., Mailloux, Z. K., & Wendler, C. L. (1987). Developmental dyspraxia: Is it a unitary function? *Occupational Therapy Journal of Research, 7*(2), 93–110.

1989

Ayres, A. J. (1989). Forward. In L. J. Miller (Ed.), Developing norm-referenced standardized tests [Special issue]. *Physical and Occupational Therapy in Pediatrics, 9* (1), xi-xii.

1991

Ayres, A. J., & Marr, D. B. (1991). Sensory Integration and Praxis Test. In A. G. Fisher, E. A. Murray, & A. C. Bundy (Eds.), *Sensory integration theory and practice* (pp. 203–229). Philadelphia: F. A. Davis.

Psychological Tests

1962

Ayres, A. J. (1962). *Ayres Space Test*. Los Angeles: Western Psychological Services.

1964

Ayres, A. J. (1964). *Southern California Motor-Accuracy Test*. Los Angeles: Western Psychological Services.

1966

Ayres, A. J. (1966). *Southern California Figure Ground Visual Perception Tests*. Los Angeles: Western Psychological Services.

Ayres, A. J. (1966). *Southern California Kinesthesia and Tactile Perception Tests*. Los Angeles: Western Psychological Services.

1968

Ayres, A. J. (1968). *Southern California Perceptual-Motor Tests*. Los Angeles: Western Psychological Services.

1972

Ayres, A. J. (1972). *Southern California Sensory Integration Tests*. Los Angeles: Western Psychological Services.

1975

Ayres, A. J. (1975). *Southern California Postrotary Nystagmus Test*. Los Angeles: Western Psychological Services.

1980

Ayres, A. J. (1980). *Southern California Motor Accuracy Test—Revised 1980*. Los Angeles: Western Psychological Services.

Ayres, A. J. (1980). *Southern California Sensory Integration Tests—Revised 1980*. Los Angeles: Western Psychological Services.

1989

Ayres, A. J. (1989). *Sensory Integration and Praxis Tests*. Los Angeles: Western Psychological Services.

Republished Articles

1959

Ayres, A. J. (1959). Proprioceptive erleichterungsmethoden. *Krankengymnastic, 11,* 191–195, 196–200, 220–225.

1967

Ayres, A. J. (1967). Types of perceptual motor deficits in children with learning difficulties. In Bilovsky, Attwell, & Jamison (Eds.), *Readings in learning disability*. New York: Selected Academic Readings.

1971

Ayres, A. J. (1971). Interrelations among perceptual-motor abilities in a group of normal children. In C. Kopp (Ed.), *Readings in early development for occupational and physical therapy students*. Springfield, IL: Charles C. Thomas.

1973

Ayres, A. J. (1973). The development of perceptual-motor abilities: A theoretical basis for treatment of dysfunction. In American Occupational Therapy Association, Inc. (Ed.), *The Eleanor Clarke Slagle Lectures, 1955-1972* (pp. 127–135). Dubuque, IA: Kendall/Hunt.

1974

Henderson, A., Llorens, L. A., Gilfoyle, E., Myers, C., & Prevel, S. (Eds.). (1974). *The development of sensory integrative theory and practice: A collection of the works of A. Jean Ayres* (pp. 167–175). Dubuque, IA: Kendall/Hunt.

Professional Films

1966

Ayres, A. J. (1966). *Perceptual-motor evaluation of a child with dysfunction.* Los Angeles: University of California, Los Angeles.

Ayres, A. J. (1966). *Perceptual-motor evaluation of a perceptually normal child.* Los Angeles: University of California, Los Angeles.

1969

Ayres, A. J., & Heskett, W. M. (1969). *Clinical observations of dysfunctions in postural and bilateral integration.* Los Angeles: University of Southern California.

Ayres, A. J., & Heskett, W. M. (1969). *A therapeutic activity for perceptual-motor dysfunction.* Los Angeles: University of Southern California.

References

Allen, S., & McDonald, M. (1995). The effect of occupational therapy on the motor proficiency of children with motor/learning difficulties: A pilot study. *British Journal of Occupational Therapy, 58*, 385-391.

American Occupational Therapy Association. (1985). Jean Ayres retires from clinical practice. *Occupational Therapy News, 39*(6), 24.

American Occupational Therapy Association. (1987). Ayres award established. *Occupational Therapy News, 41*(11), 3.

American Occupational Therapy Association. (1989a). A. Jean Ayres, PhD, OTR, FAOTA: Profession remembers eminent clinician and scholar. *Occupational Therapy News, 43*(2), 1, 10, 15.

American Occupational Therapy Association. (1989b). OT leaders Ayres and Robinson receive special tributes in Baltimore. *Occupational Therapy Week, 3*(17), 4.

Arendt, R. E., MacLean, W. E., & Baumeister, A. A. (1988). Critique of sensory integration therapy and its application in mental retardation. *American Journal on Mental Retardation, 92*(5), 401–411.

Ayres, A. J. (1949). An analysis of crafts in the treatment of electroshock patients. *American Journal of Occupational Therapy, 3*, 195-198.

Ayres, A. J. (1954). Ontogenetic principles in the development of arm and hand functions. *American Journal of Occupational Therapy, 3*, 95-99.

Ayres, A. J. (1958). The visual-motor function. *American Journal of Occupational Therapy, 12*, 130–138.

Ayres, A. J. (1960). Occupational therapy for motor disorders resulting from impairment of the central nervous system. *Rehabilitation Literature, 21*, 302–310.

Ayres, A. J. (1961a). Development of the body scheme in children. *American Journal of Occupational Therapy, 15*, 99–102.

Ayres, A. J. (1961b). The role of gross motor activities in the training of children with visual motor retardation. *Journal of the American Optometric Association, 33*, 121–125.

Ayres, A. J. (1962). *Ayres Space Test.* Los Angeles: Western Psychological Services.

Ayres, A. J. (1963a). The development of perceptual-motor abilities: A theoretical basis for treatment of dysfunction. Eleanor Clarke Slagle lecture. *American Journal of Occupational Therapy, 17,* 221–225.

Ayres, A. J. (1963b). Occupational therapy directed toward neuromuscular integration. In H. S. Willard & C. S. Spackman (Eds.), *Occupational therapy* (3rd ed.) (pp. 358–466). Philadelphia: J.B. Lippincott.

Ayres, A. J. (1964a). Perceptual motor training for children. In C. Satterly (Ed.), *Approaches to the treatment of patients with neuromuscular dysfunction: Study Course VI. Third International Conference of the World Federation of Occupational Therapists, 1962* (pp. 17–22). Dubuque, IA: William C. Brown.

Ayres, A. J. (1964b). *Southern California Motor Accuracy Test.* Los Angeles: Western Psychological Services.

Ayres, A. J. (1964c). Tactile functions: Their relation to hyperactivity and perceptual-motor behavior. *American Journal of Occupational Therapy, 18*, 6–11.

Ayres, A. J. (1965). Patterns of perceptual-motor dysfunction in children: A factor analytic study. *Perceptual and Motor Skills, 20*, 335-368.

Ayres, A. J. (1966a). Interrelation of perception, function, and treatment. *Journal of the American Physical Therapy Association, 46*, 741–744.

Ayres, A. J. (1966b). Interrelations among perceptual-motor abilities in a group of normal children. *American Journal of Occupational Therapy, 20*, 288–292.

Ayres, A. J. (1966c). Interrelationships among perceptual-motor functions in children. *American Journal of Occupational Therapy, 20*, 68–71.

Ayres, A. J. (1966d). *Southern California Figure Ground Visual Perception Tests.* Los Angeles: Western Psychological Services.

Ayres, A. J. (1966e). *Southern California Kinesthesia and Tactile Perception Tests.* Los Angeles: Western Psychological Services.

Ayres, A. J. (1967). Remedial procedures based on neurobehavioral constructs. In *Proceedings of the 1967 International Convocation on Children and Young Adults with Learning Disabilities.* Pittsburgh, PA.

Ayres, A. J. (1968a). Reading—A product of sensory integrative processes. In A. Henderson et al. (Eds.), *The development of sensory integrative theory and practice* (pp. 167–175). Dubuque, IA: Kendall/Hunt.

Ayres, A. J. (1968b). Sensory integrative processes and neuropsychological learning disability. In *Learning Disorders* (Vol. 3, pp. 41–58). Seattle, WA: Special Child Publications.

Ayres, A. J. (1968c). *Southern California Perceptual-Motor Tests.* Los Angeles: Western Psychological Services.

Ayres, A. J. (1969). Deficits in sensory integration in educationally handicapped children. *Journal of Learning Disabilities, 2,* 160–168.

Ayres, A. J. (1971). Characteristics of types of sensory integrative dysfunction. *American Journal of Occupational Therapy, 25,* 329–334.

Ayres, A. J. (1972a). Basic concepts of occupational therapy for children with perceptual-motor dysfunction. In *Proceedings of the Twelfth World Congress of Rehabilitation International.* Sydney, Australia.

Ayres, A. J. (1972b). Improving academic scores through sensory integration. *Journal of Learning Disabilities, 5,* 338–343.

Ayres, A. J. (1972c). An interpretation of the role of the brain stem in intersensory integration. In A. Henderson & J. Coryell (Eds.), *The body senses and perceptual deficit: Proceedings of the Occupational Therapy Symposium on Somatosensory Aspects of Perceptual Deficits* (pp. 81–89). Boston: Boston University.

Ayres, A. J. (1972d). *Sensory integration and learning disorders.* Los Angeles: Western Psychological Services.

Ayres, A. J. (1972e). *Southern California Sensory Integration Tests.* Los Angeles: Western Psychological Services.

Ayres, A. J. (1972f). Types of sensory integrative dysfunction among disabled learners. *American Journal of Occupational Therapy, 26,* 13–18.

Ayres, A. J. (1975a). Sensorimotor foundations of academic ability. In W. M. Cruickshank & D. P. Hallahan (Eds.), *Perceptual and learning disabilities in children* (Vol. 2, pp. 301–358). Syracuse, NY: Syracuse University Press.

Ayres, A. J. (1975b). *Southern California Postrotary Nystagmus Test.* Los Angeles: Western Psychological Services.

Ayres, A. J. (1976a). *The effects of sensory integration therapy on learning disabled children.* Los Angeles: University of Southern California.

Ayres, A. J. (1976b). *Interpreting the Southern California Sensory Integration Tests.* Los Angeles: Western Psychological Services.

Ayres, A. J. (1977a). Cluster analyses of measures of sensory integration. *American Journal of Occupational Therapy, 31,* 362–366.

Ayres, A. J. (1977b). Dichotic listening performance in learning-disabled children. *American Journal of Occupational Therapy, 31,* 441–446.

Ayres, A. J. (1977c). Effect of sensory integrative therapy on the coordination of children with choreoathetoid movements. *American Journal of Occupational Therapy, 31,* 291–293.

Ayres, A. J. (1978). Learning disabilities and the vestibular system. *Journal of Learning Disabilities, 11,* 18–29.

Ayres, A. J. (1979). *Sensory integration and the child.* Los Angeles: Western Psychological Services.

Ayres, A. J. (1980a). *Southern California Motor Accuracy Test—Revised 1980.* Los Angeles: Western Psychological Services.

Ayres, A. J. (1980b). *Southern California Sensory Integration Tests—Revised 1980.* Los Angeles: Western Psychological Services.

Ayres, A. J. (1985). *Developmental dyspraxia and adult onset dyspraxia.* Torrance, CA: Sensory Integration International.

Ayres, A. J. (1989). *Sensory Integration and Praxis Tests.* Los Angeles: Western Psychological Services.

Ayres, A. J., & Mailloux, Z. K. (1981). Influence of sensory integration procedures on language development. *American Journal of Occupational Therapy, 35,* 383–390.

Ayres, A. J., Mailloux, Z. K., & McAtee, S. (1985). An update of the Sensory Integration and Praxis Tests. *Sensory Integration Special Interest Section Newsletter, 8*(3).

Ayres, A. J., Mailloux, Z. K., & Wendler, C. L. (1987). Developmental dyspraxia. Is it a unitary function? *Occupational Therapy Journal of Research, 7*(2), 93–110.

Ayres, A. J., & Marr, D. B. (1991). Sensory Integration and Praxis Test. In A. G. Fisher, E. A. Murray, & A. C. Bundy (Eds.), *Sensory integration theory and practice* (pp. 203–229). Philadelphia: F.A. Davis.

Ayres, A. J., & Tickle, L. S. (1980). Hyper-responsivity to touch and vestibular stimuli predict positive response to sensory integration procedures in autistic children. *American Journal of Occupational Therapy, 34,* 375-381.

Benton, A. L. (1964). Developmental aphasia and brain damage. *Cortex, 1,* 40–45.

Bobath, K., & Bobath, B. (1964). The facilitation of normal postural reactions and movements in the treatment of cerebral palsy. *Physiotherapy, 50,* 246–262.

Bochner, S. (1978). Ayres, sensory integration and learning disorders: Question of theory and practice. *American Journal of Mental Retardation, 5,* 41–45.

Brodol, A. (1964). Anatomical organization and fiber connectioins of the vestibular nuclei. In W. S. Fields & B. R. Alford (Eds.), *Neurological aspects of auditory and vestibular disorders.* Springfield, MO: Charles C. Thomas.

Carrasco, R. C. (1993). Key components of sensory integration evaluation. *Sensory integration Special Interest Section Quarterly, 16* (2), 1–7.

Case-Smith, J., & Bryan, T. (1999). The effects of occupational therapy with sensory integration emphasis on preschool-age children with autism. *American Journal of Occupational Therapy, 53,* 489–505.

Case-Smith, J., & Miller, L.J. (1999). Occupational therapy with children with pervasive developmental disorders. *American Journal of Occupational Therapy, 53,* 506–513.

Cermak, S. A. (1988). The relationship between attention deficits and sensory integration disorders. *Sensory Integration Special Interest Section Newsletter, 11*(2), 1–4.

Cermak, S. A. (1991). Somatodyspraxia. In A. G. Fisher, E. A. Murray, & A. C. Bundy (Eds.), *Sensory integration theory and practice* (pp. 137–165). Philadelphia: F.A. Davis.

Cermak, S.A., (1994). What is sensory integration? *Sensory Integration Special Interest Section Quarterly, 17* (2), 2–3.

Cermak, S. A., & Henderson, A. (1990). The efficacy of sensory integration procedures: Part II. *Sensory Integration Quarterly, 18*(1), 1–5, 17.

Cermak, S. A., Morris, M., & Koomar, J. (1990). Praxis on verbal command and imitation. *American Journal of Occupational Therapy, 44*(7), 641–645.

Cermak, S. A. & Murray, E. A. (1991). The validity of the constructional subtests of the Sensory Integration and Praxis Tests. *American Journal of Occupational Therapy, 45,* 539–543.

Clark, E., Mailloux, Z., & Parham, D. (1985). Sensory integration and children with learning disabilities. In P. N. Clark & A. S. Allen (Eds.), *Occupational therapy for children* (pp. 359–405). St. Louis: C. V. Mosby.

Clements, S. D., & Peters, J. E. (1962). Minimal brain dysfunction in the school age child. *Archives of General Psychiatry, 6,* 185-197.

Committee on Children with Disabilities. (1985). School aged children with motor disabilities. *Pediatrics, 76,* 648–649.

Coster, W., Tickle-Degnan, L., & Armenta, L. (1995). Therapist-child interaction during sensory integration treatment: Development and testing of a research tool. *Occupational Therapy Journal of Research, 15*(1), 17–34.

Cratty, B. J. (1964). *Movement behavior and motor learning.* Philadephia: Lee & Febigen.

Critchley, M. (1994). *Developmental dyslexia.* London: William Heinemann Medical Books.

Cross, L. A., & Coster, W. J. (1997). Symbolic play language during sensory integration treatment. *American Journal of Occupational Therapy, 51*(10), 808–814.

Cummins, R. A. (1991). Sensory integration and learning disabilities: Ayres's factor analyses reappraised. *Journal of Learning Disabilities, 24*(3), 160–168.

Davidson, T., & Williams, B. (2000). Occupational therapy for children with developmental coordination disorder: A study of the effectiveness of a combined sensory integration and perceptual-motor intervention. *British Journal of Occupational Therapy, 63*(10), 495-499.

DeGangi, G., Sickel, R., Wiener, A., & Kaplan, E. (1996). Fussy babies: To treat or not to treat. *British Journal of Occupational Therapy, 59*(10), 457–464.

Densem, J. F., Nutall, G. A., Bushnell, J., & Horn, J. (1989). Effectiveness of a sensory integrative therapy program for children with perceptual-motor deficits. *Journal of Learning Disabilities, 22*(4), 221–229.

Dunkerley, E., Tickle-Degnan, L., & Coster, W. J. (1997). Therapist-child interaction in the middle minutes of sensory integration treatment. *American Journal of Occupational Therapy, 51*(10), 799–805.

Dunn, W. (1999). *The sensory profile.* San Antonio, TX: Therapy Skill Builders.

Dura, J. R., Mulick, J. A., & Hammer, D. (1988). Rapid clinical evaluation of sensory integrative therapy for self-injurious behavior. *Mental Retardation, 26,* 83–87.

Eccles, J. C. (Ed.) (1966). *Brain and conscious experience.* New York: Springer-Verlag.

Evan, P. R., & Peham, M. A. (1981). *Testing and measurements in occupational therapy: A review of current practice with special emphasis on the Southern California Sensory Integration Tests.* Minneapolis: University of Minnesota.

Evarts, E. V., & Thach, W. T. (1969). Motor mechanism of the CNS: Cerebrocerebellar interrelations. *Annual Review of Physiology, 31,* 451–498.

Fanchiang, S., Snyder, C., Zobel-Lachiusa, J., Loeffler, C. B., & Thompson, M. E. (1990). Sensory integrative processing in delinquent-prone and non-delinquent-prone adolescents. *American Journal of Occupational Therapy, 44*(7), 630–639.

Fay, T. (1954). The use of pathological and unlocking reflexes in the rehabilitation of spastics. *American Journal of Physical Medicine, 33,* 347–352.

Fisher, A. G. (1991). Vestibular-proprioceptive processing and bilateral integration and sequencing deficits. In A. G. Fisher, E. A. Murray, & A. C. Bundy (Eds.), *Sensory integration theory and practice* (pp. 71–107). Philadelphia: F.A. Davis.

Fisher, A. G., & Dunn, W. (1983). Tactile defensiveness: Historical perspectives, new research. A theory grows. *Sensory Integration Special Interest Section Newsletter, 6*(2), 1–2.

Fisher, A. G., & Murray, E. A. (1991). Introduction to sensory integration theory. In A. G. Fisher, E. A. Murray, & A. C. Bundy (Eds.), *Sensory integration theory and practice* (pp. 3–26). Philadelphia: F.A. Davis.

Fisher, A. G., Murray, E. A., & Bundy, A. C. (Eds.). (1991). *Sensory integration theory and practice.* Philadelphia: F.A. Davis.

Geschwind, N. (1965). Disconnexion syndromes in animals and man. *Brain*, *88*, 237–194.

Gesell, A. (1940). *The first five years of life*. New York: Harper & Row.

Gorsuch, R. L. (1983). *Factor analysis* (2nd ed.). Hillsdale, NJ: Erlbaum.

Greenspan, S. I. (1994). *Diagnostic classification of mental health and developmental disorders of infancy and early childhood*. Washington, DC: Zero to Three.

Haack, L., Short-DeGraff, M., & Hanzlik, J. (1993). Relationship of ocular motor skills to vestibular-related clinical observations. *Physical and Occupational Therapy in Pediatrics, 13,* 1–13.

Hames-Hahn, C. S., & Llorens, L. A. (1989). Impact of a multisensory occupational therapy program on components of self-feeding behavior in the elderly. *Physical and Occupational Therapy in Geriatrics*, *6*(3–4), 63–86.

Hanft, B. E., Miller, L. J., & Lane, S. J. (2000). Toward a consensus in terminology in sensory integration theory and practice—Part 3: Observable behaviors: Sensory integration dysfunction. *Sensory Integration Special Interest Section Quarterly*, *23*(3), 1–4.

Harlow, H. (1958). The nature of love. *American Psychologist*, *13*, 673–685.

High, J., Gough, A., Pennington, D., & Wright, C. (2000). Alternative assessments for sensory integration dysfunction. *British Journal of Occupational Therapy, 63*, 2–8.

Hoehn, T. P., & Baumeister, A. A. (1994). A critique of the application of sensory integration therapy to children with learning disabilities. *Journal of Learning Disabilities*, *41*, 338–350.

Humphries, T., Snider, L., & McDougall, B. (1993). Clinical evaluation of the effectiveness of sensory integrative and perceptual motor therapy in improving sensory integrative function in children with learning disabilities. *Occupational Therapy Journal of Research*, *13*, 163–182.

Humphries, T., Wright, M., McDougall, B., & Vertes, J. (1990). The efficacy of sensory integration therapy for children with learning disability. *Physical and Occupational Therapy in Pediatrics*, *10*(3), 1–17.

Kabat, H., & Knott, M. (1948). Principles of neuromuscular re-education. *Physical Therapy Review*, *28I, 107–111.*

Kavale, K., & Mattson, P. D. (1983). One jumped off the balance beam: Meta-analysis of perceptual motor training. *Journal of Learning Disabilities, 16,* 165–173.

Kephart, N. C. (1960). *The slow learner in the classroom*. Columbus, OH: Charles E. Merrill Books, Inc.

Kielhofner, G. (2002). *A model of human occupation: Theory and application* (3rd ed.). Baltimore, MD: Williams & Wilkins.

Kimball J. (1990). Using sensory integration and praxis tests to measure change: A pilot study. *American Journal of Occupational Therapy*, *44*, 603–608.

Kimball, J. G. (1993). Sensory integrative frame of reference. In P. Kramer & J. Hinojosa (Eds.), *Frames of reference for pediatric occupational therapy* pp. 87–175. Baltimore: Williams & Wilkins.

Kinnealey, M., & Wilbarger, P. (1993). Test-retest reliability fo the SIPT on high-risk children. *Sensory Integration Quarterly*, *21*(3), 1–7.

Kluver, H., & Bucy, P. C. (1939). Preliminary analysis of the functions of the *temporal* lobes in monkeys. *Archives of Neurology and Psychiatry*, 979–1000. Reprinted in: Journal of Neuropsychiatry and Clinical Neuroscience Neurology 1997 Fall 9(4) 606–620.

Knickerbocker, B. M. (1980). *A holistic approach to learning disabilities*. Thorofare, NJ: Charles B. Slack.

Knox, S., Mack, W., & Mailloux, Z. (1988). *Interpreting the sensory integration and praxis tests*. Los Angeles: Sensory Integration International.

Koomar, J. A., & Bundy, A. C. (1991). The art and science of creating direct intervention from theory. In A. G. Fisher, E. A. Murray, & A. C. Bundy (Eds.), *Sensory integration theory and practice* (pp. 251–314). Philadelphia: F.A. Davis.

Lai, J., Fisher, A., Magalhaes, L., & Bundy A. (1996). Construct validity of the Sensory Integration and Praxis Tests. *Occupational Therapy Journal of Research, 16*(2), 75–97.

Lai, J., Parham, D., & Johnson-Ecker, C. (1999), Sensory dormacy and sensory defensiveness: Two sides of the same coin? *Sensory Integration Special Interest Section Quarterly, 22*(4), 1–4.

Lane, S. J., Miller, L. J., Hanft, B. E. (2000). Toward a consensus in terminology in sensory integration theory and practice: Part 2: Sensory integration patterns of function and dysfunction. *Sensory Integration Special Interest Section Quarterly, 23*(2), 1–3.

Larson, K. A. (1982). The sensory history of developmentally delayed children with and without sensory defensiveness. *American Journal of Occupational Therapy, 36*, 590–596.

Lerer, R. J. (1981). An open letter to an occupational therapist. *Journal of Learning Disabilities, 14*, 3–4.

Luria, A. R. (1966). *Higher cortical functions in man*. New York: Basic Books.

Maslow, P., Frostig, M., Lefever, D. W., & Whittlesey, J. R. B. (1964). The Marianne Frostig Developmental Test of Visual Perception, 1963 standardization. *Perceptual and Motor Skills, 19*, 463–499.

Mason, S. A., & Iwata, B. A. (1990). Artifactual effects of sensory integrative therapy on self-injurious behavior. *Journal of Applied Behavior Analysis, 23*, 361–370.

Meleis, A. I. (1985). *Theoretical nursing: Development and progress*. Philadelphia: Lippincott.

Melzack, R., & Wall, P. D. (1965). Pain mechanisms: A new theory. *Science, 150*, 971–979.

Mercer, C. D. (1983). *Students with learning disabilities*. Columbus, OH: Merrill.

Miller, L. J., & Kinnealey, M. (1993). Researching the effectiveness of sensory integration. *Sensory Integration Quarterly, 21*(2), 1, 3–5, 7.

Miller, L. J. & Lane, S. J. (2000). Toward a concensus in terminology in sensory integration theory and practice: Part 1: Taxonomy of neurophysiological processes. *Sensory Integration Special Interest Section Quarterly, 23*, 1–4.

Miller, L. J., & McIntosh, D. N. (1998). The diagnosis, treatment, and etiology of sensory modulation disorder. *Sensory Integration Special Interest Section Quarterly, 21*, 1–3.

Miller L. J., Reisman, J., McIntosh, D.N. & Simon, J. (2001). An ecological model of sensory modulation: Performance of children with fragile X syndrome, autism, ADHD and SMD. In S. Roley, R. Schaaf, & E. Blanche (Eds.), *Sensory integration and developmental disabilities*. San Antonio, TX: Therapy Skill Builders.

Mulligan, S. (1996). An analysis of score patterns of children with attention disorders on the Sensory Integration and Praxis Tests. *American Journal of Occupational Therapy, 50*, 647–654.

Mulligan, S. (1998). Patterns of sensory integration dysfunction: A confirmatory factor analysis. *American Journal of Occupational Therapy, 52,* 819–828.

Mulligan, S. (2000). Cluster analysis of scores of children on the Sensory Integration and Praxis Tests. *Occupational Therapy Journal of Research, 20*(4), 256–270.

Murray, E. A., & Anzalone, M. E. (1991). Integrating sensory integration theory and practice with other intervention approaches. In A. G. Fisher, E. A. Murray, & A. C. Bundy (Eds.), *Sensory Integration Theory and Practice,* (pp. 354–381). Philadelphia: F.A. Davis.

Myers, P. I., & Hammill, D. D. (1982). *Learning disabilities: Basic concepts, assessment practices and instructional strategies.* Austin, TX: PRO-ED.

Nommensen, A., & Maas, F. (1993). Sensory integration and Down's syndrome. *British Journal of Occupational Therapy, 56*(12), 451–454.

O'Hara, S. C. (1998). *The effect of self-treatment on adaptability in sensory defensive adults.* Philadelphia, PA: Temple University.

Ottenbacher, K. (1982). Sensory integration therapy: Affect of effect. *American Journal of Occupational Therapy, 36,* 571–578.

Ottenbacher, K., & Short, M. A. (1985). Sensory integrative dysfunction in children: A review of theory and treatment. *Advances in Developmental and Behavioral Pediatrics, 6,* 287–329.

Parham, D. (1998). The relationship of sensory integrative development to achievement in elementary students: Four-year longitudinal patterns. *Occupational Therapy Journal of Research, 18*(3), 105-127.

Parham, L. D., & Mailloux, Z. (2001). Sensory integration. In J. Case-Smith (Ed.), *Occupational therapy for children,* pp. 329–379. St. Louis: Mosby.

Penfield, W., & Roberts, L. (1959). *Speech and brain mechanisms.* Princeton: Princeton University Press.

Piaget, J. (1952). *The origins of intelligence in children.* New York: International Universities Press.

Polatajko, H. J., Kaplan, B. J., & Wilson, B. N. (1992). Sensory integration treatment for children with learning disabilities: Its status 20 years later. *Occupational Therapy Journal of Research, 12*(6), 323–341.

Polatajko, H., Law, M., Miller, J., Schaffer, R., & Macnab, J. (1991). The effect of a sensory integration program on academic achievement, motor performance, and self-esteem in children identified as learning disabled: Results of a clinical trial. *Occupational Therapy Journal of Research, 11*(3), 155–176.

Posthuma, B.W. (1983). Sensory integration: Fact or fad. *American Journal of Occupational Therapy, 37,* 343–345.

Pribram, K. H. (1961). Limbic system. In D. E. Sheer (Ed.), *Electrical stimulation of the brain.* Austin, TX: University of Texas Press.

Reisman, J. (1993). Using a sensory integrative approach to treat self-injurious behavior in an adult with profound mental retardation. *American Journal of Occupational Therapy, 47,* 403–411.

Robichaud, L., Hebert, R., & Desrosiers, J. (1994). Efficacy of a sensory integration program on behaviors of inpatients with dementia. *American Journal of Occupational Therapy, 48,* 355-360.

Roley, S., Schaaf, R., & Blanche, E. (Eds.). (2001). *Sensory integration and developmental disabilities.* San Antonio, TX: Therapy Skill Builders.

Rood, M. (1954). Neurophysiologic reactions as a basis for physical therapy. *Physical Therapy Review, 34,* 444–449.

Royeen, C. B. (1998). Editorial: Four areas of sensory integrative scholarship for the next millennium. *Occupational Therapy International 5*(4), 49–251.

Royeen, C. B., & Fortune, J. C. (1990). TIE: Touch Inventory for Elementary School Aged Children. *American Journal of Occupational Therapy, 44,* 165-170.

Royeen, C. B., & Lane, S. J. (1991). Tactile processing and sensory defensiveness. In A. G. Fisher, E. A. Murray, & A. C. Bundy (Eds.), *Sensory integration theory and practice* (pp. 108–133). Philadelphia: F.A. Davis.

Schaffer, R. (1984). Sensory integration therapy with learning disabled children: A critical review. *Canadian Journal of Occupational Therapy, 51*(2), 73–77.

Schilder, P. (1964). *Contributions to developmental neuropsychiatry.* New York: International Universities Press.

Sieben, R. I. (1977). Controversial medical treatments of learning disabilities. *Academic Therapy, 13,* 133–147.

Soper, G., & Thorley, C. (1996). Effectiveness of an occupational therapy program based on sensory integration theory for adults with severe learning disabilities. *British Journal of Occupational Therapy, 59*(10), 475-482.

Sperry, R. W., & Gazzaniga, M. S. (1967). Language following surgical disconnection of the hemispheres. In C. H. Millikan & F. L. Darley (Eds.), *Brain mechanisms underlying speech and language.* New York: Grune & Stratton.

Stallings-Sahler, S. (1993a). Enhancing reimbursement for occupational therapy services using sensory integration procedures. *Sensory Integration Special Interest Section Newsletter, 16*(4), 4–8.

Stallings-Sahler, S. (1993b). Prenatal cocaine exposure and infant behavioral disorganization. *Sensory Integration Special Interest Section Newsletter, 16*(3), 1–4.

Stallings-Sahler, S., Anzalone, M., Bryze, K., Carrasco, R., & Pettit, K. (1993). Results of the 1003 Sensory Integration Special Interest Section Reimbursement Survey. *Sensory Integration Special Interest Section Newsletter, 16*(4), 1–3.

Stonefelt, L. L., & Stein, F. (1998). Sensory integrative techniques applied to children with learning disabilities: An outcome study. *Occupational Therapy International, 5*(4),252–272.

Thomas, J. (1995). AOTA efforts result in new sensory integration code for 1995 CPT. *Sensory Integration Special Interest Section Newsletter, 18*(3), 1.

Tickle-Degnan, L. (1988). Perspectives on the status of sensory integration theory. *American Journal of Occupational Therapy, 42*(7), 427–433.

Tickle-Degnan, L., & Coster, W. (1995). Therapeutic interaction and the management of challenge during the beginning minutes of sensory integration treatment. *Occupational Therapy Journal of Research, 15*(2), 122–141.

Trevarthen, C. B. (1968). Two mechanisms of vision in primates. *Psychologische Forschung, 331,* 299–337.

Vargas, S., & Camilli, G. (1999). A meta-analysis of research on sensory integration treatment. *American Journal of Occupational Therapy, 53*(2), 189–198.

Walker, K. F. (1991). Sensory integrative therapy in a limited space: An adaptation of the Ayres Clinic design. *Sensory Integration Special Interest Section Newsletter, 14*(3), 1, 2, 4.

Walker, K. F., & Burris, B. (1991). Correlation of Sensory Integration and Praxis Test Scores with Metropolitan Achievement Test scores in normal children. *Occupational Therapy Journal of Research, 11*(5), 307–310.

Wilbarger, P. (1984, September). Planning an adequate "sensory diet"- application of sensory processing theory during the first year of life. *Zero to Three*, pp. 7–12.

Wilbarger, P., & Wilbarger, J. L. (1990). *Defensiveness in children: An intervention guide for parents and other caregivers*. Hugo, MN: PDP Products.

Wilson, B., & Kaplan, B. (1994). Follow-up assessment of children receiving sensory integration treatment. *Occupational Therapy Journal of Research, 14*(4), 244–266.

Wilson, B., Kaplan, B., Fellowes, S., Gruchy, C., & Faris, P. (1992). The efficacy of sensory integration treatment compared to tutoring. *Physical and Occupational Therapy in Pediatrics, 12*(1), 1–36.

Wincent, M., & Engel, J. (1995). Vestibular and proprioceptive abilities in children experiencing recurrent headaches. *Occupational Therapy International, 2*(2), 98–107.

Mary Reilly

Julia Van Deusen

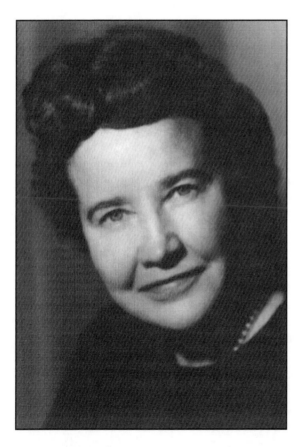

Man, through the use of his hands as they are energized by mind and will, can influence the state of his own health. (Reilly, 1962, p. 2)

Thi his oft-referenced quote from Reilly has been a guiding principle for occupational therapy. Reilly's belief in this thesis as central to the profession's survival led her to express this in her practice, education, research, and theory development, and also eventually resulted in her separation from the field. Nonetheless, her words are echoed and often cited by other occupational therapists and occupational scientists in subsequent theories related to human occupation.

Biographical Sketch

Mary Reilly was born in Boston in 1916. A major early influence shaping her scholarly career was her experience at Girls' Latin High School (W. West, personal communication, July 7, 1987). She became interested in occupational therapy (OT) while working as a camp counselor earning money for college tuition. There she became fascinated by stories of patients related by a fellow employee, an occupational therapist. Somehow, arts and crafts as media were never mentioned, so it was with much surprise, on beginning OT training, that Reilly encountered her first craft lessons (W. West, personal communication, July 7, 1987). She obtained her certificate in OT from the Boston School of Occupational Therapy in 1940 and for her first job chose to work with patients with cerebral palsy at a Crippled Children's Program in Michigan (Occupational Therapy Yearbook, 1957). Experience with these patients, as well as with soldiers with brain injuries at Letterman Army Hospital (Reilly 1956b), led to her early studies on the relevance of the central nervous system (CNS) to occupational therapy. Her sophisticated knowledge of neurodevelopmental principles and their application to OT was apparent even at this early stage.

During her years with the U.S. Army Medical Department (1941–1955), Reilly came to realize that a focus only on the CNS ignored the necessary emphasis on the development of patient skills and competence. Reilly's work with the Army began when she was appointed chief occupational therapist at Lovell General and Convalescent Hospital, Fort Devens, Massachusetts. From 1944 to 1946, she was OT consultant to the Service Command Surgeon's Office, Fourth Service Command, Atlanta, Georgia. In this position, she supervised OT at 2 convalescent, 11 general, and 6 regional and station hospitals. She also provided technical assistance for a War Department Technical Manual, a medical supply catalogue, and an apprentice-training course of study. For "outstanding devotion to duty and superior achievement," she was granted the Meritorious Civilian Service Award ("Meritorious," 1947).

In 1951 and 1955, Reilly obtained, respectively, a bachelor's degree from the University of Southern California (USC) and a master's degree from San Francisco State College in California. In 1959, she earned her doctorate of education degree from the University of California at Los Angeles (UCLA), where she wrote her dissertation on a theoretical basis of planned change in professional education. Following her doctoral work, she was made chief of the Rehabilitation Department of the Neuropsychiatric Institute at UCLA (Reilly, 1966b; *Yearbook*, 1972).

At UCLA, Reilly met the social scientist M. Brewster Smith, who had a major influence on her scholarly work. Basic ideas relevant to Reilly's work were Smith's views on intrinsic motivation and competence. He proposed that attitudes of self-respect and hopefulness are highly relevant to competence and that human beings are capable of actively constructing their lives in a dignified manner (Smith, 1974). In his foreword to Reilly's (1974c) book *Play as Exploratory Learning*, Smith concured with her underlying premises and expressed hope that "the efforts of Dr. Reilly and her collaborators will turn out to be a part of a new stream of interest in play as a scientific problem, and as a therapeutic and educational strategy" (Smith, 1974, p. 5). Although claiming the social psychology perspective of Smith as her primary influence, Reilly also credited the contributions of other psychologists, such as Jerome Bruner, Robert White, and David McClelland; vocational theorists, such as Donald Super and Anne Roe; and the founders of OT, such as Adolph Meyer (M. Reilly, comments on unpublished student paper, August 9, 1986).

Reilly began to associate with USC students while she was still at UCLA. After she assumed a full-time position as director of graduate programs in the OT department at USC, she influenced the work of her graduate students, which was to have a major impact on the field of OT.

Over the years, Reilly has received a number of honors for her creative scholarly activities. She is a fellow of the American Occupational Therapy Association (AOTA) and was awarded the

Eleanor Clarke Slagle Lectureship for 1961. She was named a charter member of the Academy of Research of the American Occupational Therapy Foundation (AOTF) in 1983, being cited for her exemplary contributions to "the development of a generic paradigm for practice" (AOTF, 1983). When she retired in 1977, she became a professor emeritus of USC. She also found an intellectual "home" at Oxford University in England, where she occasionally studied, lectured, and consulted (W. West, personal communication, July 7, 1987).

In her retirement years, Reilly has lost faith in the field of OT because she feels it has placed the interests of the profession over those of the chronic patient—that patient most in need of OT services (Reilly, 1984). Without benefit of the occupational behavior (OB) approach, the chronic patient is at high risk of becoming "a member of the hard core unemployable poor" ("To Treat," 1968). In fact, although Reilly has continued her interest in scholarly activity, she has abandoned the field because she perceives the reductionistic point of view as still inappropriately dominating OT (W. West, personal communication, July 7, 1987).

An early contributor to the professional literature (Licht & Reilly, 1943; Reilly & Barton, 1944), Reilly has been a colorful and creative figure in the field of OT. Her development of the paradigm of occupational behavior is one of the most significant influences on the evolution of the OT profession. When introducing a number of proposals for "modernizing" the field into congruence with OB thinking, Reilly stated, "To the rational who value the continuity of civilization, tradition means pouring the old wine of knowledge into the new bottles of contemporary issues and problems" (Reilly, 1971, p. 243). Reilly has succeeded in doing just that.

Theoretical Concepts

Foundations

The "occupation" in occupational therapy has been emphasized by Reilly from the time of her earliest scholarly work. In 1943, she wrote that the essential difference between occupational therapy and physical therapy (PT) was not that OT treatment is active and PT treatment is passive, but rather that OT's purpose is to help the patient integrate the fundamental motions elicited by PT into total activities (Licht & Reilly, 1943). This core concept of occupational functioning as the goal of treatment underlies all of Reilly's research. Addressing occupational therapists' use of splinting, she wrote, "I shall attempt to explore what I believe my role should be. This I shall do via a process of rational thinking based upon some soul searching" (Reilly, 1956a, p. 118). Drawing on OT's unique perspective based on observations of patient functioning, she concluded that appropriate orthopedic devices enabled patients to assume "their rightful place in life" (Reilly, 1956a, p. 132), that is, their occupational roles.

In her early writings, Reilly explored OT for individuals with physical disabilities (Licht & Reilly, 1943; Reilly, 1956a, 1956b). Her knowledge of neurophysiology made her realize that for those with recent brain injuries, participation in activities of daily living must be delayed; however, she never abandoned the central concept that patients must eventually perform movements voluntarily in occupational behavior (Reilly, 1956b).

Believing that the domain of OT is promotion of life satisfaction through occupational (work) and recreational roles, Reilly proposed to OT educators criteria for a curriculum designed to foster practice in performance of these roles (Reilly, 1958). According to Reilly, disease and injury can profoundly disrupt the self-actualization that one ordinarily obtains as worker and recreator, and OT restores the patient to these roles. A curriculum to support OT practice would use qualitative, quantitative, and historical perspectives to promote the critical thinking of students. Course content would include growth and development, neurophysiology, and psychology (Reilly, 1958).

In 1960, when Reilly first addressed the role of research, OT research was in its infancy. She felt that research, as well as educational programming, must address the central domain of occupational therapy. She argued that OT research should focus on such variables as achievement, creativity, and patterns of aptitudes, interests, and abilities relating to activities as a whole, rather than dealing with a specific modality, such as arts and crafts (Reilly, 1960).

Having long advocated the individual's need for productive and creative occupation as the core concept of occupational therapy,

Reilly was presented the opportunity to refine this concept as the Eleanor Clarke Slagle lecturer at the 1961 AOTA conference. Drawing on historical literature in the field, she formulated the central founding belief of OT as the previously quoted hypothesis "that man, through the use of his hands as they are energized by mind and will, can influence the state of his own health" (Reilly, 1962, p. 2). The major implication of this hypothesis is that the individual can manually and creatively "deploy his thinking, feelings, and purposes to make himself at home in the world and to make the world his home" (Reilly, 1962, p. 2).

In her Slagle lecture, Reilly considered the value of this hypothesis and whether 20th-century America was the time and place for its testing through OT practice. She argued that human beings have an intrinsic need to master and improve their environment through skills acquired in their various life roles, and that they suffer dysfunction and dissatisfaction if this need is blocked by disease or injury. Reilly proposed that the unique content of the OT body of knowledge was the nature of productive and creative occupation, particularly from a developmental perspective. According to Reilly, the treatment process should focus on work satisfaction and "the ability to experience pleasure in achievement, to tolerate the frustrations of struggle, to sustain the burden of routine tasks, and to maintain the level of aspiration within the reality level of work skills" (p. 7). The goal of the OT process is for patients to engage actively with their life role tasks. Treatment techniques should address the dysfunctions and difficulties people experience on coping with play, work, and school situations (Reilly, 1962). Reilly closed her Slagle lecture by reiterating the grand purpose of occupational therapy—to help patients influence the state of their own health—but she did not predict whether the field could or would be able to fulfill this mandate.

Published in the *American Journal of Occupational Therapy* (Reilly, 1962) and reprinted in Canada (Reilly, 1963), Reilly's Slagle lecture had a profound impact on the field. As her paradigm of OB evolved, it was fleshed out by her graduate students and cited and used throughout the United States and Canada (Madigan & Parent, 1985; Matsutsuyu, 1983; Woodside, 1976). In her position at USC, Reilly was also able to develop an OT graduate curriculum based on her occupational behavior point of view (Reilly, 1969a, 1969b).

Parameters of the Paradigm

Reilly (1969a) named four concepts as central to her paradigm: (a) the human need to be competent and to achieve, (b) the developmental aspects of work and play, (c) the nature of occupational role, and (d) the relationship of health and human adaptation. Although Reilly's work was not organized according to these concepts, they are clearly discernible in both her writings and those of her graduate students.

The basic premise underlying the OB paradigm is that human beings have a vital need to produce, to create, to master, and to improve their environment—that is, to be competent and to achieve in their daily occupation. And because human beings need to be competent, they also need to function in occupational roles, which are the vehicles for competency (Reilly, 1962). In the process of meeting their need for achievement, human beings acquire interests, abilities, skills, and habits of cooperation or competition that support their various occupational roles throughout the life span. Reilly broadly defined occupational roles to include preschooler, student, housewife, and retiree, as well as paid worker (Reilly, 1969a). Occupational choice is a key point in the occupational role developmental process, providing a bridge between the skills and habits of the child and the mature roles of the adult (Matsutsuyu, 1983).

It was Reilly's plan in building the OB paradigm to describe the aptitudes, abilities, interests, and motivational states supporting occupational roles at each stage of the developmental process (Reilly, 1969a). Only when normal roles could be understood at each stage would it be possible to identify and address occupational role dysfunction (Reilly, 1969b).

Reilly views the health of human beings in terms of level of adaptation to their environment rather than freedom from pathology. Occupational role dysfunction is the domain of OT. It is the responsibility of the occupational therapist to evaluate and facilitate the adaptive skills of patients who are occupationally dysfunctional. This responsibility entails maximizing the healthy behaviors of patients (Reilly, 1966b). A major hypothesis of the OB paradigm is that children's play, social recreation, and even chores are critical to the development of the adaptive skills necessary for competence in the complex work and daily living roles of adults. Play is a safe area for the child or adult who is occupationally dysfunctional to accumulate successful graded experiences for adaptation to life roles (Reilly, 1966a, 1966b).

Whether the patient is an adult or a child, the goal of OT is to assess the developmental level of the patient's occupational roles and to foster appropriate growth. Emphasis is placed on environmental support for achievement and an appropriate balance of daily activity. The occupational therapist becomes the advocate for patients to practice a healthy balance of work, rest, and play within the OT clinic, the institution as a whole, and eventually within the larger community environment (Reilly, 1966a, 1966b).

Reilly found the constructs of open systems theory and hierarchy useful in guiding her paradigm development because of their interdisciplinary nature and complexity (Reilly, 1969a, 1974b). Viewing occupational behavior from these perspectives allowed for both longitudinal and cross-sectional approaches to investigation.

Florey (1981) succinctly reviewed the constructs of open systems theory and hierarchy as they relate to the OB paradigm. The human being can be conceived of as an open system that evolves and undergoes different forms of growth and development. As an open system, the human maintains itself in relation to its environment via a process of input, throughput, and output of energy or matter. Growth or change, as applied to human skills, may occur in terms of amount or complexity of skill.

The concept of hierarchy relates to the process of change over time. This process is orderly but dynamic: Behavior changes from simple to complex and from less to more autonomous. Higher levels of behavior direct lower levels. However, lower levels serve to constrain the higher ones in such a way that a change at any level of the hierarchy will affect all levels. Thus, newer skills can emerge from the recombination, reorganization, and transformation of more primitive skills (Florey, 1981).

Work–Play Continuum

According to Reilly (1974a), "Play serves the function of adaptation by facilitating man's manipulatory and social skills and serves society by socializing the aggression of its members" (p. 113). An action and an attitude are both involved in play. The action must be voluntary, and the attitude is one of amusement, fun, and pleasure (Takata, 1969). The label given to play changes as the person ages: "play" becomes "recreation" for adults and "leisure" for the retired. Examples of activity that may be play are music, dramatics, games, and crafts (Reilly, 1974a, p. 60).

Because Reilly proposed play as the instrument by which dysfunctional patients could experience achievement and learn healthy adaptation to their environment, her major work concerned the investigation of play (Reilly, 1974a, 1974b). Analyzing play from the perspectives of the evolutionary biologists, psychologists, anthropologists, and sociologists, she concluded that play is "a behavior in search of an explanation" (Reilly, 1974a, p. 115).

Reilly described play as one of three subsystems of the imagination system of learning (see Figure 6.1). The other two subsystems are myth and dream. Although the other subsystems use words or visual images, play uses rules as symbols to represent reality. Through "doing" in play, human beings learn the rules of the hows and whys of objects in their environments. The result is the development of skills leading to competency and the mastery of the real world (Reilly, 1974b).

Within the play subsystem of the imagination, Reilly posed a hierarchy of three subsystems: exploration, competency, and achievement. Intrinsically motivated play that is undertaken for the pure pleasure of doing it is termed exploratory. It is associated with sensory, aesthetic, and novel experiences. Developmentally,

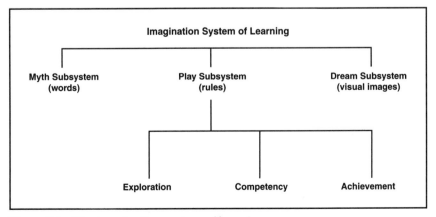

Figure 6.1. The imagination system of learning.

it is the early childhood stage of play. Although Reilly initially described the attitude developed by exploratory play as trust (Reilly, 1974b), she later posited that this stage of play generates an attitude of curiosity (M. Reilly, comments on unpublished student paper, August 9, 1986).

The competency stage of play comes developmentally later than exploration. It involves persistence and practice for task mastery. Although Reilly originally believed that it led to an attitude of self-confidence (Reilly, 1974b), she later described it as engendering hope (M. Reilly, comments on unpublished student paper, August 9, 1986).

The third phase of play behavior is termed achievement because it focuses on competitive performance and has a standard of excellence. Competition may be with self or with others (Reilly, 1974b). Reilly described achievement behavior as leading to an attitude of altruism (M. Reilly, comments on unpublished student paper, August 9, 1986). At this stage of play, the human has gained control over his or her environment. "The man who has played his way gradually and safely towards the skillful mastery of his world" is now free to show concern for others (Reilly, 1974b, p. 148).

The results of Reilly's intensive interest in play were twofold: (a) she derived a number of "rules of thumb" about play to encourage others to pursue this line of investigation, and (b) a number of her graduate students chose to study play as their thesis projects. Before Reilly's major publication, several students had already explored this area and thus contributed to the volume on play edited by her (Hurff, 1974; Knox, 1974; Michelman, 1974; Shannon, 1974; Takata, 1974).

Elaboration of Theory by Reilly's Students

Because the OB paradigm was only in an early stage of development, the studies by Reilly's students made major contributions to it. These studies were exploratory; they drew up principles of relevance to occupational therapy and described clinical applications in the areas of the work–play continuum, motivation and environment, and temporal adaptation.

Work–Play Continuum

Takata's research on play (1969, 1971, 1974, 1980) extended Reilly's research in this area. His six principles on play (Takata, 1971) guided the studies of other graduate students working under the direction of Reilly (Florey, 1981). These principles are as follows:

1. Play is spontaneous, pleasurable, complex behavior.
2. Play involves sensory, motor, mental, or a combination of all three processes.
3. Play can involve exploration, experimentation, imitation, and repetition.
4. Play integrates the child's internal and external worlds.
5. Play has temporal and spatial limits.
6. Play follows a developmental sequence. (Takata, 1971, p. 283)

Robinson (1977) developed the concept of the construct of rule. Rules organize information from the environment. Play is the arena where this learning can occur—where information on space, time, and interpersonal relations can be processed for daily living skills. Concepts of curiosity and conflict are key to understanding rule learning through play.

Michelman (1969, 1971, 1974) was interested in the relationship between art experiences and symbolic and creative development. From an extensive review of the literature, Michelman identified a six-step symbolic developmental sequence starting with scribbling and culminating in representational works.

Florey (1969, 1971) identified four principles from her study of childhood play as the critical arena for the development of intrinsic motivation:

1. Play is spare-time learning.
2. Play involves action on human and nonhuman objects.
3. Environmental conditions affect play. For example, anxiety inhibits and novelty facilitates play.
4. Constitutional deficits may interfere with play satisfactions.

Drawing on Reilly's ideas about the developmental nature of work and play, Florey also discussed variables critical for fostering intrinsic motivation in the older child and adult.

Florey's major contributions to the OB literature were a review of Reilly's position on play for an OT textbook (Florey, 1985) and an analysis of the studies on play done under Reilly's guidance (Florey, 1981). Florey categorized these studies according to the principles identified by Takata and provided information on their relevance to OT practice.

Other studies of play include those of Zorn (1969), who studied games as an arena for the development and practice of cognitive skills, and DeRenne-Stephan (1980), who used a systems approach to analyze imitation as a critical mechanism of play.

Because play is the antecedent to work, occupational behavior addresses the entire developmental continuum of play and work (Reilly, 1969a). Reilly urged the study of work–play phenomena in their environmental context. Although Reilly herself did not investigate the work part of the continuum as intensely as she addressed play, several of her graduate students focused on the aspects of OB more directly related to work.

Shannon (1970, 1972b, 1977) and Matsutsuyu (1971) shared and disseminated Reilly's view of the importance of the work-play phenomena for occupational therapy. Occupational choice, occupational role, and socialization are important concepts because humans being become socialized into their occupational roles (Matsutsuyu, 1971).

Shannon's work-play model (Shannon, 1970, 1972b) emphasized the kinds of work–play–social skills necessary for the adaptation of persons with disabilities to their environments. These work–play–social skills should be central to OT whether programming involves prevention, maintenance, or restoration. Shannon's (1970) model was based on six premises:

1. The human being is activity-oriented, and this activity consists of work and time free from work (maintenance activities and play).

2. A balance of rest, play, and work appropriate to each individual's needs is required for positive physical and mental health.

3. A deficiency in learning how to work or to play creates the potential for maladaptive behavior.

4. Inability to work or play leads to mental illness.

5. The hospital environment can contribute to the deterioration of work–play skills.

6. The primary objective for the hospitalized patient is restoration of function for resumption of daily living. (p. 112)

Although acknowledging the nature of the work–play continuum, Shannon showed particular interest in work adjustment programming for young men in the military (Shannon, 1970, 1972a, 1974). He identified the developmental tasks of adolescence, concluding that a common element was that of choice. Occupational choice involves a series of developmental stages spanning childhood play and adult work roles and ends in selection of an occupation. Shannon cited Eli Ginzberg's stages of the development of occupational choice (Shannon, 1972a). Briefly, these stages are a pretend, fantasy period based only on interests; a tentative stage in which alternative vocational possibilities are weighed; and a final stage when a single, realistic choice is made.

True to the open systems perspective, Shannon also reviewed environmental influences on occupational choice. Occupational therapy can facilitate the adolescent choice process by providing activities that foster self-discovery and decision making, that enable experimentation in work roles and the development of occupational skills, and that promote constructive use of time free from work.

Pezzuti (1979) centered her discussion of occupational choice on the female adolescent. She concurred with Shannon on the developmental nature of the process from the exploratory play of early childhood through the final phase of occupational choice. She argued, however, that women's dual role options—homemaker and paid worker—complicate their occupational choice process. The development of occupational choice includes three elements: (a) opportunity for a genuine choice; (b) exposure to appropriate work role models and role playing; and (c) participation in play activity for development of skills, values, interests, and cognitive realization.

Pezzuti found that the attitudes and skills that contribute to a sound occupational choice growth process at various life stages are trust (infancy); a sense of competence within immediate surroundings and motor development (early childhood); identification with role models and mastery of self-help skills (childhood); and rudiments of organizational, social, and work skill competencies (school age). By adolescence, a sense of competence in roles, independence from parents, and occupational choice should occur (Matsutsuyu, 1971).

A second work concept receiving the attention of Reilly's students was that of occupational role. Moorhead (1969) made a major contribution in this area, identifying the common elements among the various occupational roles, such as worker, homemaker, and retiree. These roles all serve as vehicles for self-identification and for identification within society. Early occupational roles—player, student, and others—influence adult occupational behavior.

Moorhead (1969) provided a list of variables critical to occupational role performance. Autonomy and independence variables include a realistic perception of one's own strengths and weaknesses and an ability to make firm decisions and manage time. Motivation and orientation to one's interests and satisfactions and appreciation of alternatives are implementation variables. Maintenance variables include standards and stability of work task behavior, performance under stress, interpersonal competence, work-play-rest balance, and ability to handle role conflicts. Moorhead (1969) also developed four categories for analyzing occupational role development: learning and socialization in childhood roles, issues around occupational choice, influences of environment on patterns of achievement and failure, and course of adult occupational mobility or solidification.

Reilly's students also build on each other's work. For example, Matsutsuyu (1971) cited Schmaltz's thesis project on the place of the socialization process in learning occupational role. The OT setting should facilitate role maintenance, learning, and relearning. Maintenance focuses on keeping intact daily living skills active. If a patient is assessed as able to learn new roles, occupational role development should be emphasized. If occupational role dysfunction is present, relearning may be the goal.

Motivation and Environment

A crucial concept of the OB paradigm is human motivation. Because of its importance, this concept was addressed repeatedly by Reilly's students (Bell, 1975; Burke, 1977; Florey, 1969; Sharrott & Cooper-Fraps, 1986). Motivation cannot be understood apart from environment.

Florey (1969) proposed that intrinsic motivation was the kind of motivation most relevant to occupational therapy. "Intrinsic motivation builds toward self-reward in independent action that underlies competent behavior" (Florey, 1969, p. 320). Satisfaction in completion of the activity itself is intrinsically motivating.

Because competence breeds competence, Florey (1969) described in detail the environmental conditions that foster competence in children and adults. Childhood play is vital to the development of intrinsic motivation. Environmental factors critical to play are the presence of humans and of novel nonhuman objects among familiar objects. The environment should allow for exploration, repetition, and imitation of competent role models, and should be free of such stresses as hunger, fear, and pain. For the older child, the environment should provide tools, instruction for useful productivity, and opportunity to relate to peers and to adult models of sportsmanship and craftsmanship. In adulthood, intrinsic motivation is related to achievement. Tasks should present challenges within the adult's range of abilities. The environment should foster responsibility for outcome and present feedback on results.

For some individuals, when there is a standard for excellence, competition fosters achievement (Bell, 1975). Therefore, competitive behavior needs a task-related, self-related, or other-related standard of excellence (Bell, 1975; Florey, 1969). Bell (1975) used the interrelationship between risk taking and competition to identify individuals for whom competition would be motivating.

Under Reilly's guidance, Burke's (1977) graduate thesis elaborated on the concept of personal causation—that human beings are motivated to interact effectively with their environment—as a means of understanding human motivation. This internal motivation is directed primarily toward producing environmental change. Feedback on the effectiveness of current behavior provides guidance for future behavior. Thus, adaptation to life's endless challenges can occur and humanity survives. Four theoretical statements by Burke (1977) underlie the concept of personal causation:

1. Success leads to feelings of success, which lead to more success.

2. Individuals who perceive they have control over their environments show active behaviors.

3. A belief that one has skills to address obstacles generates a sense of control.

4. A feeling of worth accompanies use of one's own resources to change one's environment. (p. 256)

Sharrott and Cooper-Fraps (1986) associated lack of intrinsic motivation with dysfunction in occupational behavior and presented two criteria—lack of satisfaction to self and lack of satisfaction to society—for determining such dysfunction. People can become dysfunctional if they do not derive satisfaction from their occupational roles, or if their role performance does not meet society's standards.

Reilly (1966a) was probably the first vocal environmental manager in the field of OT. Addressing the 1965 AOTA conference, she stated,

> We should be the first to realize that a hospital environment should be a place where the patient's daily living skill could be improved because of the environment and not despite it; and that the homes and the jobs or schools are progressive extensions of the same concepts. (1966a, p. 224)

Although little of the work addressing the OB paradigm could avoid the environmental context, several of Reilly's students chose to address this topic directly. Gray (1972) described conditions or practices within a hospital environment that can negatively affect such daily living (work–play) skills as self-care skills, social skills, and general or specific work skills. She also described those practices affecting loss of time, leisure time, and decision-making skills. Some practices cited are failure of staff to serve as appropriate role models, lack of patient evaluation in the specified skill area, and lack of encouragement for patients to practice skills in the hospital setting.

Parent (1978) reviewed the literature on the effects of sensory and perceptual deprivation and of immobilization and social isolation. The demonstrated impact of deprivation and isolation on the hospitalized patient provides support for the OT position that meaningful occupation is essential to maintaining hospitalized patients' functioning.

Klavins (1972) emphasized the importance of cultural influences on patient behaviors in occupational therapy. "As part of the human environment, culture is that special way of life which characterizes it" (Klavins, 1972, p. 176). Work-play behaviors are influenced by the values held by one's cultural group. Therapists must know, accept, and work within the value and belief structures of patients from a variety of cultural backgrounds.

Drawing on the research from the field of environmental psychology, Dunning (1972) developed a classification system for study of environments through analysis of their components: space, people, and tasks. She analyzed the space component in terms of territoriality, privacy, crowding, and objects in the environment; the people component in terms of social role relationships and social distance; and the task component in terms of potential use of objects and space, given their presence, availability, desirability, and feasibility. Dunning designed a grid showing the givens, possibility for change, and preference for change. She applied her analysis to psychiatric outpatients.

Temporal Adaptation

Although time is not a part of the physical environment, it is "the inescapable boundary for human existence and activity" (Kielhofner, 1977, p. 237), so that it is, in a sense, one's surroundings. Kielhofner (1977) treated the concept of temporal adaptation in depth as part of his master's work with Reilly. He derived seven propositions relevant to OT as a preliminary framework for the generation of treatment strategies and demonstrated their utility through discussion of case histories.

The first proposition describes the cultural basis of every person's perspective toward time. The second proposition states that the formal learning of the cultural notions of time is only part of the temporal training begun in childhood. Kielhofner argued that there are three levels of learning through which each person acquires a unique temporal frame of reference: the formal, the technical, and the informal. The third proposition incorporates Reilly's notion of life spaces and a temporal order to daily living. Time is organized around the life spaces of existence (self-maintenance), subsistence (work), and discretionary time (recreation and leisure). Health in relation to this aspect of time means a balance of life spaces consistent with the values, interests, and goals of an individual and of his or her society. The fourth proposition states that time for each individual is organized around his or her social roles, although these roles should not be considered as unchanging. Proposition five defines time use as a function of a person's internalized interests, values, and goals. According to proposition six, because habits are intimately linked with temporal functioning, they are the basic structures that order daily behavior in time. Finally, in proposition seven, Kielhofner proposed that the temporal dysfunction of patients may be a more difficult problem to address than pathology per se. The goal of achieving temporal adaptation is applicable to all dysfunctional categories of patients.

Application to Occupational Therapy

Educational Needs

For occupational therapists to base service on the OB paradigm, their educational training must be based on the OB perspective. The master's entry-level curriculum and postprofessional curriculum at USC, which Reilly developed, was based on that perspective in order to conceptualize from a frame of reference to better explain and measure OT and to challenge old values (Reilly, 1969a). The USC curriculum included content from the biological system of medical science, the personality system of the psychological sciences, and the social system of the social sciences. The medical sciences were part of the curriculum, but because of the fundamental difference between medicine's goal of reducing illness and occupational therapy's goal of reducing the incapacities resulting from illness, medicine was not a major focus. She believed that OT must decrease its "passive dependence upon the medical field" (Reilly, 1969a, p. 299). Emphasis was placed on the behavioral sciences because occupational therapy's major concern is the identification and treatment of occupational role dysfunction. Reilly made the behavioral science content relevant by selecting from many disciplines—anthropology, psychology, sociology, social geography, psychiatry, economics, political science, and law—those portions dealing with human behavior (Reilly, 1969a). Social psychology, particularly the developmental aspects of human achievement, was a core curricular area because the development of healthy adaptive behavior is a basic part of the OB paradigm (Reilly, 1969b). The rich heritage that Reilly provided continues to influence all levels of educational curricula offered in the Department of Occupational Sciences at USC.

Clinical Application

Without clinical application, a paradigm can have no value for a profession concerned with patient treatment. Reilly's OB paradigm has evolved along with OT service over the years. The best illustration of this symbiosis is Reilly's original psychiatric program at the Neuropsychiatric Institute (NPI) at UCLA (Reilly, 1966b). The NPI program was designed both to serve as a teaching model and to provide OT service to 100 psychiatric patients.

> The NPI model assumed as its foundation and first specification the need (1) to examine the life roles of patients relative to community adaptation; (2) to identify the various skills which support them; and (3) to create an environment where the relevant rehabilitative behavior could be evoked and practiced. (Reilly, 1966b, p. 62)

Occupational therapists functioned in clinician, administrator, and teacher roles. Evaluation of the NPI program showed that OT was an important service in the restoration of healthy adaptive behavior.

The NPI program was structured according to five principles.

1. Occupational behavior is developmentally acquired.

2. Patient programming should be graded from craft work in the OT clinic to work in the larger institutional environment to work in the community.

3. Occupational therapy must provide realistic decision-making arenas for the patients.

4. Because basic needs of patients in areas of food, shelter, and safety are met by other services in the hospital, OT should emphasize programming to meet cognitive, aesthetic, and self-realization needs of patients.

5. Occupational therapy should engineer a normal daily pattern of work, play, and rest for the lives of the patients and tailor programs to their abilities, interests, ages, and occupational roles.

Application of the Paradigm by Others

Assessment

From its inception, the OB paradigm has been intimately linked to OT practice through the development of assessment tools for clinical use. Line (1969) considered the case method to be the clinical problem-solving vehicle that was consistent with the OB paradigm (Line, 1969). Line evaluated the case methods of several disciplines and selected that of business administration as the model for OT. This method allows the professional to gain an understanding of the problem and develop a plan to solve it that maximizes patient assets and minimizes weaknesses. The case method as a problem-solving vehicle for OT was piloted by the OT graduate students at USC. The frame of reference was human adaptation to role expectations in work and play roles. Data were collected by direct observation, tests, interviews, and history taking, and were classified according to structure, function, expectancies, patterns of success and failure, and prior learnings and learning style. The data thus collected were organized into social, activities of daily living, and disease adaptation categories. Analysis of data led to problem definition and development of a plan of action. That plan seemed to be the weakest component in the pilot study for application of the OB method to occupational therapy.

The case method approach confirmed the need for assessment tools relevant to the OB point of view. Many of Reilly's graduate students conducted extensive literature searches to support the development of such tools. The purpose of their work was not to create rigorous psychometric instruments, but rather to develop tools to guide the data collection phase of clinical problem solving by a professional person knowledgeable about OB. Thus, the descriptions of the assessment tools were often illustrated with applications to patient case material. The flexibility of this approach to assessment allowed emphasis to be placed on the individual differences observable in human occupational behavioral dysfunction.

Various approaches to assessments devised by Reilly's graduate students, are briefly described in the following paragraphs. The reader is referred to the references for the detailed information necessary for clinical application.

Takata (1969) developed the Play History to identify the quality and quantity of play in children with multiple handicaps. It can be used to obtain a play deficit diagnosis. Matsutsuyu (1969) based her 80-item Interest Checklist on six propositions gleaned from a literature review. Interests (a) are family influenced, (b) evoke affective responses, (c) are choice states, (d) can be manifested in effective action, (e) can sustain action, and (f) reflect self-perception. Matsutsuyu's assessment tool also included a special interest section and a leisure-time history.

After an extensive review of the literature on interests, Borys (1974) investigated an indirect approach to interest study. She compared values of subjects showing a low interest in daily living (minimal activity participation, low curiosity, and low risk taking) to those with high interest. Low-interest subjects gave greater value to security, whereas high-interest subjects gave greater value to self-development and contributing to others. Thus, one of the measures of values evaluated in this study (the Buhler Life Goals Inventory) had utility for OT in terms of daily living interests.

Michelman (1969) developed a sequential growth gradient as a means of evaluating symbolic and creative development. She developed a brief checklist for assessing creative growth. Knox's (1974) Play Scale, which was based on normal behaviors of the child from birth to 6 years, assessed the developmental level of space management, material management, imitation, and participation.

Hurff's (1980) Play Skills Inventory assessed the individual's readiness to move into adolescence in sensory, motor, perceptual, and intellectual areas.

Pezzuti's (1979) self-evaluative tool provided information on the developmental task level of female adolescents.

Occupational choice and role were concerns of other assessments. Shannon (1974) designed the Inventory of Occupational Choice Skills with a companion rating scale. Black's (1976) Adolescent Role Assessment identified deficiencies in the occupational choice process by examining such issues as childhood-play, adolescence-socialization, school, peers, adolescence-occupational choice, and adulthood-work.

Moorhead (1969) developed an occupational history format centered around an analysis of childhood roles, the issue of occupational choice, patterns of achievement and failure, and occupational role mobility. Related to this assessment was a screening tool, the Occupational Role History (Florey & Michelman, 1982). This semistructured interview format contained questions about worker–homemaker roles and school. Role status could be classified as functional, temporarily impaired, or dysfunctional. Vause-Earland (1991) included these two tools in her study titled "Perceptions of Role Assessment Tools in the Physical Disability Setting."

Zorn (1969) provided guidelines to determine cognitive level.

Bell's (1975) five-question interview asked the participant to select low-risk, intermediate-risk, and high-risk items. An intermediate-risk score indicated that competition would motivate competent performance.

Dunning (1972) and Gray (1972) developed tools emphasizing the environment. Dunning's tool, based on her environmental grid, assessed the interaction between the patient and the environment. Gray identified the presence of depersonalizing conditions in the hospital environment.

Treatment

The breadth of the clinical applicability of the OB paradigm has been demonstrated by its application to other cultures and to diagnostic groups other than psychiatric inpatients. During the 1970s, the Canadian inpatient psychiatric service at the McMaster University Medical Center organized its OT program to be consistent with Reilly's OB paradigm. Subsequent developments of the Canadian model of occupational performance expanded upon Reilly's base (Woodside, 1976). Also, Kielhofner and Burke's (1977) model of human occupation germinated from OB.

According to the OB paradigm, deficits in OB result from genetic or environmentally elicited gaps in occupational skill development and from the effects of illness or institutionalization. It is the task of OT to fill the gaps or counteract the effects of illness.

Treatment goals include maintenance, correction, or new learning of occupational behaviors. Through assessment, development, and patterns of work–play skills, OB strengths and weaknesses and current and potential environments can be identified. Therapist attitudes that foster occupational behaviors include respect for the patient and faith in the patient's ability to succeed and live his or her own life. The occupational therapist needs to be the patient's advocate in changing the environment to support OB.

Woodside (1976) suggested five treatment guidelines:

1. Select and use activities that are interesting and challenging for each patient.

2. Use activity that reflects the developmental stages from playing with the activity to learning under a teacher to independent performance.

3. Provide the patient with guidance and feedback.

4. Teach general, transferable work skills such as relating to authority figures, rather than specific work skills.

5. Make the OT clinic a laboratory for human productivity. (p. 13)

Although originating with psychiatric patients, the OB paradigm has been clinically applied to several other occupationally dysfunctional populations. With young men considered to be juvenile delinquents, Paulson (1980) focused the OB approach on goal-oriented tasks in the problem areas of daily living skills, occupational social behaviors, and prevocational skills. The success rate, as indicated by active participation in vocational training, was 80%.

The OB approach also was found to be applicable to a young adult with mild mental retardation (Webster, 1980). Webster described a 20-year-old female who was assessed for her interests, abilities, skills, and values. Her assets and weaknesses were identified in terms of developmental level in the occupational choice process. To further development, treatment goals addressed her weaknesses, such as deficient money management skills.

Heard (1977) discussed the application of OB concepts to an adolescent with a chronic physical disability. She identified three critical points for the use of concepts of role in treating OT patients in the clinic. Roles cannot be fulfilled without the skill mastery that leads to automatic routines or habits. Role progression organizes daily living, and the ease of occupational role acquisition depends on the adaptive nature of the individual. Heard's assessment of a 17-year-old female with cerebral palsy revealed her strengths and deficits. Through OT programming, this patient was able to acquire the worker role of salesperson.

Conclusion

Reilly has had a powerful influence on the development of the profession of occupational therapy. Her work has generated numerous studies by students who have refined her theories, applied them clinically, and developed assessment tools for clinical use. Perhaps the most far-reaching consequence of Reilly's work has been the model of human occupation developed by two of her students, Kielhofner and Burke (1980). Chapter 7 includes discussion of this model.

Bibliography

1943

Licht, S., & Reilly, M. (1943). The correlation of physical therapy and occupational therapy. *Occupational Therapy and Rehabilitation, 22*, 171–175.

1944

Reilly, M., & Barton, W. E. (1944). Do's and don'ts in military occupational therapy. *Occupational Therapy and Rehabilitation, 23*, 121–123.

1956

Reilly, M. (1956). The role of the therapist in protective and functional devices. *American Journal of Occupational Therapy, 10*, 118–132, 133.

Reilly, M. (1956). Therapeutically influenced recovery. *American Journal of Occupational Therapy, 10*, 229–232.

1958

Reilly, M. (1958). An occupational therapy curriculum for 1965. *American Journal of Occupational Therapy, 12*, 293–299.

1960

Reilly, M. (1960). Research potentiality of occupational therapy. *American Journal of Occupational Therapy, 14*, 206–209.

1962

Reilly, M. (1962). Occupational therapy can be one of the great ideas of 20th century medicine. The Eleanor Clarke Slagle lecture. *American Journal of Occupational Therapy, 16*, 1–9.

1963

Reilly, M. (1963). The Eleanor Clarke Slagle Lecture. *Canadian Journal of Occupational Therapy, 30*, 5–19.

1966

Reilly, M. (1966). The challenge of the future to an occupational therapist. *American Journal of Occupational Therapy, 20*, 221–225.

Reilly, M. (1966). A psychiatric occupational therapy program as a teaching model. *American Journal of Occupational Therapy, 20*, 61–67.

1969

Reilly, M. (1969). The educational process. *American Journal of Occupational Therapy, 23*, 299–307.

Reilly, M. (1969). Selecting human development knowledge for occupational therapy. In W. L. West (Ed.), *Occupational therapy functions in interdisciplinary programs for children. Proceedings of the Conference, The Training Function of Occupational Therapy in University-Affiliated Centers* (pp. 64–75). Rockville, MD: Department of Health, Education, and Welfare.

1971

Reilly, M. (1971). The modernization of occupational therapy. *American Journal of Occupational Therapy, 25*, 243–246.

1974

Reilly, M. (1974). Defining a cobweb. In M. Reilly (Ed.), *Play as exploratory learning* (pp. 57–116). Beverly Hills, CA: Sage.

Reilly, M. (1974). An explanation of play. In M. Reilly (Ed.), *Play as exploratory learning* (pp. 117–149). Beverly Hills, CA: Sage.

Reilly, M. (Ed.). (1974). *Play as exploratory learning*. Beverly Hills, CA: Sage.

1977

Reilly, M. (1977). A response to: Defining occupational therapy: The meaning of therapy and the virtues of occupation. *American Journal of Occupational Therapy, 31*, 673.

1984

Reilly, M. (1984). The issue is—The importance of the client versus patient issue for occupational therapy. *American Journal of Occupational Therapy, 38*, 404–406.

References

American Occupational Therapy Foundation. (1983). Ayres, Reilly, Yerxa named to Academy of Research. *Occupational Therapy Journal of Research, 3*, 185–187.

Bell, C. H. (1975). Competition as a motivational incentive. *American Journal of Occupational Therapy, 29*, 277–279.

Black, M. M. (1976). Adolescent Role Assessment. *American Journal of Occupational Therapy, 30*, 73–79.

Borys, S. S. (1974). Implications of interest theory for occupational therapy. *American Journal of Occupational Therapy, 28*, 35–38.

Burke, J. P. (1977). A clinical perspective on motivation: Pawn versus origin. *American Journal of Occupational Therapy, 31*, 254–258.

DeRenne-Stephan, C. (1980). Imitation: A mechanism of play behavior. *American Journal of Occupational Therapy, 34*, 95–102.

Dunning, H. (1972). Environmental occupational therapy. *American Journal of Occupational Therapy, 26*, 292–298.

Florey, L. L. (1969). Intrinsic motivation: The dynamics of occupational therapy theory. *American Journal of Occupational Therapy, 23*, 319–322.

Florey, L. L. (1971). An approach to play and play development. *American Journal of Occupational Therapy, 25*, 275–280.

Florey, L. L. (1981). Studies of play: Implications for growth, development and for clinical practice. *American Journal of Occupational Therapy, 35*, 519–524.

Florey, L. L. (1985). Major theoretical approaches to pediatric occupational therapy. Reilly: An explanation of play. In P. N. Clark & A. S. Allen (Eds.), *Occupational therapy for children* (pp. 36–38). St. Louis: Mosby.

Florey, L. L., & Michelman, S. M. (1982). Occupational role history: A screening tool for psychiatric occupational therapy. *American Journal of Occupational Therapy, 36*, 301–308.

Gray, M. (1972). Effects of hospitalization on work-play behavior. *American Journal of Occupational Therapy, 26*, 180–185.

Heard, C. (1977). Occupational role acquisition: A perspective on the chronically disabled. *American Journal of Occupational Therapy, 31*, 243–247.

Hurff, J. M. (1974). A play skills inventory. In M. Reilly (Ed.), *Play as exploratory learning* (pp. 267–283). Beverly Hills, CA: Sage.

Hurff, J. M. (1980). A play skills inventory: A competency monitoring tool for the 10 year old. *American Journal of Occupational Therapy, 34*, 651–656.

Kielhofner, G. (1977). Temporal adaptation: A conceptual framework for occupational therapy. *American Journal of Occupational Therapy, 31*, 235–242.

Kielhofner, G., & Burke, J. P. (1977). Occupational therapy after 60 years: An account of changing identity and knowledge. *American Journal of Occupational Therapy, 31*, 675–689.

Kielhofner, G., & Burke, J. P. (1980). A model of human occupation: Part I, Conceptual framework and content. *American Journal of Occupational Therapy, 34*, 572–581.

Klavins, R. (1972). Work-play behavior: Cultural influences. *American Journal of Occupational Therapy, 26*, 176–179.

Knox, S.H. (1974). A play scale. In M. Reilly (Ed.), *Play as exploratory learning* (pp. 247–266). Beverly Hills, CA: Sage.

Licht, S., & Reilly, M. (1943). The correlation of physical therapy and occupational therapy. *Occupational Therapy and Rehabilitation, 22*, 171–175.

Line, J. (1969). Case method as a scientific form of clinical thinking. *American Journal of Occupational Therapy, 23*, 308–313.

Madigan, M. J., & Parent, L. H. (1985). Preface. In G. Kielhofner (Ed.), *A model of human occupation: Theory and application* (pp. vii–x). Baltimore: Williams & Wilkins.

Matsutsuyu, J. S. (1969). The Interest Checklist. *American Journal of Occupational Therapy, 23*, 323–328.

Matsutsuyu, J. S. (1971). Occupational behavior: A perspective on work and play. *American Journal of Occupational Therapy, 25*, 291–294.

Matsutsuyu, J. S. (1983). Occupational behavior approach. In H. L. Hopkins & H. D. Smith (Eds.), *Willard and Spackman's occupational therapy* (6th ed., pp. 129–134). New York: Lippincott.

Meritorious Civilian Service Awards. (1947). *American Journal of Occupational Therapy, 1*, 33.

Michelman, S. (1969). Research in symbol formation and creative growth. In W. L. West (Ed.), *Occupational therapy functions in interdisciplinary programs for children. Proceedings of the Conference, The Training Function of Occupational Therapy in University-Affiliated Centers* (pp. 88–110). Rockville, MD: Department of Health, Education, and Welfare.

Michelman, S. (1971). The importance of creative play. *American Journal of Occupational Therapy, 25*, 285–290.

Michelman, S. (1974). Play and the deficit child. In M. Reilly (Ed.), *Play as exploratory learning* (pp. 157–207). Beverly Hills, CA: Sage.

Moorhead, L. (1969). The occupational history. *American Journal of Occupational Therapy, 23*, 329–334.

Occupational therapy yearbook. (1957). New York: American Occupational Therapy Association.

Parent, L. H. (1978). Effects of a low-stimulus environment on behavior. *American Journal of Occupational Therapy, 32*, 19–25.

Paulson, C. P. (1980). Juvenile delinquency and occupational choice. *American Journal of Occupational Therapy, 34*, 565–581.

Pezzuti, L. (1979). An exploration of adolescent feminine and occupational behavior development. *American Journal of Occupational Therapy, 33*, 84–91.

Reilly, M. (1956a). The role of the therapist in protective and functional devices. *American Journal of Occupational Therapy, 10*, 118–132, 133.

Reilly, M. (1956b). Therapeutically influenced recovery. *American Journal of Occupational Therapy, 10*, 229–232.

Reilly, M. (1958). An occupational therapy curriculum for 1965. *American Journal of Occupational Therapy, 12*, 293–299.

Reilly, M. (1960). Research potentiality of occupational therapy. *American Journal of Occupational Therapy, 14*, 206–209.

Reilly, M. (1962). Occupational therapy can be one of the great ideas of 20th century medicine. The Eleanor Clarke Slagle Lecture. *American Journal of Occupational Therapy, 16*, 1–9.

Reilly, M. (1963). The Eleanor Clarke Slagle Lecture. *Canadian Journal of Occupational Therapy, 30*, 5–19.

Reilly, M. (1966a). The challenge of the future to an occupational therapist. *American Journal of Occupational Therapy, 20*, 221–225.

Reilly, M. (1966b). A psychiatric occupational therapy program as a teaching model. *American Journal of Occupational Therapy, 20*, 61–67.

Reilly, M. (1969a). The educational process. *American Journal of Occupational Therapy, 23*, 299–307.

Reilly, M. (1969b). Selecting human development knowledge for occupational therapy. In W. L. West (Ed.), *Occupational therapy functions in interdisciplinary programs for children. Proceedings of the Conference, The Training Function of Occupational Therapy in University-Affiliated Centers* (pp. 64–75). Rockville, MD: Department of Health, Education, and Welfare.

Reilly, M. (1971). The modernization of occupational therapy. *American Journal of Occupational Therapy, 25*, 243–246.

Reilly, M. (1974a). Defining a cobweb. In M. Reilly (Ed.), *Play as exploratory learning* (pp. 57–116). Beverly Hills, CA: Sage.

Reilly, M. (1974b). An explanation of play. In M. Reilly (Ed.), *Play as exploratory learning* (pp. 117–149). Beverly Hills, CA: Sage.

Reilly, M. (Ed.). (1974c). *Play as exploratory learning.* Beverly Hills, CA: Sage.

Reilly, M. (1984). The issue is—The importance of the client versus patient issue for occupational therapy. *American Journal of Occupational Therapy, 38*, 404–406.

Reilly, M., & Barton, W. E. (1944). Do's and don'ts in military occupational therapy. *Occupational Therapy and Rehabilitation, 23*, 121–123.

Robinson, A. L. (1977). Play: The arena for acquisition of rules for competent behavior. *American Journal of Occupational Therapy, 31*, 248–253.

Shannon, P. D. (1970). Work adjustment and the adolescent soldier. *American Journal of Occupational Therapy, 24*, 111–115.

Shannon, P. D. (1972a). The adolescent experience. *American Journal of Occupational Therapy, 26*, 284–287.

Shannon, P. D. (1972b). Work-play theory and the occupational therapy process. *American Journal of Occupational Therapy, 26*, 169–172.

Shannon, P. D. (1974). Occupational choice: Decision-making play. In M. Reilly (Ed.), *Play as exploratory learning* (pp. 285–314). Beverly Hills, CA: Sage.

Shannon, P. D. (1977). The derailment of occupational therapy. *American Journal of Occupational Therapy, 31*, 229–234.

Sharrott, G. W., & Cooper-Fraps, C. (1986). The theories of motivation in occupational therapy: An overview. *American Journal of Occupational Therapy, 40*, 249–257.

Smith, M. B. (1974). Foreword. In M. Reilly (Ed.), *Play as exploratory learning* (pp. 5–8). Beverly Hills, CA: Sage.

Takata, N. (1969). The play history. *American Journal of Occupational Therapy, 23*, 314–318.

Takata, N. (1971). The play milieu: A preliminary appraisal. *American Journal of Occupational Therapy, 25,* 281–284.

Takata, N. (1974). Play as a prescription. In M. Reilly (Ed.), *Play as exploratory learning* (pp. 209–246). Beverly Hills, CA: Sage.

Takata, N. (1980). Introduction to a series: Occupational behavior research for pediatric practice. *American Journal of Occupational Therapy, 34,* 11–12.

To treat not only the injury, but also the man . . . (1968). *Tufts Alumni Review, 14,* 22–23.

Vause-Earland, T. (1991). Perceptions of role assessment tools in the physical disability setting. *American Journal of Occupational Therapy, 45,* 26–31.

Webster, P. S. (1980). Occupational role development in the young adult with mild mental retardation. *American Journal of Occupational Therapy, 34,* 13–18.

Woodside, H. (1976). Dimensions of the occupational behavior model. *Canadian Journal of Occupational Therapy, 43,* 11–14.

Yearbook. (1972). New York: American Occupational Therapy Association.

Zorn, J. A. (1969). Research in cognitive assessment. In W. L. West (Ed.), *Occupational therapy functions in interdisciplinary programs for children. Proceedings of the Conference, The Training Function of Occupational Therapy in University-Affiliated Centers* (pp. 111–120). Rockville, MD: Department of Health, Education, and Welfare.

Gary Kielhofner

Patricia Scott, Rosalie J. Miller, and Kay F. Walker

· ·

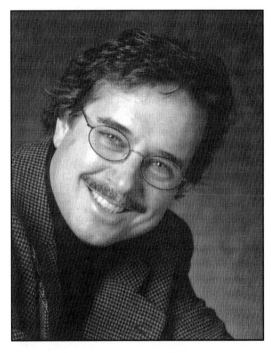

The real challenge for occupational therapy in the coming decades will not be to establish itself as the purveyor of science, but to use science to advance and document our practice. This will require a new approach to the development of occupational therapy knowledge in which theoreticians, researchers, practitioners, and clients work in partnership to shape the nature of practice. (G. Kielhofner, personal communication, October 22, 2001)

Gary Kielhofner, teacher, mentor, scholar, researcher, and writer, is best known for developing of the model of human occupation (MOHO). The central feature of this conceptual model is the importance placed on personal meaning and value of therapy in the context of the individual's life course. Kielhofner stresses the need to work closely with the individual to change from a maladaptive to an adaptive life course. His work has become widely read and discussed by occupational therapists and students, dating from the 1977 publication of his master's thesis in the *American Journal of Occupational Therapy*. Kielhofner has endeavored to document a theory that would provide direction and coherence to occupational therapy (OT) treatment. He and his colleagues have developed theory and researched how the theory was supported by practice. They have developed assessments to assist the clinician in gathering data needed to understand the client's function and dysfunction and to plan intervention that is most appropriate and meaningful in the individual's life situation. Throughout his career, Kielhofner has engaged in collaborative writing and research with colleagues, educators, clinicians, and graduate students in the United States and other countries. He has challenged researchers and educators to combine efforts with therapists and service recipients to validate assumptions about the role of occupation and the methods of implementing occupation-based practice to restore meaningful and satisfying lifestyles. Information regarding MOHO publications, research, and assessments is disseminated through the MOHO clearinghouse Web site (http://www.uic.edu/ahp/OT/MOHOC/).

Biographical Sketch

Childhood

Gary Kielhofner was born in 1949 in Oran, Missouri, a rural area on the northern edge of the Ozarks. He grew up on a 200-acre farm that his great-grandmother and great-grandfather (who came from Alsace-Lorraine, France) cleared from homestead woods. The local community was quite homogeneous and predominantly Catholic, with strong French and German ties. Kielhofner lived with his four sisters, paternal grandparents, mother and father, and an aunt. He worked on the farm before and after school and, like his father and grandfather before him, was expected to take over the farm.

When he was about 10, an incident happened that had a significant influence on him and his career choice. His grandparents were in a serious automobile accident. His grandmother, a vibrant, active woman in her 50s, sustained multiple fractures in one leg. She was in and out of the hospital for 27 months and stayed in a hospital bed in the family living room each time she was discharged. At the end of that long period, her leg was amputated, leaving about a 10-inch stump. She received only a few sessions of training with a prosthesis from a staff whose attitude was that "here was this mechanical thing she could try out. She fell a couple of times and that was it" (G. Kielhofner, personal communication, March 6, 1987). She spent the rest of her life in a wheelchair.

The experience of seeing his grandmother in a hospital bed and wheelchair, and observing the failure of her rehabilitation, not only had a powerful impact on Kielhofner's life, but also influenced his later thinking about OT theory. He came to realize that the context of the prosthesis was not defined in meaningful terms for his grandmother, as in "You've got to struggle with this situation and if you hang in there, ultimately you will be able to walk and go back to a lifestyle you had before and do all the things you've always done" (G. Kielhofner, personal communication, March 6, 1987).

Schooling

Also around the age of 10, Kielhofner felt a calling to become a Catholic priest. At 14 he went to live at St. Vincent's College, a high school seminary run by the Vincentian Order. He spent the next 4 years studying in the demanding classical tradition and living a disciplined life. He graduated in 1967 and entered the novitiate in Santa Barbara, California. Two years later, after a period of inner turmoil and searching, he left the seminary. He finished his college studies at St. Louis University in 1971 and graduated with a bachelor's degree in psychology. While in college at St. Louis, he was active in the peace movement and did volunteer work with rehabilitation patients at the Jewish Hospital. In his senior year, he was drafted. He applied for and was granted conscientious objector status (G. Kielhofner, personal communication, March 6, 1987). As his alternative service commitment, he arranged to work full time for half-time pay as director of recreation and an aide in OT at the Jewish Hospital in St. Louis. He described this job:

> I had no idea of what occupational therapy was, and I still had plans to go on and be a clinical psychologist. What the occupational therapists learned quickly was that I was good with my hands, so they started having me do things such as cutting out splint materials and working with patients in woodworking and leatherwork. There was no other male in the department, and we had a lot of young male spinal cord injured patients from rural Missouri. They were farm kids. They related to me, and the occupational therapists had me do a lot of work with them. (G. Kielhofner, personal communication, March 6, 1987)

Kielhofner was excited about the combination of using his hands to do things and working with patients. The head of that OT department, Sandy Liemer (now Malone), encouraged him to become an occupational therapist. In 1972, he entered the OT program at Washington University in St. Louis while still working at the hospital on evenings and weekends. At the end of his first year of the program, he went to the 1973 American Occupational Therapy Association (AOTA) Conference in Los Angeles. He was so impressed with Mary Reilly, the University of Southern California (USC) faculty and graduate students, and the USC philosophy that was a strong influence at that conference that he transferred to the basic master's program at USC.

> In the course of those two years Mary Reilly persuaded me to her essential theme, which was that occupational therapy needs to define what its business is, and that its business is dealing with people's everyday occupational problems and using occupation as a therapeutic media, and all that that means. (G. Kielhofner, personal communication, March 6, 1987)

Reilly had a tremendous influence on Kielhofner, as she had on many of her students. She helped him identify his strengths and weaknesses, and she demanded more of him than anyone had before. While writing his thesis, Kielhofner felt pushed to his limits, doing seemingly endless rewrites. He commented, "I remember times when I was so discouraged that I would think about 'what else can I do besides being an occupational therapist because I am never going to make it, it's impossible'" (G. Kielhofner, personal communication, March 6, 1987).

Kielhofner's master's thesis (1975) presented a history of occupational therapy and the beginnings of the model of human occupation, which he conceptualized as being in harmony with that history. Janice Burke, another master's student at USC, and Kielhofner became friends and enjoyed lengthy discussions about Reilly's theories and ideas of occupational behavior. After graduation in 1975, they coauthored the article (Kielhofner & Burke, 1977) "Occupational Therapy After 60 Years: An Account of Changing Identity and Knowledge" that evolved from the historical perspective encouraged in their graduate study.

Work

Kielhofner worked at the NeuroPsychiatric Institute (NPI) of the University of Southern California, Los Angeles, as a staff occupational therapist and coordinator of training from 1975 to 1979. From 1977 to 1979, he was also an assistant clinical professor in the OT department at USC. During his last 3 years at NPI, he worked on a doctorate in public health and wrote his dissertation, "Evaluating Deinstitutionalization: An Ethnographic Study of Social Policy" (Kielhofner, 1980a). In 1977 he married Nancy Croutt, the head nurse on the adolescent psychiatry ward at NPI. In 1979, he moved to Richmond, Virginia, where he took the position of associate professor and later director of graduate studies in the OT department at Virginia Commonwealth University (VCU). In 1982 Kielhofner's daughter, Kimberly, was born, and in 1984 he had a son, Kristian.

Kielhofner worked at VCU for 5 years until 1984. During that time he gave more than 40 scholarly presentations and workshops, edited one book and coauthored a second, and authored or coauthored more than 15 articles. In addition, in 1981 he received the National Merit Award for Outstanding Achievement from the American Public Health Association, and in 1983 he was made a fellow of the AOTA and received the Award of Merit for registered occupational therapists from the Virginia Occupational Therapy Association. In 1984, he was inducted as a charter member of the Academy of Research of the American Occupational Therapy Foundation (AOTF). During this time he also served on several national committees of the AOTA.

In 1984, Kielhofner moved to Boston, where he served for 2 years as associate professor in the OT department at Sargent College of Boston University. During that time he continued his extensive publications and workshop presentations.

Although he was not considering the position of chair of an academic department as a possible career move, he was approached by a colleague about an opening at the University of Illinois at Chicago (UIC). The opportunity to work in a setting with unusually rich resources and to influence persons as a mentor was attractive. He also wanted the challenge of trying to provide leadership as a scholar, in addition to being a manager. The position offered the opportunity to be in charge of both academic and clinical settings because, as head of the department, he would also be responsible for OT clinical services in the University of Illinois Hospital. The challenge of bringing academic and clinical pursuits closer was very enticing. In the fall of 1986, he became a tenured associate professor and head of the Department of Occupational Therapy in the College of Associated Health Professions at UIC. He continues as chair and is now both a full professor of OT and a professor of community health sciences in the School of Public Health at UIC.

In 1988, Kielhofner received the A. Jean Ayres Award from the AOTF for contributions to theory development. In 1991, he was the first occupational therapist to be awarded a fellowship from the Japanese Society for the Promotion of Science. It funded him to serve as keynote speaker to the 25th anniversary conference of the Japanese Occupational Therapy Association and to consult throughout Japan.

Professional Outlook

In practice at the NPI in the 1970s, Kielhofner worked hard to find creative ways to apply Reilly's concepts of occupational behavior (OB). He and Burke "started moving to do this intermediate theory that was between Reilly's occupational behavior paradigm, and what we called a model of practice" (G. Kielhofner, personal communication, March 6, 1987). He feels that some people misunderstood their efforts and thought they were trying to replace Reilly's generic OB theoretical formula with their model. However, many of Reilly's students before them had made significant strides in translating OB concepts to make them more applicable to practice. Similarly, Kielhofner and Burke integrated their ideas into a workable model (Table 7.1), which, after rejections for both presentation and publication, was finally published in the *American Journal of Occupational Therapy* in a series of four articles in 1980 (Kielhofner, 1980b, 1980c; Kielhofner & Burke, 1980; Kielhofner, Burke, & Igi, 1980).

Kielhofner considers the model of human occupation to be the centerpiece of his theoretical work (G. Kielhofner, personal communication, June 30, 1992).

I think the model sort of evolved and matured the way a lot of deductive theories have. We started with a set of ideas that we inherited from a tradition and tried to put them into coherent statements of relationships. Now we're in the process of trying

Table 7.1
The Model of Human Occupation

The model presents a series of theoretical arguments as to how the individual is motivated to act in a certain way. These arguments are organized to express the relationship between a number of concepts. These concepts are organized into three interacting subsystems which interact with the environment to produce behavior.

Human Occupation—The doing of work, play, or activities of daily living within a temporal, physical and socio-cultural context that characterizes most of human life.

Subsystems

Volition—A pattern of thoughts and feelings by the individual as he or she makes choices, experiences success or failure, and makes personal sense about what is happening around him or her.

Habituation—An internalized, variable predisposition to act in a certain way, guided by habits and roles.

Performance—Physical, intellectual, and social abilities that supply resources for action.

Note. Definitions from "The Model of Human Occupation: An Overview of Current Concepts," by G. Kielforner and K. Forsyth, 1997, *British Journal of Occupational Therapy, 60,* pp. 103–110.

> to link it to the empirical world . . . through research and test-
> ing. (G. Kielhofner, personal communication, March 6, 1987)

Kielhofner's efforts to revise, change, and correct the model have
involved the influence of mentors and colleagues, the collaboration with others in research and publications, and his own writing. Dialogue and debate with colleagues have helped him to examine his ideas. Gerry Sharrot, who died in 1986, was a friend
and colleague who shared Kielhofner's strong sense of playful-
ness about ideas. Sharrot was important to Kielhofner because
he analyzed Kielhofner's work critically, helping him become
aware of subtle issues underlying his thinking.

> I felt safer knowing he would help scout out flaws in my ideas,
> and he understood my insistence on the absolute right to dis-
> agree with myself after I had written something. His death is
> not only a loss to me personally but also to the profession.
> (G. Kielhofner, personal communication, June 3, 1987)

Kielhofner acknowledges that in his early years in the field
he put forth his ideas fairly dogmatically. Then he began to seek
to become more open and flexible in his thinking, drawing both
from research findings and from dialogue and debate with others in the field, such as Sharrot. As he said, "I'm realizing more
and more that there are very few black and white things in life"
(G. Kielhofner, personal communication, March 6, 1987).

Kielhofner states that he enjoys working with other therapists and developing collaborative relationships. For example,
while living in Boston, he was as a member of a group of theorists and researchers, including Cheryl Mattingly, who met to
discuss the possibilities of a clinical reasoning study. This planning committee initiated the AOTF-funded study that ultimately led to Mattingly and Fleming's (1994) work on clinical
reasoning in the profession. After Kielhofner moved to Chicago,
Mattingly completed her doctoral work at UIC and further developed the implications of the clinical reasoning study, a subject
that Kielhofner integrated into his work. More recently, he has
lectured and consulted in Japan, has spent much time in Scan-
dinavia, and is currently dissertation adviser to students in doctoral programs in Sweden, much of this work resulting in published doctoral dissertations. When asked if a lesson is to be

learned from delivery of health in other nations, Kielhofner responded,

> I had the good fortune to observe health care and occupational therapy in many different contexts. So much could be said but the following are some of my observations. From Scandinavia I have learned socialized health care that guarantees universal access is the only humane system. From South America I have learned that occupational therapy can be closely tied to human rights issues and the notions of liberation from oppression. From many parts of Europe, I've seen how therapy can be better tied to local culture and society. (G. Kielhofner, personal communication, September 28, 2001)

Kielhofner is a prolific writer who attributes his productivity to a passion for writing.

> I find it extremely exciting to formulate ideas and organize them into a written record. I also feel compelled to write because so much of occupational therapy wisdom exists in an oral tradition and has never been labeled and organized. (G. Kielhofner, personal communication, June 3, 1987)

His work, often written with coauthors, has appeared in 20 different journals. He also has made numerous oral presentations around the world.

In reflecting on his work, he hopes that by the time he leaves the field, the tradition of clinical research will have contributed an empirically sound practice model to the profession. However, he considers his model as only a portion of his work and he also sees his model as one among many that serve to guide practice. As he stated, "My work has been varied and multifaceted. . . . I have been concerned with both the broad sweep of occupational therapy knowledge development and with the development of one specific model" (G. Kielhofner, personal communication, June 30, 1992).

During the 1990s, his work was aimed at clarifying the model and developing assessment methodology to enable therapists to establish the therapeutic alliance necessary for effecting change. When asked to identify one accomplishment he was most proud of from the 1990s, Kielhofner identified his "mission" to connect theory to practice. He wrote, "I'm on a mission now to create knowledge in a way that moves to practice. I think it's a structural problem in how we generally create knowledge separate from practice" (G. Kielhofner, personal communication, September 9, 2001). Regarding future directions, he said,

> In the next decade (2000–2010), I plan to focus my attention on increasing both the empirical support for and the application for the model of human occupation. My focus will be on developing more and more specificity about the model's use in practice. I am working in several venues with practitioners to achieve this. Furthermore, I plan to continue research that demonstrates the value of this model in practice. (G. Kielhofner, personal communication, October 22, 2001)

Theoretical Concepts

Temporal Adaptation

Kielhofner conceptualizes time as a key determinant of how people sequence their selection of activities and maintain habits, and since his first published article on temporal adaptation, time has remained a central concept in the model. In 1977, Kielhofner won the Cordelia Meyers Award for "New Writer of the Year" from the *American Journal of Occupational Therapy* for his article "Temporal Adaptation: A Conceptual Framework for Occupational Therapy." Developed from his graduate study with Mary Reilly, this article described the concept of time and its meaning in organizing human activity. He presented a temporal frame of reference as a culturally determined perspective that is modified in action by each individual's own values, interests, and goals, which are naturally inclined toward a rhythm of self-maintenance, work, and play. Habits are the structures for organizing time in daily behavior, and social roles determine to a large degree what habits will be formed (Kielhofner, 1977).

In the 1980s, Kielhofner no longer saw temporal adaptation as a separate concept and incorporated it into the model of human occupation. He considered this concept to be a stepping-stone in his own thinking and a part of the history and development of the model (G. Kielhofner, personal communication,

March 6, 1987). Subsequently, Kielhofner (1995b) integrated the concept of temporal adaptation into what he calls temporality. He explained that human experience cannot be understood outside of the context of time. The personal meaning an individual attaches to an occupation is influenced by the time in which it takes place along with the way that life events are occurring in time. He still presents time as having impact in two spheres: (a) the use of time and (b) the occurrence of events over time and the influence of time on perception and choice. Modifications of the concept of temporal organization is an example of how Kielhofner has repeatedly refined and, as needed, redefined concepts in an effort to provide clarity, validation, and utility of his work. His concept of time can be understood in his citation of Adolph Meyers: "Time reveals itself as a vacuum, inviting us to fill it with doing" (Kielhofner, 2002b, p. 1).

Model of Human Occupation

Before describing the model of human occupation, we discuss the evolution of ideas about the nature of change from a systems perspective. This system-based thinking was central to the development of the model.

Evolution of Beliefs About the Nature of Change

In his first edited book (1983), Kielhofner's writings reflected the incorporation of general systems theory (GST), which had challenged traditional scientific thinking in the 1960s. He embraced GST as a departure from knowledge based on cause–effect explanations, stating that "reductionistic science begins with cause and effect empiricism and culminates in linear causal explanations," and this explanation assumes "that all the parts and their relationships can ultimately be reconstituted into an understanding of the whole" (p. 59). According to this perspective, "systems are conceptualized as irreducible organized patterns or configurations, rather than collections of parts" (p. 59) and are open systems of "network dynamics, gestalt functions, [and] autoregulaton" (p. 58).

In the mid-1990s, Kielhofner's writing incorporated dynamic systems theory and open systems theory in addition to GST, and he defined a system as a complex of elements that interact together to constitute a logical whole with a purpose or function. According to Kielhofner, GST seeks to explain properties across phenomena regardless of the type of system studied, and open systems theory describes these properties in living systems interacting with the environment. Additionally, dynamic systems theory, developed in the physical sciences, seeks to explain the dynamics within systems that result in the emergence and reorganization of a new, higher order, functional state of the system, arising from a former state of disorganization, or "chaos." This "order out of chaos" is achieved through the cooperation of separate properties in the system and has been referred to as "chaos theory." Dynamic systems theory has been applied to human behavior and, in the model of human occupation, is helpful in explaining adaptive behavior as a response that seeks to stabilize and maintain integrity of the human system (chaos theory) (Kielhofner & Forsyth, 1997) and in clarifying that the task and the environment are the stimuli to which the human system elicits spontaneous, ever-changing behaviors (dynamic systems theory).

In his most recent book, Kielhofner (2002b) developed these concepts further and described the principles of "emergence"—the "spontaneous occurrence of complex actions coming out of the interactions of several components without the benefit of a central controller" (p. 35)—and "heterarchy,"—the idea "that parts of any system will interact with each other in ways that depend on the situation" and "each component contributes something to the total dynamic" (p. 35). He gives the example of grasping a glass in which the hand spontaneously conforms to the object being grasped (emergence), and the central nervous system, the musculoskeletal system, the tactile system, and the environment (object to be grasped) contribute to the heterarchy for performance of this simple motor behavior. These concepts maintain and strengthen early descriptions (Barris, Kielhofner, & Watts, 1983) of how behavior cannot be understood outside the context of the usual environment and how life events that affect the individual at any point in time exert pressure on the individual to adapt to the situational environment.

Development of the Model

In the first of four seminal articles on the model of human occupation (Kielhofner, 1980b, 1980c; Kielhofner & Burke, 1980;

Kielhofner et al., 1980), Kielhofner and Burke (1980) stated: "The model presented here is preliminary and exploratory and thus incomplete. It will require substantial empirical validation and conceptual refinement. It is presented to stimulate, rather than confine, thinking in OT" (p. 573). This statement made in 1980 describes the ongoing development of the model. In the book, *A Model of Human Occupation: Theory and Application*, which Kielhofner edited, he and Burke provided the initial details and elaborated on the subsystem components that had been defined earlier (Kielhofner & Burke, 1985). Since that time, a second edition was published in 1995 and a third in 2002. These detailed revisions, as well as the research publications, reflect progress in empirical validation and revision of both the content of and the interaction among concepts in the model.

A basic assumption, which Kielhofner and Burke attributed to Reilly, is that

> all human occupation arises out of an innate, spontaneous tendency of the human system—the urge to explore and master the environment. The model is based on the assumption that occupation is a central aspect of the human experience. It is Man's innate urge toward exploration and mastery and his consequent ability to symbolize that makes him unique among animals. (Kielhofner & Burke, 1980, p. 573)

This interaction of the person with the environment is occupational behavior (OB). The model of human occupation seeks to explain how individuals make choices for participation in society based on their interests, values, and the environment around them. These choices occur relative to their physical capacity, their beliefs about their ability to succeed, and the degree of pleasure that will be experienced. Occupational identity, including the roles and habits associated with it, develops through doing activities over time. The resulting model seeks to explain human behavior as the interaction of three subsystems—volition, habituation, and performance—within the context of the individual's usual environment.

Human Subsystems

The volitional subsystem directs choice of an action, the habituation subsystem organizes activity to produce action, and the performance subsystem produces the skilled action to carry out the action. Actions are based on choice, are contextual to the environment in which they occur, and provide feedback to the individual. In the original conceptualization of the model, actions were described as "doing," the output as the behavior, as moderated by the person (human system) in response to influences of the environment.

The volitional subsystem comprises three aspects: (a) a sense of personal causation, which is the sense one has of one's efficacy—the ability to do the things that are valued and important—including the expectation one has about his or her likelihood of success or failure in the ability to direct one's own life; (b) interests, which are those things one finds pleasurable and satisfying; and (c) values, which are commitments and convictions that guide the sense of right and wrong (Kielhofner & Forsyth, 1997). As a result of volition, the individual makes occupational choices and establishes an occupational identity.

The habituation subsystem organizes behavior into patterns and roles. Its function is to allow for the efficient performance of routine behavior. By developing habits and internalizing role expectations, this subsystem produces patterns of action from a preconscious, automatic level, thus freeing attention for the person to respond to other environmental stimuli. Through habituation, the individual develops habit maps, which guide routine repetitive behaviors, and role scripts, which influence ways of acting that are both expected and socially relevant. The result of this subsystem is occupational participation.

The performance subsystem includes the mind (through processing of thoughts), the brain (through patterned messaging of the nervous system), and the body (with its musculoskeletal, neurological, cardiopulmonary, and other systems), which provide the material needed to perform the skills, which in turn are the basic abilities for action. The performance subsystem is thus the resource for occupational performance.

Development of Subsystems

The human infant enters the world as a totally undifferentiated open system (except at the cellular and organ levels). The first activity of this new human system is exploration. As the baby explores, it begins to develop skills. As these skills are repeated and practiced and the child develops competency and mastery (e.g., ability to place blocks on top of one another, ability to grasp a spoon), combinations of skills are put together and routinized into habits (e.g., brushing teeth, feeding self, dressing, walking, riding a bicycle). As time is spent in practicing the skills needed to perform an occupation, such as riding a bicycle, less attention is needed to perform the action. As the skill becomes habituated, attention becomes available to develop other skills. The child begins to develop an understanding of expectations for his or her behavior in certain roles (e.g., family member, sibling, friend, student). Finally, as the child is exploring and developing skills and habits, things are discovered that he or she likes to do or does not enjoy, and so interests develop. Through the interaction that the child has with the environment (physical and social) during exploration and development of competency and mastery, a sense of personal causation or a self-perception of how effective he or she is within the environment is developed. Through interaction with the environment—including family, community, and culture—the child develops values.

Kielhofner and Burke (1980) suggested that occupational therapy can take what has been learned about the various performance components (much of that information coming from the use of a reductionism perspective) and put it within the larger context of the system. Components of performance can be seen as being motivated and directed by habits and roles (habituation) and by values, interests, and sense of personal causation (volition).

The three subsystems—volition, habituation, and performance—organize and regulate the output of the human system. Each contributes to the output in a different way. The volition subsystem has the greatest degree of freedom; it is the level at which action is freely and consciously chosen. The habituation subsystem represents automatic and routine behavior. It regulates the output of the system into regular and predictable patterns. The performance subsystem organizes output at the lowest level, governing small patterns of skilled action (Kielhofner, 1995b).

These subsystems act in concert with each other, working together as one until pressure is placed on one system over another. An environmental event, such as peer pressure placed on a teen to try drugs, stresses the volitional subsystem. In this example, the person is faced with making a decision that stems from the challenge of values (it is wrong to take drugs) in tension with roles (these are my friends and I want to be an accepted part of the group). The volitional subsystem's specification of personal choice must resolve the tension between perceptions of what is right and good (values) and the internalized set of role expectations.

In prior work, Kielhofner understood the system as working with the rules of general systems, where the lower levels constrain higher ones. Under a hierarchical system, for instance, for the person who is paraplegic, the lower (performance) subsystem would constrain the higher ones (volition and habituation), no matter how motivated he or she was to learn to water ski. That is because, as Kielhofner previously believed, the motor performance component would be unable to function in the necessary ways. However, because the higher subsystems direct and organize the lower ones and because change can happen more quickly at higher levels than at lower ones, the person could decide to adapt the activity and learn to use a water sled.

Dynamic systems theory understands the relationship between the subsystems as having different levels of environmental demand that call the subsystems into play at different times. Using the previous example, if highly motivated (volition), the person would call on his or her cognitive problem-solving skill (performance) to plan an adaptive response to the environmental challenge. The occupational form of "water skiing" could be performed using a water sled. Conversely, if faced with the situation in which the person lacked interest, he or she would simply move attention to another, more motivating challenge.

As Kielhofner moved forward with his work, he addressed this concept of motivation as an important factor: "Motivation is still linked to volition. I see volition in existential terms. Essential questions to all of us are, what do we do well, like and value" (G. Kielhofner, personal communication, September 9, 2001).

Environmental Influences

The environment consists of objects, people, and events with which the system (the person) interacts, influenced by the culture of which that person is a part. Kielhofner and Burke's (1980) original conceptualization was that, "The open system interacts with the environment by way of a process of input, throughput, output, and feedback. The system represents Man, and the interaction of the system with the environment is human occupation" (pp. 573–574).

Kielhofner also suggested that this person–environment system changes and develops, and the three systems (volition, habituation, and performance), conceptualized as being located within the person, drive the balance of work and play through the lifetime. In the 1985 book, *A Model of Human Occupation*, Kielhofner stated that this process is explained through "blending of the occupational behavior and development perspectives in occupational therapy" (p. 77). He illustrated this concept, shown in Figure 7.1, and called it an "occupational lifespan theory" (Kielhofner, 1980b). This is the original graphic associated with the model of human occupation.

Kielhofner, in his more recent work, has presented a new graphic to explain motivators of performance and the conditions that contribute to behavior (see Figure 7.2).

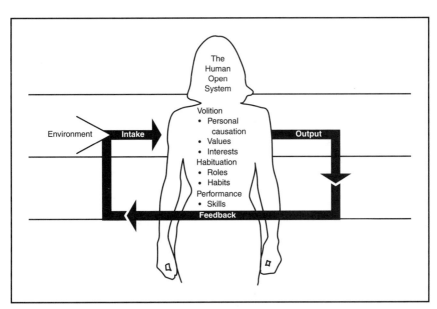

Figure 7.1. Open system representing human occupation. *Note.* From *A Model of Human Occupation: Theory and Application* (p. 35), by G. Kielhofner (Ed.), 1985, Baltimore: Williams & Wilkins. Copyright 1985 by Williams & Wilkins. Reprinted with permission.

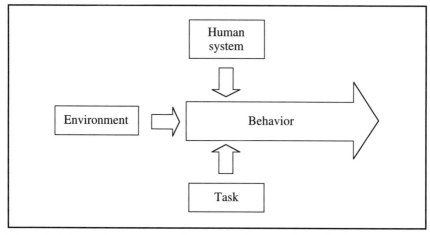

Figure 7.2. Behavior emanates from conditions to which the human system, the task, and the environment contribute. *Note.* From "The Model of Human Occupation: An Overview of Current Concepts," by G. Kielhofner and K. Forsyth, 1977, *British Journal of Occupational Therapy 60,* p. 103. Copyright 1997 by the College of Occupational Therapists. Reprinted with permission.

> While musculoskeletal integrity, cognitive capacity, motivation and other factors internal to the person are important to performance, they do not cause performance or behavior directly. Rather, the human system, the task and the environment together contribute to determine occupational performance. (Kielhofner & Forsyth, 1997, p. 103)

The difference is that in the early graphic (Figure 7.1), the person is portrayed as considering input from the environment, whereas in the more recent version (Figure 7.2), the person is motivated to perform in specific ways by environmental influences. This more recent portrayal of the role of the environment includes two components, physical and social, as well as the environmental impact—that is, the "opportunity, support, demand, and constraints" and the "interaction between features of the environment and characteristics of the person" (Kielhofner, 2002b, p. 103). To explain how the environment provides contextual influence, Kielhofner addresses occupational forms and occupational behavior settings.

Occupational Forms *Occupational forms*, a term first articulated by Nelson (1988, 1994) was adapted and redefined by Kielhofner (1995b) as "rule-bound sequences of action which are at once coherent, oriented to a purpose, sustained in collective knowledge, culturally recognizable and named" (p. 102). These occupational forms are "a way of doing something that is generated and stored in the cultural collective" (p. 102). When using the model of human occupation in practice, the understanding of occupational forms enables the therapist to appreciate individual motivations. Occupational forms, as convention for doing, have a set of rules. Appreciation for these rules assists the therapist in understanding how one individual may shun while another may seek engagement in a given activity, such as a bridge game. A therapist may notice that a number of individuals on the unit indicated interest in playing bridge on their interest checklist. The therapist arranges for a card table to be set up in a common area with cards and a score pad. The presence of the necessary objects presents an opportunity, and four people start playing. Soon one member of the foursome becomes agitated, insists the rest of the group does not know what they are doing, and storms off. The therapist finds out that the woman became agitated because the people she generally plays bridge with are very serious about a set of rules and behaviors not shared by the unit participants. The chatter from other card players interfered with this woman's attention, and she made mistakes. The need to adapt to the occupational forms of the card game challenged her performance system, resulting in her sense of inefficacy.

Occupational Behavior Setting The term *occupational behavior setting* refers to the "composite of spaces, objects, occupational forms, and/or social groups that cohere and constitute a meaningful context for performance" (Kielhofner, 1995b, p. 104). The importance of these settings is that they afford and press for behavior. If one does not have access to an occupational behavior setting, occupational performance is not elicited. For example, a man returning home from a cardiac rehabilitation hospital is restricted from driving for a period of months. Although he used to join the same friends for lunch every day and bowling once a week, the driving limitation has restricted access to occupational behavior settings (lunch and bowling with friends) that this man highly valued. He has lost contact with a social group and access to performance within a strongly habituated and valued activity.

Development of Change

In describing sources of motivation toward play, Reilly (1974) stated, "The readiness state of curiosity, it is speculated, has three hierarchical stages, namely exploratory, competency, and achievement" (p. 145). Kielhofner expanded on Reilly's three stages of motivation—exploration to competency to achievement—as the aspects of the volitional subsystem that internally drive the other two subsystems (habituation and performance) to change. Through exploration, one develops skills; through pursuing competence, one organizes habits; and through striving for achievement, one develops competent role behaviors (Kielhofner, 1980b). Thus, one explores and develops skills; then, motivated by the desire for competency, one develops habits; and, finally, motivated by the internal desire to attain a role in the social group—to achieve—together with the external demands of that group for certain behavior, one develops role behavior. This role behavior, when internalized, consists of a collection of role scripts, which guide occupational performance (Kielhofner & Forsyth, 1997). These three stages—exploration, competency, and mastery—"represent states of optimal arousal and involvement with the environment" (Kielhofner, 1985, p. 64). The states of occupational dysfunction that Kielhofner delineated represent stress and a lack of productive involvement with environment.

Occupational Dysfunction

Kielhofner conceptualized three states of increasing occupational dysfunction, starting with inefficiency, which results "when there is an interference with performing meaningful activity accompanied by dissatisfaction with performance. Sources of inefficiency may be environmental constraints, disease processes, or imbalanced lifestyles" (Kielhofner, 1985, p. 69). The second state of occupational dysfunction is incompetence, which is characterized by

> a major loss or limitation of skills, a failure or disruption of self-confidence and satisfaction, and inability to routinely and

adequately perform the tasks of everyday living associated with occupational roles. It may result from marginal learning due to poor environments, from disease or from a life-style, which erodes system organization. (Kielhofner, 1985, p. 71)

Helplessness is the third stage of occupational dysfunction. Kielhofner describes this as

total or nearly total disruption of occupational performance coupled with extreme feelings of ineffectiveness, anxiety and/ or depression. A state of helplessness may result from some traumatic episode, which suddenly renders a healthy person totally dependent, or from a lifelong series of negative experiences. (Kielhofner, 1985, p. 72)

In this hierarchical model, it is critical to determine at which level behaviors are disrupted and to begin with the lowest level of motivation. One must then manage the total environment of therapy so that the person is encouraged to explore.

The patient or client is not only the focus but also the instrument of therapy. Through engaging in directed occupations, the person begins to change their role scripts, more importantly their motivation to do things differently, to adapt, through engagement in a series of meaningful and satisfying activities. (Kielhofner, 1985, p. 74)

Once the patient's motivation has been engaged and exploration has begun, it is important to change the environment so that competence can be elicited. Then, once the patient has achieved a point of mastery, the demands of the environment must be "integrated with existing skills and habits to reach achievement of valued goals" (Kielhofner, 1980c, p. 737).

Application to Occupational Therapy

Assumptions

Three assumptions underlie the application of the MOHO in practice. As Kielhofner stated,

Reilly points out that occupational therapy is directed toward enabling man to fulfill his innate need for "occupation and . . . the rich and varied stimuli that solving life problems provides him." According to this primary assumption, humans are occupational creatures who cannot be healthy in the absence of meaningful occupation.

Reilly has also stated the second assumption: "Man, through the use of his hands as they are energized by mind and will, can influence the state of his own health." According to this assertion, occupation can shape the health of a person, and can thus serve as a means to health. The first two assumptions assert that occupation is both a basic human activity essential to health and a healing process.

A third assumption is that for occupational therapy to be instrumental as a means to an end, it must embody the characteristics of the end itself. This means that occupational therapy must be true "occupation." Therapy must embody the characteristics of purposefulness, challenge, accomplishment, and satisfaction that make up every occupation. Therefore, a theory of occupation is critical to practice.

The idea that, by engaging in occupation designed as therapy, man can restore, increase, and maintain his ability as an occupational creature is the foundation of occupational therapy. A theory of human occupation serves to justify the field's commitment to occupation as a worthy goal for therapy. It also demonstrates how therapy should be organized and carried out. (Kielhofner, et al., 1980, pp. 777–778)

Assessment

Kielhofner believes that effective therapy occurs when the therapist can identify the individual's existential view of him- or herself and then engage the person in meaningful occupations that allow participation in things he or she does well, likes, and values. His work with narrative, and incorporation of the narrative in assessment, reflects how the therapist in practice can obtain this essential information about the factors that motivate an individual to achieve meaningfulness in the therapeutic process (Barrett, Beer, & Kielhofner, 1999; Kielhofner & Mallinson, 1995; Mallinson, Kielhofner, & Mattingly, 1996). Assessment is a continual process of obtaining and thinking about data according to the MOHO (Kielhofner & Mallinson, 1995). Questions to consider include, "Is this person's habit pattern contributing to their substance abuse? How has the onset of chronic pain affected this person's enjoyment of previous interests? . . . Does this child hesitate to move because of the anxiety of being out of control?" (Kielhofner, 1995b, p. 189).

Given the contextual nature of human behavior, Kielhofner emphasized that assessment and treatment are interrelated. He specified four types of data gathering (Kielhofner, 1995b):

1. Therapists observe, through informal and formal structured assessment, what the person does

2. The person provides data to the therapist through verbal or written means

3. Therapists gain information from family, other staff, employers, co-workers or relevant others

4. Therapists observe the physical and social environment in which the person lives and performs. (p. 190)

A vitally important area of research is determining the reliability and validity of tests or assessment instruments used to measure model variables. This determination is a long-term process because many studies need to be done with any one instrument before it can be used with confidence. The Model of Human Occupation Clearinghouse, established by Kielhofner and colleagues in 1989, has been instrumental in the validation of clinically relevant tools for use in the specification of occupational dysfunction and the establishment of treatment approaches. Brief descriptions of the assessments available on the clearinghouse Web site (http://www.uic.edu/ahp/OT/MOHOC/) appear in Table 7.2. Although providing full descriptions of these instruments is beyond the scope of this chapter, a review of three instruments illustrates how the more recent assessments direct data gathering for ordinal ratings as well as understanding of the person's priorities. The three assessments selected for their prominence in the literature are the Assessment of Communication and Interaction Scales (ACIS; Forsyth, Lai, & Kielhofner, 1999; Forsyth, Salamy, Simon, & Kielhofner, 1998), the Worker

Table 7.2

Decription of Assessments Listed on MOHO Clearinghouse Web Site

Assessment	Appropriate Population	Description
Assessment of Communication and Interaction Skills	Adults with communication difficulties	Evaluates communication and interaction skills to accomplish daily occupations. Highlights the impact of communication deficits on task performance. Physicality and information exchange items.
Occupational Performance History Interview–II	Adults who can reflect upon and talk about their life history	Semi-structured interview and rating scales: Occupational Identity, Occupational Competence, and Occupational Behavior Settings. Guides clinical practice by eliciting life narrative.
The Occupational Questionnaire	Adults who can complete a written, 24-hour log	Self-report of typical or actual daily occupational activities over a 24-hour period. Ratings of personal experience in competency, value, and enjoyment in activities. Classification of activities as work, daily living, recreation, and rest tasks. Guides clinical practice by providing a visual record of time spent in activities, and of confidence and satisfaction in daily activities.
Occupational Self-Assessment	Adults and adolescents with cognitive skills to think abstractly and realistically appraise themselves	Self-report form that is easily and quickly administered. Explores a client's performance, habits, roles, volition, interests, and environment. Guides clinical practice by identifying a client's perception of his or her strengths and weaknesses, as well as priority goal areas.
The OT Psychosocial Assessment of Learning	Elementary students who are having difficulty meeting school expectations and roles in the classroom	Observational and descriptive (interview) assessment that evaluates volition, habituation, and environmental fit in the classroom setting. Assists clinicians in identifying a child's strengths and limitations within the school environment.

(continues)

Table 7.2. *Assessments Continued.*

Assessment	Appropriate Population	Description
The Pediatric Volitional Questionnaire–Revised	Preschoolers with cognitive or verbal difficulties	Play-based observational assessment designed to evaluate volition. Motivation, personal causation, values, and interests items. Guides practice by providing information about volition and recommends various environments.
The School Setting Interview	Students with physical disabilities able to communicate enough to discuss school experiences	Semistructured interview to assess student–environment fit. Identifies need for accommodations. Guides clinical practice by providing suggested interview questions; facilitates the impact of the physical and social environment on occupational performance, habits, meaning, and values.
The Volitional Questionnaire	Adults with cognitive or verbal difficulties	Assesses volition through observation. Evaluates motivation, values, and interests in three environmental areas: work, leisure, and activities of daily living. Guides clinical practice by providing information suggesting various contexts that enhance motivation and choice, and recommends supports to facilitate exploration.
The Work Environment Impact Scale	Adult workers with recent or current work experience	Semistructured interview that evaluates features in the work environment that support or impede occupational performance. Designed to be used with persons having difficulty on the job or persons whose work has been interrupted by injury or illness. The impact of the work setting on the person's performance, satisfaction, and well-being is evaluated with a 17-item scale. Guides clinical practice by indicating potential environmental barriers related to work task performance, job task/description, and objects used (tools, supplies, etc.), which may delay return to work.

(continues)

Table 7.2 Assessments *Continued.*

Assessment	Appropriate Population	Description
Worker Role Interview	Injured workers	Semistructured interview used during an initial evaluation. Evaluates injured workers in personal causation, values, interests, roles, habits, and perception of environmental support. Guides practice to focus on the effects of injury on the client, life outside of work, past and present work experience, and plans for return to work.
Pediatric Interest Profiles	Children or adolescents from age 6 to 21 years who may be at risk for play-related problems	Age-appropriate surveys to assess play and leisure through self-report and interview. Three levels of profiles: Kid Play Profile, Preteen Profile, and Adolescent Leisure Interest Profile.
National Institutes of Health Activity Record	Adolescents or adults with ability to read each question	Performance-based questionnaire that is most useful when it is necessary to quantify and identify changes in participation in role information on how the client feels about daily activities (meaningful, enjoyable), as in psychosocial disorders, and when disability results in changed role activities, perception about performance (difficulty, how well done), pain, and level and patterns of physical activity and rest.
Role Checklist	Adolescents and adults	A self-report checklist that seeks information about a person's past, present, and future occupational roles and identifies the degree to which the person values each role.
Assessment of Motor and Process Skills	5-year-olds through older adults with functional limitations on instrumental activities of daily living	Structured, observational evaluation that includes instrumental activities of daily living (IADLs) that vary in complexity. It evaluates the underlying motor and process skills needed to complete everyday tasks.

(continues)

Table 7.2 *Assessments Continued.*

Assessment	Appropriate Population	Description
Assessment of Occupational Functioning	Elders in inpatient settings; persons with schizophrenia or alcohol dependence	A semistructured, self-report instrument designed to yield qualitative and quantitative information about how a person is functioning relative to key components of the model of human occupation.
Occupational Circumstances Analysis Interview and Rating Scale	Broad range of clients with psychiatric or physical disabilities and who are able to participate in an interview	Semistructured interview, rating scale, and summary form to gather, analyze, and report data on occupational adaptation.
The Model of Human Occupation Screening Tool	Broad range of clients	Screening of occupational performance and comprehensive evaluation using various methods of data collection.

Note. Retrieved August 2003 from http://www.uic.edu/ahp/OT/MOHOC/assessments.html

Role Interview (WRI; Haglund, Karlsson, Kielhofner, & Lai, 1997; Velozo, et al., 1999; Velozo, Kielhofner, & Lai, 1998), and the Occupational Performance History Interview—Second Edition (OPHI–II; Kielhofner, et al., 1998; Kielhofner, Mallinson, Forsyth, & Lai, 2001; Lai, Haglund, & Kielhofner 1999; Mallinson, Mahaffey, & Kielhofner, 1998).

Assessment of Communication and Interaction Skills

The ACIS is an observational assessment designed to obtain information about how the individual communicates and interacts, and the impact of any problems on task performance. The ACIS is structured to recognize the importance of interests and values in the initiation of communication and interaction. The format includes observational rating scales with 22 skill items in three domains: physicality, information exchange, and relations. Physicality, the way the person responds physically to others and presents him- or herself, is observed in behaviors such as eye contact, posturing and appearance. Information exchange addresses the way a person speaks, the tone of his or her voice, and the manner in which he or she participates in a conversation. Relations, the manner in which the person has interchanges with others, is noted in collaboration, respect, and conformity to social norms. Knowledge of MOHO is essential for clinicians to meaningfully use the instrument and interpret the results. An example of an item in the information exchange domain (Shares: Gives out factual or personal information) is provided in Table 7.3.

Research on the ACIS includes a study by Forsyth et al. (1999). In this study, 52 occupational therapists, trained to administer the instrument, completed 244 ACIS batteries on 117 people with a variety of psychiatric diagnoses including schizophrenia, depression, eating disorders, and autism. Rasch analysis of the items' ability to measure both the constructs and the breadth of performance in the ACIS revealed that all but three items "fit" the Rasch model and reflected therapists' comfort and understanding in the use of these domains. This fit demonstrates internal, construct, and personal response validity of the ACIS. For the three items that did not fit the scales, clarification or deletion was suggested. While recommendations for revision were presented, the utility of the ACIS was supported.

Table 7.3

Example of Item from Information Exchange Domain of the
Assessment of Communication and Interaction Skills (ACIS)

Sample Item	Shares: Gives out factual or personal information.
Rating	**Criteria**
4—Readily and consistently shares, which supports ongoing social action.	• Identifies needs and/or contributes information and personal experiences in a manner appropriate to the situation. • Information does not offend others.
3—Questionable ability sharing; however, there is no disruption in ongoing social action.	• Observer questions appropriateness of information contributed. • Observer questions hesitation to give out factual information.
2—Ineffective sharing ability that impacts ongoing social action.	• Delays in sharing or fails to share factual information, which impacts social action. • Shares appropriate factual information, which impacts social action.
1—Deficit in sharing ability causes an unacceptable delay or breakdown in social action.	• Avoids sharing information when opportunity occurs (e.g., opts to "pass" on one's turn). • Refuses to/does not share information requiring therapist or social partner intervention. • Information shared may offend others causing an unacceptable delay.

Note. Adapted from *A User's Guide to the Assessment of Communication and Interaction Skills (Version 4.0) ACIS* (p. 38), by K. Forsyth, M. Salamy, S. Simon, and G. Kielhofner, 1998, Chicago: Model of Human Occupation Clearinghouse. Copyright 1998 by The Model of Human Occupation Clearinghouse. Adapted with permission.

Worker Role Interview

The Worker Role Interview is designed for use in conjunction with a more broad-scope test such as the Occupational Circumstances Analysis Interview and Rating Scale (OCAIRS; Model of Human Occupation Products, 2002) or the OPHI–II. The WRI, first developed by Velozo et al. (1998), is described by Velozo et al. (1999). This instrument, appropriate for injured workers, collects information about personal causation, interests, roles, habits, and perception of environmental support. It includes items that assist therapists to assess the client's ability and to make recommendations regarding return to work. Both the issue of appropriateness for return to work and the needed abilities are considered. A sample item about the individual's commitment to work as well as the importance placed on work from the values section of this instrument is provided in Table 7.4.

Table 7.4
Example of Values Item from Worker Role Interview (WRI)

Sample Item	Commitments to Work: The client's commitment to work and importance placed on work.
Rating	**Criteria**
4—Strongly supports: Item strongly supports the client returning to previous employment.	• Client historically has demonstrated a strong commitment to his/her job and to being a worker and continues to value work.
3—Supports: Item supports the client returning to previous employment.	• Client historically has shown a moderate level of commitment to return to work. While this commitment is not at a high level, it is adequate enough to support the client in returning to his/her job.
2—Interferes: Item interferes with the client returning to previous employment.	• Client historically has demonstrated weak commitment to his/her job and/or circumstances now appear to have reduced to how valuable work is for him/her.
1—Strongly interferes: Item strongly interferes with the client returning to previous employment.	• Client historically has demonstrated little or no commitment to working or presently sees limited value in working.

Note. Adapted from *A User's Guide to Worker Role Interview (Version 9.0) WRI* (p. 24), by C. Velozo, G. Kielhofner, and G. Fisher, 1998, Chicago: Model of Human Occupation Clearinghouse. Copyright 1998 by The Model of Human Occupation Clearinghouse. Adapted with permission.

Occupational Performance History Interview—Second Edition

Kielhofner views the concept of narrative as an integral resource for a therapist to understand how an individual's life events unfold in an ongoing process. Through understanding the individual's narrative, the therapist can better understand the person. This understanding enables the therapist to select intervention strategies to motivate the person and engage him or her in therapeutic change (Helfrich, Kielhofner, & Mattingly, 1994). Narratives can be used to help people to make sense out of their own circumstances, to motivate people to live their lives as unfolding life stories, and to establish guidelines to continue or remake these life stories as the individual desires. Kielhofner and Mallinson (1995) suggested guidelines for structuring questions in ways that will elicit the information needed to formulate these narratives (see Table 7.5).

Table. 7.5
Interview Guidelines for Narrative

Techniques Likely To Record Responses	Techniques To Elicit Information To Record Responses
Let the person determine the direction of the interview	Redirect the interviewee if he or she strays from the topic
Ask the person to expand or elaborate on an answer	Interrupt long responses
Make sure the person has finished what he or she wants to say before moving on	Make sure you get all the information needed to fill out the form
Show genuine interest in the person's point of view	Make sure you clarify; obtain the type of information you need to be accurate
Ask about changes in the direction of the person's life	Ask about goals while in therapy
Ask questions about specific events or circumstances	Ask about personal motivational qualities

Note. Based on "Gathering Narrative Data Through Interviews: Empirical Observations and Suggested Guidelines," by G. Kielhofner and T. Mallison, 1995, *Scandinavian Journal of Occupational Therapy, 2*, pp. 63–68.

The OPHI–II is used to rate an individual's performance and to generate a personal narrative and a graph of significant points in the person's life. An example of the graph is shown in Figure 7.3. The therapist collects information about occupational identity, occupational competence, and occupational behavior settings. An example of the item "Identifies a desired occupational lifestyle" on the occupational identity scale is given in Table 7.6.

Table 7.6

Example of Occupational Identity Scale Item from *Occupational Performance History Interview–Second Edition*

Sample Item Rating	Identifies a desired occupational lifestyle. Criteria
4—Exceptionally competent occupational functioning	• Extremely committed to current lifestyle. • Strong feelings about how to live life. • Identifies a strongly preferred future occupational lifestyle. • Identifies one or more very meaningful occupations. • Clear idea of priorities for structuring/filling time.
3—Appropriate, satisfactory occupational functioning	• Identifies a desired future lifestyle with some misgivings/dissatisfaction. • Adequate idea of priorities for structuring/ filling time. • Identifies one or more occupations that are somewhat important/meaningful. • Basically happy with current occupational lifestyle.
2—Some occupational dysfunction	• Trouble identifying desired future occupational lifestyle. • Major misgivings/dissatisfaction with current occupational lifestyle. • Difficulty identifying how to structure/fill time. • Trouble identifying/Lost enthusiasm for] current meaningful occupations.
1—Extremely occupationally dysfunctional	• Extremely unhappy with current lifestyle/routines. • Cannot identify a future meaningful lifestyle. • Cannot identify occupations that excite/fulfill. • Cannot envision how to structure/fill time.

Note. Adapted from *A User's Manual for the Occupational Performance History Interview (Version 2.0) OPHI–II* (p. 165), by G. Kielhofner et al., 1998, Chicago: Model of Human Occupation Clearinghouse. Copyright 1998 by The Model of Human Occupation Clearinghouse. Adapted with permission.

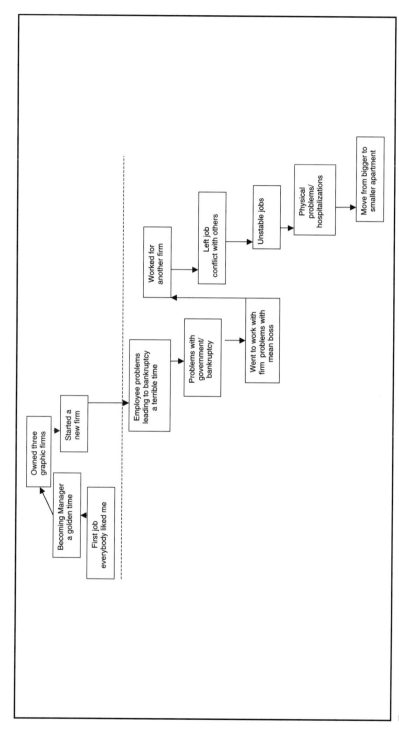

Figure 7.3. Narrative graph showing significant points in a person's life. *Note.* From: *A User's Manual for the Occupational Performance History Interview (Version 2.0) OPHI-II* (p. 94), by G. Kielhofner et al., 1998, Chicago: Model of Human Occupation Clearinghouse. Copyright 1998 by The Model of Human Occupation Clearinghouse. Reprinted with permission.

The initial development of the OPHI was supported by an AOTF grant in 1987 in an effort to develop a tool for practitioners across practice areas to assess occupational performance (Lynch & Bridle, 1993). Henry and Mallinson (1999) found that practitioners with grounding in the model of human occupation more reliably administered the OPHI. This finding supported the use of assessment and treatment relative to theory. The OPHI has undergone extensive revision (Mallinson et al., 1998), culminating in the OPHI–II (Kielhofner et al., 1998).

In a construct validity study (Mallinson et al., 1998), Rasch analysis revealed that the OPHI had three, separate constructs: occupational competence, occupational identity, and occupational behavior settings. (Table 7.7 describes the three constructs.) In a subsequent validity study (Kielhofner et al., 2001), scales of these three constructs were found to be valid across age, diagnosis, culture, and language.

The ACIS, WRI, and OPHI–II all provide rating scales. They are semistructured, with questions designed to elicit information. The commonalities of these assessments enable the therapist to assess the individuals they treat in the areas delineated in the model of human occupation. Use of these instruments requires therapists to be familiar with the MOHO and is very helpful to the therapist who is trying to understand function and dysfunction according to the model.

Intervention

The model of human occupation offers a conceptual basis for therapists to understand failure of occupational adaptation and to work to influence change; it does not specifically describe application of the model and treatment techniques. In this model, the therapist is portrayed as a guide who uses theory-driven conceptualizations of function and dysfunction to identify the direction in which a person is headed. The therapist seeks to engage the person to make the choices, actions, and decisions in a positive direction. Instead of treatment specifics, Kielhofner (1995b, pp. 253–267) offers a set of principles to guide intervention:

1. Therapy is an event that comes into a life in progress and must be understood and undertaken in that context.

Table 7.7

Items Associated with Competence, Identity,
and Occupational Behavior Settings Scales of the
Occupational Performance History Interview–II

Occupational Competence	Occupational Identity	Occupational Behavior Settings
Maintains satisfying lifestyle	Identifies a desired occupational lifestyle	Major productive role—social group
Participates in interests	Has interests	Leisure—social group
Works towards goals	Has personal goals and projects	Home life—social group
Fulfills role expectations	Has commitments and values	Major productive role—occupational forms
Meets personal performance standards	Recognizes identity and obligations	Leisure—occupational forms
Organizes time for responsibilities	Expects success	Home life–occupational forms
Fulfilled roles (past)	Appraises abilities and limitations	Major productive role—space and objects
Achieved satisfying lifestyle (past)	Accepts responsibility	Leisure–space and objects
Maintained habits (past)	Found meaning and satisfaction in lifestyle (past)	Home Life—space and objects
	Felt effective (past)	

Note. From "Psychometric Properties of the Second Version of the Occupational Performance History Interview (OPHI–II)," by G. Kielhofner, T. Mallinson, K. Forsyth, and J. Lai, 2001, *American Journal of Occupational Therapy, 55,* p. 262. Copyright by the American Occupational Therapy Association, Inc. Reprinted with permission.

2. The focus for change should be the action of process underlying the human system.

3. Change does not simply mean more or less; it means a different organization.

4. Change can and should occur in many aspects of the human system simultaneously.

5. Change is often disorderly.

6. Therapy should involve experimentation to find the best solutions.

7. The only tool that a therapist has at their disposal is to change the relevant environment to support or precipitate a change in the human system.

8. Changes in skill (as opposed to underlying capacity) should be the primary target of therapy.

9. Change in performance can involve learning to call upon different configurations of skills.

10. Occupations have a powerful influence on changes in skill.

11. Habits and roles are naturally resistant to change since their basic function is to preserve patterns of behavior; sustained practice is necessary to cement change in habituation.

12. Habituation organizes behavior for specific ecologies; new habits must often be learned in new ecologies.

13. The loss of roles and habits require swift replacement.

14. Acquiring a new role script and related habits is a process of socialization and negotiation.

15. Volitional anticipation, experience, interpretation, and choice are at the core of what is referred to as meaning of therapy.

16. Volitional change means finding a direction for one's personal narrative.

In the third edition of *A Model of Human Occupation: Theory and Application* (2002b), Kielhofner presents 16 chapters on client-centered approaches and case illustrations that follow the theoretical arguments of the model laid out in the first 10 chapters of the book. This configuration of theory and application is typical of earlier editions of this guidebook on application of the model.

In a study of validity and utility of Kielhofner's model, Munoz, Lawlor, and Kielhofner (1993) investigated how the model components were useful in assisting therapists to define and treat problems in occupational functioning and to define adaptive functioning. Therapist participants had more than 2 years of experience in a psychiatric setting, had formal education and/or additional training in the MOHO, and were self-identified as having been influenced by the model in their practice. Participants were asked to rank the usefulness of the major concepts addressed by the model, to identify other practice models used in conjunction with MOHO, and to identify the need for conceptual change.

The overall categories were ranked on a scale of 0 (*not used in practice*) to 4 (*essential to practice*). Findings revealed that general category average ratings—Interests, 3.54; Habits, 3.48; Roles, 3.48; Environmental System, 3.44; and Values, 3.32—were seen as more useful than the specifiers within the categories. Temporal Orientation, Perceived Incumbency, and Objects were ranked as categories only sometimes or rarely used. These findings clarify how therapists use the model.

Many therapists have published articles describing their use of MOHO in clinical practice for assessing and intervening in the occupational functioning of patients, including those with borderline personality disorder (Salz, 1983), those with multiple personality disorder (Sepiol & Froehlich, 1990), hospice patients (Tigges & Sherman, 1983), patients in chronic pain (Gusich, 1984), native Canadians (Wieringa & McColl, 1987), adolescents with diabetes (Curtin, 1991); young adults in psychiatry (Kielhofner & Brinson, 1989); adults with codependency (Neville-Jan, Bradley, Bunn, & Gheri, 1991); adults with alcoholism (Scaffa, 1991), adults in a day hospital (Gusich & Silverman, 1991), adults with HIV infection and AIDS (Pizzi, 1990), immigrant women in Canada (Khoo & Renwick, 1989), elders (Burton, 1989a, 1989b), and persons with Alzheimer's disease (Borell, Sandman, & Kielhofner, 1991; Oakley, 1987). The model has also been used to investigate adolescents' development (Blakeney, 1985); adults' anger (Grogan, 1991a, 1991b); child psychiatry (Baron, 1991; Sholle-Martin, 1987; Sholle-Martin & Alessi, 1990), adolescent psychiatry (Lancaster & Mitchell, 1991; Sholle-Martin, 1987), and early intervention (Schaaf & Mulrooney, 1989). These are a sample of the articles that have been published. For a complete list, the reader is referred to the MOHO Clearinghouse Web site (http://www.uic.edu/ahp/OT/MOHOC/).

Ethical Aspects of Assessment and Treatment

Aside from practical aspects of assessment and treatment, Kielhofner (1995b) emphasized the ethical responsibility inherent in intervention and the incumbent requirement to understand the interface of various forces in an individual's life. He noted that in the gathering and interpreting of data, therapists make moral judgments, and he referred to the work of Mattingly and Fleming (1994) on moral reasoning. This moral reasoning is reflected in the decisions therapists make as to (a) the best interests of the client and (b) a future state of affairs that is preferable to the current one.

Kielhofner (1993) wrote, "If we claim responsibility for the occupational welfare for members of society, we are also obligated as professionals to collect data on how social structures make possible or prevent adaptive occupational behavior" (p. 251). To exemplify this, Kielhofner (1993) took a stand that functional assessment "is often to determine what freedoms a person will and will not have, what roles he or she may take on, what activities he or she may do, and what benefits or resources he or she will receive" (p. 248).

He pointed out the variety of factors that affect performance and addressed the moral part of functional assessment. Functional assessment of work includes what a person can and cannot do (functional capacity), how this capacity influences what the person should and should not be doing according to his or her life circumstances (functional significance), and how this capacity and significance relate to what other interested parties want or expect from this person (functional interface). Factors of functional capacity, functional significance, and functional interface must all be considered before functional status can be determined (Kielhofner, 1993).

Thus, in the MOHO, data gathering is critical for the occupational therapist to develop an understanding of the status of the volitional, habituation, and performance subsystems and the individual's story, reflected through the ongoing narrative of the plots, twists, and turns of his or her life. From this information, the therapist develops a picture of the individual's level of occupational function or dysfunction. Intervention is then aimed at influencing a particular subsystem thereby effecting change.

In his work, "A Meditation on the Use of Hands," Kielhofner (1995a) described how individuals make choices as they adapt and readapt, and emphasized the need for therapists to understand and respect the fact that the loss or compromise of automatic, habituated movements can corrode an individual's sense of competence. This loss of competence challenges the individual's belief system. Consider the following scenario developed by Patricia Scott, the first author of this chapter:

> A young girl growing up depended on her mother to braid her long hair. Eventually the girl took over the task, both hands behind her head, fingers flying as she braided her own hair. The process of getting her own hair in order became important as the girl found straggling hair to be inconvenient and annoying. Over time, her hands developed intelligence, and she could even braid her hair on the sidelines of a soccer game while cheering for her teammates.
>
> The same girl, now a woman 50 years later, sits slumped in a wheelchair with tears running down her cheek. Her hair is disheveled, falling in her face. She just tried to bring both hands back to braid her hair, but her left arm stayed limp on the side of her chair. She mourns the loss of such a simple, automatic activity.

This passage illustrates a part of the story that reflects the woman's perception of the path her life has taken.

The model of human occupation specifies the components that motivate and organize performance. In his work on creating occupational life, Kielhofner (2002b) referred to defining events, in this case a stroke that changed the woman's story into one where simple activities, such as braiding one's hair, create a sense of incompetence. To understand this story, one must obtain information from a number of sources to identify the circumstances that changed the individual's life from an adaptive cycle to a maladaptive one. As shown previously in Figure 7.3, the OPHI–II includes a section in which the therapist graphs critical life events to ascertain a pattern and better understand the trajectory in which an individual is headed. When the integrity of the human system is compromised, the therapist's challenge is to achieve an understanding of how an individual system is disrupted and can be meaningfully restored, and then to structure participation in a series of occupations with the intent to restore and develop the individual's belief that he or she can perform the occupation. Although the individual's performance may differ from before the illness, elements that are important and valuable to the individual may be retained.

A qualitative study (Borrell, Gustavsson, Sandman, & Kiel-hofner, 1994) highlights the economic pressure on therapists to involve people in groups versus individual treatment. In this study, 4 elders with Alzheimer's disease, living independently in their own homes, attended a day treatment program. One objective of the program was to promote this independence. Engagement in activity was considered to be a critical component of day treatment, as was compliance with a group activity program that was controlled and structured by the staff. This environment had an impact on the way the elders responded by constraining individual initiative and spontaneity. These 4 individuals, otherwise capable of independent action and decision making, acted in a passive manner, in compliance with the staff's expectations.

Establishing the parameters of therapeutic activities prior to assessing individuals' needs can lead to routinized treatment, exemplified by the use of "canned" treatment goals and protocols in attempts to reduce a preconceived notion of deficits. For example, loss of initiative is a classic symptom of depression. The therapist's treatment plan may therefore address the decrease in initiative. Initiative is understood in the model of human occupation as pressure from the environment to "do" something. The quality of this doing is dependent on motivation, which is tied to an individual's interests, values, and goals. The therapist, therefore, cannot design an effective strategy to improve initiation without determining what is motivating for each individual. As Rogers and Kielhofner (1985) wrote, "The choice to effectively occupy oneself comes from a sense of personal freedom. The patient must ultimately will the action, which is undertaken as part of the clinical process, or else true change cannot result" (p. 145).

Theory Validation and Research

Research on Basic Aspects of the Model

Investigations on the model of human occupation include five types of research studies (Kielhofner, 2002b): content validity, correlative, comparative, prospective, and qualitative. We briefly define (using definitions given by Portney & Watkins, 2000) and provide one or more examples of each. For abstracts of 80 research studies published since 1980, most from 1999 through 2001, the reader is referred to the third edition of *A Model of Human Occupation* (Kielhofner, 2002b). New research is being generated and the most up-to-date complete list of publications is found on the MOHO Clearinghouse Web site (http://www.uic.edu/ahp/OT/MOHO/).

Construct validity refers to the extent to which a theoretical concept is measured by a test instrument. The process of construct validity includes definition of what is and what is not included in the construct, and what behaviors manifest or do not manifest the construct, or what dimensions would result in high or low scores on a test. An example of this type of study is the concept of occupational identity that was delineated in an investigation of the OPHI when it became clear that occupational adaptation reflected two concepts: occupational identity and competence (Mallinson et al., 1998).

Correlative studies are descriptive studies that investigate the relationship of model variables and test whether they are related in the way the model suggests. Such studies test the relationship between the human system and the environment. For example, life satisfaction in 79 elder adults was significantly correlated with meaningfulness of activities but not with age and length of retirement (Gregory, 1983). Elliott and Barris (1987) found a positive relationship between life satisfaction and the number and value of roles performed by 185 noninstitutionalized elders. In an investigation of the volition subsystem, activity pattern, and life satisfaction of 60 elders, positive correlations were found among degree of interests, value, and personal causation, and life satisfaction was more influenced by time spent in work and leisure than by time spent in activities of daily living and rest (Smith, Kielhofner, & Watts, 1986). In contrast to these relationships, a study of 129 elders living independently found no significant correlations between life satisfaction and value, interests, and personal causation (Knapp, 1983).

Comparative studies help to differentiate the presence or absence of a variable in two groups of individuals or in separate concepts of a theory. Comparative studies of different groups of individuals ascertain whether groups differ on selected variables as the model predicts. For example, comparisons of volitional and habituation subsystems yielded significant group differences in a number of studies: 50 adults 18 to 25 years of age, 25 with and 25 without alcoholism, differed in the habituation subsystem (Scaffa, 1981); 37 adolescents in psychiatric facilities and 36 high school students differed in locus of control, in self-esteem, and in potency of interests and value placed on roles and number of present roles (Smyntek, Barris, & Kielhofner, 1985); and 10 high school students, 10 adolescents hospitalized for psychosocial problems in conjunction with a primary medical diagnosis, and 10 adolescents hospitalized with a primary psychosocial diagnosis differed in locus of control (Barris et al., 1986). In contrast to these findings, no significant differences were found in selected volitional traits of 10 employed and 18 unemployed young adults with mental retardation (Lyons, 1983) or in locus of control, values, and perceptual motor skills between 15 delinquent and 15 nondelinquent adolescents (Lederer, Kielhofner, & Watts, 1985).

Prospective studies assess how well the construct or test results predict future performance. Thus, these studies are used to predict to what extent a current measure of a MOHO concept would predict some status of that concept in the future. For example, volition predicted compliance with home exercise programs in 62 outpatients in upper extremity rehabilitation (Chen, Neufeld, Feely, & Skinner, 1999), whereas number of roles and leisure values predicted physical activity levels in 140 adult women (Rust, Barris, & Hooper, 1987).

Qualitative studies (Kielhofner, 1982a, 1982b) seek to explore and describe phenomena or aspects of a theory as they occur in their natural state and help, in this case, to test assumptions of the model of human occupation (i.e., Does development of adjustment to disability actually occur the way the model would suggest?) and to look at apparent relationships of observations. In studies in 1994, Kielhofner and colleagues (Helfrich & Kielhofner, 1994; Helfrich et al., 1994) articulated how the individual's life story is operationalized in volitional narratives. In a longitudinal study of retirees in Sweden, Jonsson, Josephsson, and Kielhofner (2001) and Jonsson, Kielhofner, and Borell (1997) explored how volitional narrative helps to understand the changes in life events that unfold over time. Sixteen men and 16 women were randomly selected from a group of 63-year-old workers, who were within 2 years of the expected retirement age of 65. They were interviewed about their thoughts, plans, and expectations about retirement, as well as their valuing of work and overall opinion of what life would be like as a retiree. The researchers generated stories and used comparative analysis to assess attitudes about retirement as stable, progressive, or regressive in regard to the direction the quality of life would take, and attitudes about other activities as potential replacements for work. Two years later, a follow-up of 29 participants found that for 20 people, the anticipated events had taken place, whereas for 9 participants, their anticipated events were shaped by life events, personal actions, and unexpected experiences in retirement. The implications of these findings to occupational therapy reinforce both the stability of the individual's occupational expectations and opportunities for change given therapeutic intervention. The strength of a longitudinal design and the plan for a third follow-up make a positive move in the direction of establishing validity for the constructs of the model, as well as shedding insight on the types of events that influence a change in anticipation of outcome.

The contradictory and limited findings of studies can be attributed to several factors, including extant status of the validity and reliability of assessment tools when the studies were done. Second, tools used that were developed outside the tradition of the model of human occupation may not measure the appropriate variables within the model. Third, some studies, such as those that were master's research projects, may have limited control for variables, number of subjects, and subject selection procedures. Studies of the efficacy of the model conducted prior to the 1990s were limited by too little testing of postulates with too few subjects and with inadequately developed testing instruments.

Research on Applications of the Model

In addition to research on basic MOHO attributes, Kielhofner (2002b) categorized several types of investigations of the use of the model in practice: test development, therapeutic reasoning, therapy processes, and therapy outcomes. Test development involves the examination of psychometric properties of instruments and is exemplified in the refinement and revisions of the OPHI (Henry & Mallinson, 1999; Kielhofner et al., 2001; Lynch & Bridle, 1993; Mallinson et al., 1998), which were discussed earlier in this chapter.

Investigating how the model influences therapeutic reasoning provides insights into the impact of the model on the therapist's thinking in the conduct of the therapeutic process. In a qualitative study of 4 therapists, Fossey (1996) described the therapists' clinical reasoning, interactive reasoning, and professional values in the use of a semistructured tool for client interview (the OPHI) with clients in a psychiatric day hospital.

The studies of therapy processes seek to determine what goes on in therapy that does or does not effect change. An example is Barrett et al.'s (1999) qualitative study of a single client over several months that revealed the influence of the client's narrative on the directions in the therapy process.

Outcome studies seek to determine the efficacy of the model for use in therapy and answers the question as to whether the use of the concepts leads to the desired results. For example, DeForest, Watts, and Madigan (1991) examined the issue of resonance—that change in one part of the system affects other parts—by testing whether development of new performance subsystem skills can have a positive impact on the volitional system. They found that participants experienced positive changes in their belief in their skills (volitional system), apparently through their successful performance in craft activities.

Knowledge for the Profession

In the preface to *Conceptual Foundations of Occupational Therapy* (1997), Kielhofner wrote, "I have struggled throughout my professional life with the problem of how we might properly think about the range of knowledge within occupational therapy" (p. viii). He explained that this has been such a strong concern of his because it has a direct impact on professional identity.

> Professional identity is founded on the paradigmatic constructs, viewpoint, and values that bind members of a profession together and give the profession a public identity. While each occupational therapist's identity comes from a unique set of personal experiences, it is ultimately shaped by the profession's paradigm. (p. 303)

Kielhofner (1997) proposed a three-layered sphere to visualize the organization of the field's knowledge. The central core of this sphere is the *paradigm*—the assumptions, point of view, and values shared by all occupational therapists. "It influences what problems the therapist addresses, how those problems are conceived, and what methods the therapist employs to resolve the problems" (p. 21). Surrounding the core is the layer called *conceptual practice models*. Whereas the paradigm is general and gives coherence to the whole profession in all its diversity, practice models "provide specific prescriptions for practice" (p. 22): biomechanical, cognitive disabilities, cognitive–perceptual, group work, human occupation, motor control, sensory integration, and spatiotemporal adaptation. The outside band, termed *related knowledge of the field*, consists of information and techniques from other fields "to support practice, research and other activities of the field" (p. 25).

In the late 1980s and early 1990s, concerns were raised about whether the location of professional OT training programs in graduate research universities, academic health centers, and other colleges would continue. Many OT academic programs were functioning as professional schools. Kielhofner saw a challenge in the development of an academic discipline through research and theory development. He felt this need was imminent if OT education were to continue to be offered at the college and university level.

> We've got to be able to argue to the academic community that we have an academic discipline or we will not remain in universities . . . we will only be in community colleges. To me, the survival of the occupational therapy university system is more critical right now than, for example, whether we survive in acute care practice or whether we survive in schools as practitioners. Those things will evolve and change over time. If we have an academic discipline and the professional status of being in the university we will always be able to go out and make our way in practice arenas. (G. Kielhofner, personal communication, March 6, 1987)

His thinking in 1992 about this issue was powerfully stated as follows:

> Occupation pervades life, is necessary for the maintenance of the human collective, and determines the course of individual lives. As such, it is a powerful force in human existence and a

unique part of what it means to be human. In this regard, I share the enthusiasm of the proponents of occupational science for the possibility of the emergence of a distinct discipline organized around the study of occupation in human life. (1992, p. 288)

Kielhofner feels that OT knowledge must be organized in such a way as to incorporate both basic and applied science. Such knowledge will further the capabilities of the profession to address and solve problems of individuals with disability, and therefore meet very real societal needs. Kielhofner asserts that practice is the reason for OT's professional existence, and that research and theory must therefore serve practice.

I think the basic sciences are learning the lesson of relevance. I would hate to see our scholars so wooed by the sirens of the hallowed academic halls that we forget the hard lessons of relevance gleaned by generations of therapists laboring in clinics with persons who have such pressing problems. (G. Kielhofner, personal communication, August, 1992)

In the end it may be most appropriate to identify occupational therapy scholarship as occupational therapy science, which incorporates both a basic occupational science and an applied therapeutic science (both reflected in conceptual models of practice). They are dual and interrelated elements of the knowledge that will be necessary for the future of occupational therapy. (Kielhofner, 1992, p. 289)

In June 2002, Kielhofner (2002a) addressed the 50th anniversary meeting of the World Federation of Occupational Therapists in Stockholm, Sweden, and criticized the manner in which he and other OT scholars had been working outside of the accumulating knowledge. He spoke of how his travels and collaboration with therapists had led him to the realization that theory is only useful as it addresses the needs of therapists in the practice arena. He advocated for the "scholarship of practice" whereby researchers, educators, therapists, and service recipients must collaborate if the profession is to thrive.

In his presentation, he cited numerous examples of clients' experiences of OT as being humiliating, undignified, and depressing. Kielhofner expressed concern for the practice of the profession and questioned the reason for the gap between the values in the field and experiences of practice recipients. He questioned the manner in which he (and other developers and scribes of theory and knowledge) had been working out of the ivory towers of academia rather than in alliance with practitioners. He was critical of those in the profession who believe that the field has made great strides in scholarship to guide and direct practice. He put responsibility for the failure of solid healthful occupation-based practice, where it exists, on the scholars who are not developing knowledge to guide such practice. He was most critical of himself. Although the presentation was met with mixed reactions, the international audience of several thousand gave Kielhofner a standing ovation.

For the first edition of this book, Kielhofner spoke to Rosalie Miller of his frustration when his grandmother, at the age of 57, lost her leg in a car accident. He talked about the failure of the rehabilitation effort to reengage her into a new life story and how she was essentially lost to her disabling condition. He talked about his exposure to the field of OT and the fact that he sensed that his grandmother's fate could have been different. He turned to writing, given the experience that much of his professional knowledge was inaccessible except through contact with his mentors. Gary Kielhofner has become one of the most prolific writers in the profession. In a treatise on the state of the profession, he suggested a repaving of the road he is traveling as he continues his professional journey. The comments he made in June 2002 reflect thoughts that have been brewing over time. When I (Scott) first started revising this chapter, I asked him, in October 2001, to describe the direction he saw his work going. He replied,

> My work is focusing on strategies that bring practice, theory, and research together. I believe we must forge new ways of creating knowledge that bridges the gap between knowledge development and knowledge application. My aim is to develop ways to make these processes seamless. What first attracted me to occupational therapy and what continues to intrigue me most is what happens in the therapeutic moment. Theory development and research must focus on the process of therapy and its outcomes. That's where my own work is focused now. (G. Kielhofner, personal communication, October 22, 2001)

Bibliography

1975

Kielhofner, G. (1975). *The evolution of knowledge in occupational therapy: Understanding adaptation of the chronically disabled.* Unpublished master's thesis, University of Southern California, Los Angeles.

1976

Cromwell, F. S., & Kielhofner, G. (1976). An educational strategy for occupational therapy community service. *American Journal of Occupational Therapy, 30,* 629–633.

1977

Kielhofner, G. (1977). Temporal adaptation: A conceptual framework for occupational therapy. *American Journal of Occupational Therapy, 31,* 235–242.

Kielhofner, G., & Burke, J. P. (1977). Occupational therapy after 60 years: An account of changing identity and knowledge. *American Journal of Occupational Therapy, 31,* 675–689.

1978

Kielhofner, G. (1978). General systems theory: Implications for theory and action in occupational therapy. *American Journal of Occupational Therapy, 32,* 637–645.

1979

Gillette, N., & Kielhofner, G. (1979). The impact of specialization on the professionalization and survival of occupational therapy. *American Journal of Occupational Therapy, 33,* 20–28.

Kielhofner, G. (1979). Temporal adaptation: A conceptual framework for occupational therapy. In O. Payton (Ed.), *Research: The validation of clinical practice* (pp. 210–222). Philadelphia: F. A. Davis. (Reprinted from *American Journal of Occupational Therapy,* 1977, *31,* 235–242)

Kielhofner, G. (1979). The temporal dimension in the lives of retarded adults: A problem of interaction and intervention. *American Journal of Occupational Therapy, 33,* 161–168.

1980

Kielhofner, G. (1980). *Evaluating deinstitutionalization: An ethnographic study of social policy.* Unpublished doctoral dissertation, University of Southern California, Los Angeles.

Kielhofner, G. (1980). A model of human occupation: Part two. Ontogenesis from the perspective of temporal adaptation. *American Journal of Occupational Therapy, 34,* 657–663.

Kielhofner, G. (1980). A model of human occupation: Part three. Benign and vicious cycles. *American Journal of Occupational Therapy, 34,* 731–737.

Kielhofner, G., & Burke, J. P. (1980). A model of human occupation: Part one. Conceptual framework and content. *American Journal of Occupational Therapy, 34,* 572–581.

Kielhofner, G., Burke, J., & Igi, C. H. (1980). A model of human occupation: Part four. Assessment and intervention. *American Journal of Occupational Therapy, 34,* 777–788.

Kielhofner, G., & Takata, N. (1980). A study of mentally retarded persons: Applied research in occupational therapy. *American Journal of Occupational Therapy, 34,* 252–258.

1981

Kielhofner, G. (1981). An ethnographic study of deinstitutionalized adults: Their community settings and daily life experiences. *Occupational Therapy Journal of Research, 1,* 125–142.

Kielhofner, G., & Miyake, S. (1981). Therapeutic use of games with mentally retarded adults. *American Journal of Occupational Therapy, 35,* 375–382.

1982

Chao, R., Clark, F., & Kielhofner, G. (1982). Development of time concepts in mentally retarded adults and its relationship to mental age. In *Proceedings of the Annual Piagetian Conference.*

Kielhofner, G. (1982). A heritage of activity: Development of theory. In *American Journal of Occupational Therapy, 36,* 723–730.

Kielhofner, G. (1982). Qualitative research: Part one. Paradigmatic grounds and issues of reliability and validity. *Occupational Therapy Journal of Research, 2,* 67–79.

Kielhofner, G. (1982). Qualitative research: Part two. Methodological approaches and relevance to occupational therapy. *Occupational Therapy Journal of Research, 2,* 150–164.

Kielhofner, G. (1982). Theoretical foundations of occupational therapy. *Proceedings of the World Federation of Occupational Therapy* (pp. 1265–1272).

Kielhofner, G., Barris, R., & Watts, J. (1982). Habits and habit dysfunction: A clinical perspective for psychosocial occupational therapy. *Occupational Therapy in Mental Health, 2,* 1–22.

Vandenberg, B., & Kielhofner, G. (1982). Play in evolution, culture, and individual adaptation: Implications for therapy. *American Journal of Occupational Therapy, 36,* 20–28.

1983

Barris, R., Kielhofner, G., & Watts, J. (1983). *Psychosocial occupational therapy: Practice in a pluralistic arena.* Laurel, MD: RAM Associates.

Kielhofner, G. (Ed.). (1983). *Health through occupation: Theory and practice in occupational therapy.* Philadelphia: F. A. Davis.

Kielhofner, G. (1983). Occupation. In H. Hopkins & H. Smith (Eds.), *Willard and Spackman's occupational therapy* (6th ed.). Philadelphia: Lippincott.

Kielhofner, G. (1983). "Teaching" retarded adults: Paradoxical effects of a pedagogical enterprise. *Urban Life, 12,* 307–326.

Kielhofner, G., Barris, R., Bauer, D., Shoestock, B., & Walker, L. (1983). A comparison of play behavior in nonhospitalized and hospitalized children. *American Journal of Occupational Therapy, 37,* 305–312.

Kielhofner, G., & Nelson, C. (1983). A study of patient motivation and cooperation/participation in occupational therapy. *Occupational Therapy Journal of Research, 3,* 35–46.

1984

Kielhofner, G. (1984). An overview of research on the model of human occupation. *Canadian Journal of Occupational Therapy, 51,* 59–67.

Kielhofner, G. (1984). A paradigmatic view of rehabilitation. In *Proceedings of the Second International Conference on Rehabilitation Engineering,* Ottawa, Canada.

Kielhofner, G., & Barris, R. (1984). Mental health occupational therapy: Trends in literature and practice. *Occupational Therapy in Mental Health, 4,* 35–50.

1985

Barris, R., & Kielhofner, G. (1985). Generating and using knowledge in occupational therapy: Implications for professional education. *Occupational Therapy Journal of Research, 5,* 113–124.

Barris, R., Kielhofner, G., & Bauer, D. (1985). Educational experience and changes in learning and value preferences. *Occupational Therapy Journal of Research, 5,* 243–256.

Barris, R., Kielhofner, G., & Bauer, D. (1985). Learning preferences, values, and student satisfaction. *Journal of Allied Health, 14,* 13–23.

Barris, R., Kielhofner, G., Levine, R. E., & Neville, A. (1985). Occupation as interaction with the environment. In G. Kielhofner (Ed.), *A model of human occupation: Theory and application* (pp. 42–62). Baltimore: Williams & Wilkins.

Kielhofner, G. (1985). The demise of diffidence: An agenda for occupational therapy. *Canadian Journal of Occupational Therapy, 52,* 165–171.

Kielhofner, G. (1985). The model of human occupation: Ett hjalpmedel for kliniskt uerksamma arbetsterapeuter (C. Henriksson, Trans.). *Arbetsterapeuten (Swedish Journal of Occupational Therapy), 17,* 18–23.

Kielhofner, G. (Ed.). (1985). *A model of human occupation: Theory and application.* Baltimore: Williams & Wilkins.

Kielhofner, G. & Burke, J. P. (1985). Components and determinats of human occupation. In G. Kielhofner (Ed.), *A model of human occupation: Theory and application* (pp. 12–41). Baltimore: Williams & Wilkins.

Lederer, J., Kielhofner, G., & Watts, J. (1985). Values, personal causation and skills of delinquents and non-delinquents. *Occupational Therapy in Mental Health, 5,* 59–77.

Neville, A., Kriesberg, A., & Kielhofner, G. (1985). Temporal dysfunction in schizophrenia. *Occupational Therapy in Mental Health, 5*(1), 1–20.

Oakley, F., Kielhofner, G., & Barris, R. (1985). An occupational therapy approach to assessing psychiatric patients' adaptive functioning. *American Journal of Occupational Therapy, 39,* 147–154.

Rogers, J. C., & Kielhofner, G. (1985). Treatment planning. In G. Kielhofner (Ed.), *A model of human occupation: Theory and application* (p. 140). Baltimore: Williams & Wilkins.

Smyntek, L., Barris, R., & Kielhofner, G. (1985). The model of human occupation applied to psychosocially functional and dysfunctional adolescents. *Occupational Therapy in Mental Health, 5,* 21–40.

1986

Barris, R., & Kielhofner, G. (1986). Beliefs, perspectives, and activities of psychosocial occupational therapy educators. *American Journal of Occupational Therapy, 40,* 535–541.

Barris, R., Kielhofner, G., Burch-Martin, R., Gelinas, I., Klement, M., & Schultz, B. (1986). Occupational function and dysfunction in three groups of adolescents. *Occupational Therapy Journal of Research, 6,* 301–317.

Duellman, M. K., Barris, R., & Kielhofner, G. (1986). Organized activity and the adaptive status of nursing home residents. *American Journal of Occupational Therapy, 40,* 618–622.

Harrison, H., & Kielhofner, G. (1986). Examining reliability and validity of the preschool play scale with handicapped children. *American Journal of Occupational Therapy, 40,* 167–173.

Kielhofner, G. (1986). A review of research on the model of human occupation: Part one. *Canadian Journal of Occupational Therapy, 53*, 69–74.

Kielhofner, G. (1986). A review of research on the model of human occupation: Part two. *Canadian Journal of Occupational Therapy, 53*, 129–134.

Kielhofner, G. (1986). A response to Sharrott's "An analysis of occupational therapy theoretical approaches for mental health." *Occupational Therapy in Mental Health, 5*, 17–23.

Kielhofner, G., & Barris, R. (1986). Organization of knowledge in occupational therapy: A proposal and a survey of the literature. *Occupational Therapy Journal of Research, 5*, 67–84.

Kielhofner, G., & Barris, R. (1986). Response to commentary: Organization of knowledge in occupational therapy: A proposal and a survey of the literature. *Occupational Therapy Journal of Research, 6*, 183–190.

Kielhofner, G., Harlan, B., Bauer, D., & Maurer, P. (1986). The reliability of an historical interview with physically disabled respondents. *American Journal of Occupational Therapy, 40*, 551–556.

Kielhofner, G., & Nelson, C. (1986). The nature and implications of shifting patterns of practice in physical disabilities occupational therapy. *Occupational Therapy in Health Care, 3*, 187–198.

Oakley, F., Kielhofner, G., Barris, R., & Reichler, R. (1986). The role checklist: Development and empirical assessment of reliability. *Occupational Therapy Journal of Research, 6*, 157–170.

Smith, N., Kielhofner, G., & Watts, J. (1986). The relationships between volition, activity pattern, and life satisfaction in the elderly. *American Journal of Occupational Therapy, 40*, 278–284.

Watts, J. H., Kielhofner, G., Bauer, D., Gregory, M., & Valentine, D. (1986). The assessment of occupational functioning: A screening tool for use in long-term care. *American Journal of Occupational Therapy, 40*, 231–240.

1988

Barris, R., Kielhofner, G., & Watts, J. (1988). *Bodies of knowledge in psychosocial practice*. Thorofare, NJ: Charles B. Slack.

Barris, R., Kielhofner, G., & Watts, J. (1988). *Occupational therapy in psychosocial practice*. Thorofare, NJ: Charles B. Slack.

Barris, R., Oakley, F., & Kielhofner, G. (1988). The role checklist. In B. Hemphill (Ed.), *Mental health assessment in occupational therapy* (2nd ed., pp. 73–79). Thorofare, NJ: Charles B. Slack.

Kielhofner, G. (1988). Occupational therapy base in occupation. In H. Hopkins & H. Smith (Eds.), *Willard and Spackman's occupational therapy* (7th ed.). Philadelphia: Lippincott.

Kielhofner, G., & Henry, A. (1988). Development and investigation of the Occupational Performance History Interview. *American Journal of Occupational Therapy, 42*, 489–498.

Kielhofner, G., & Henry, A. (1988). Use of an occupational history interview in occupational therapy. In B. Hemphill (Ed.), *Mental health assessment in occupational therapy* (2nd ed., pp. 59–71). Thorofare, NJ: Charles B. Slack.

1989

Fisher, A. G., Kielhofner, G., & Davis, C. (1989). Research values of occupational and physical therapists. *Journal of Allied Health, 18*, 143–156.

Kaplan, K., & Kielhofner, G. (1989). *The occupational case analysis interview and rating scale*. Thorofare, NJ: Charles B. Slack.

Kielhofner, G., & Brinson, M. (1989). Development and evaluation of an aftercare program for young chronic psychiatrically disabled adults. *Occupational Therapy in Mental Health, 9,* 1–25.

Kielhofner, G., & Nicol, M. (1989). The model of human occupation: A developing conceptual tool for clinicians. *British Journal of Occupational Therapy, 52,* 210–214.

1990

Boyle, M. A., Dunn, W., & Kielhofner, G. (1990). Funding for research and training in professional occupational therapy education programs from 1985 to 1987. *Occupational Therapy Journal of Research, 10,* 334–342.

1991

Borell, L., Sandman, P., & Kielhofner, G. (1991). Clinical decision making in Alzheimer's disease. *Occupational Therapy in Mental Health, 11,* 111–124.

Kielhofner, G., & Fisher, A. (1991). Mind–brain relationships. In A. Fisher, E. Murray, & A. Bundy (Eds.), *Sensory integration: Theory and practice* (pp. 30–38). Philadelphia: F.A. Davis.

Kielhofner, G., Henry, A., Walens, D., & Rogers, E. (1991). A generalizability study of the Occupational Performance History Interview. *Occupational Therapy Journal of Research, 11,* 292–306.

1992

Kielhofner, G. (1992). *Conceptual foundations of occupational therapy*. Philadelphia: F.A. Davis.

Kielhofner, G. (1992). The future of the profession of occupational therapy: Requirements for developing the field's knowledge base. *Journal of the Japanese Occupational Therapy Association, 11,* 112–129.

1993

Kielhofner, G. (1993). Functional assessment: Toward a dialectical view of person–environment relations. *American Journal of Occupational Therapy, 47,* 248–251.

Munoz, J., Lawlor, M., & Kielhofner, G. (1993). Use of the model of human occupation: A survey of therapists in psychiatric practice. *Occupational Therapy Journal of Research, 13,* 117–139.

1994

Borell, L., Gustavsson, A., Sandman, P., & Kielhofner, G. (1994). Occupational programming in a day hospital for patients with dementia. *Occupational Therapy Journal of Research, 14,* 4.

Helfrich, C., & Kielhofner, G. (1994). Volitional narratives and the meaning of occupational therapy. *American Journal of Occupational Therapy, 48,* 319–326.

Helfrich, C., Kielhofner, G., & Mattingly, C. (1994). Volition as narrative: Understanding motivation in chronic illness. *American Journal of Occupational Therapy, 48,* 311–317.

1995

Kielhofner, G. (1995). A meditation on the use of hands. *Scandinavian Journal of Occupational Therapy, 2,* 153–166.

Kielhofner, G., (Ed.). (1995). *A model of human occupation: Theory and application* (2nd ed.). Baltimore: Williams & Wilkins.

Kielhofner, G., & Mallinson, T. (1995). Gathering narrative data through interviews: Empirical observations and suggested guidelines. *Scandinavian Journal of Occupational Therapy, 2,* 63–68.

1996

Chern, J., Kielhofner, G., de las Heras, C., & Magalhaes, L. (1996). The volitional questionnaire: Psychometric development and practical use. *American Journal of Occupational Therapy, 50,* 516–525.

Mallinson, T., Kielhofner, G., & Mattingly, C. (1996). Metaphor and meaning in a clinical interview. *American Journal of Occupational Therapy, 50,* 338–346.

1997

Corner, R., Kielhofner, G., & Lin, F. L. (1997). Construct validity of a work environment impact scale. *Work, 9*(1), 21–34.

Haglund, L., Karlsson, G., Kielhofner, G., & Lai, J. (1997). Validity of the Swedish version of the Worker Role Interview. *Scandinavian Journal of Occupational Therapy, 4,* 23–29.

Jonsson, H., Kielhofner, G., & Borell, B. (1997). Anticipating retirement: The formation of narratives concerning an occupational transition. *American Journal of Occupational Therapy, 51,* 49–56.

Kielhofner, G., & Forsyth, K. (1997). The model of human occupation: An overview of current concepts. *British Journal of Occupational Therapy, 60,* 103–110.

Kielhofner, G. (1997). *Conceptual foundations of occupational therapy* (2nd ed.). Philadelphia: F.A. Davis.

1998

Forsyth, K., Salamy, M., Simon, S., & Kielhofner, G. (1998). *A user's guide to the Assessment of Communication and Interaction Skills (Version 4.0) ACIS.* Chicago: Model of Human Occupation Clearinghouse.

Kielhofner, G., & Barrett, L. (1998). Meaning and misunderstanding in occupational forms: A study of therapeutic goal setting. *American Journal of Occupational Therapy, 52,* 345–353.

Kielhofner, G., & Barrett, L. (1998). Theories derived from occupational behavior perspectives. In *Willard & Spackman's occupational therapy* (9th ed., pp. 525–535). Philadelphia: Lippincott.

Kielhofner, G., Mallinson, T., Crawford, C., Nowak, M., Rigby, M., Henry, A., & Walens, D. (1998). *A user's manual for the Occupational Performance History Interview (Version 2.0) OPHI–II.* Chicago: Model of Human Occupation Clearinghouse.

Mallinson, T., Mahaffey, L., & Kielhofner, G. (1998). The Occupational Performance History Interview: Evidence for three underlying constructs of occupational adaptation. *Canadian Journal of Occupational Therapy, 65,* 219–228.

Olson, L. M., & Kielhofner, G. (1998). *Work readiness: Day treatment for persons with chronic disabilities.* Chicago: Model of Human Occupation Clearinghouse.

Velozo, C. A., Kielhofner, G., & Lai, J. (1998). The use of Rasch analysis to produce scale-free measurement of functional ability. *American Journal of Occupational Therapy, 53,* 83–90.

1999

Barrett, L., Beer, D., & Kielhofner, G. (1999). The importance of volitional narrative in treatment: An ethnographic case study in a work program. *Work: A Journal of Prevention, Assessment, & Rehabilitation, 12*(1), 79–82.

Forsyth, K., Lai, J., & Kielhofner, G. (1999). The Assessment of Communication and Interaction Skills (ACIS): Measurement properties. *British Journal of Occupational Therapy, 62,* 69–74.

Kielhofner, G. (1999). From doing in to doing with: The role of environment in performance and disability. *Toimintaterapeutti, 1,* 3–9.

Kielhofner, G. (1999). Guest-editorial. *Work: A Journal of Prevention, Assessment & Rehabilitation, 12*(1), 1.

Kielhofner, G., Braveman, B., Baron, K., Fischer, G., Hammel, J., & Littleton, M. (1999). The model of human occupation: Understanding the worker who is injured or disabled. *Work: A Journal of Prevention, Assessment & Rehabilitation, 12*(1), 3–11.

Kielhofner, G., Lai, J. S., Olson, L., Haglund, L., Ekbadh, E., & Hedlund, M. (1999). Psychometric properties of the Work Environment Impact Scale: A cross-cultural study. *Work: A Journal of Prevention, Assessment & Rehabilitation, 12*(1), 71–77.

Lai, J., Haglund, L., & Kielhofner, G. (1999). Occupational Case Analysis Interview and Rating Scale: An examination of construct validity. *Scandinavian Journal of Caring Sciences, 13,* 276–273.

Mentrup, C., Niehaus, A., & Kielhofner, G. (1999). Applying the model of human occupation in work-focused rehabilitation: A case illustration. *Work: A Journal of Prevention, Assessment & Rehabilitation, 12*(1), 61–70.

Peterson, E., Howland, J., Kielhofner, G., Lachman, M. E., Assmann, S., Cote, J., & Jette, A. (1999). Falls self-efficacy and occupational adaptation among elders. *Physical and Occupational Therapy in Geriatrics, 16*(1/2), 1–16.

Velozo, C. A., Kielhofner, G., Gern, A., Lin, F., Azhar, F., Lai, J., & Fisher, G. (1999). Worker Role Interview: Toward validation of a psychosocial work-related measure. *Journal of Occupational Rehabilitation, 9,* 153–168.

2000

Jonsson, H., Josephsson, S., & Kielhofner, G. (2000). Evolving narratives in the course of retirement: A longitudinal study. *American Journal of Occupational Therapy, 54,* 463–470.

2001

Braveman, B., Sen, S., & Kielhofner, G. (2001). Community-based vocational rehabilitation. In M. Scaffa (Ed.), *Occupational therapy in community-based practice settings* (pp. 139–162). Philadelphia: F. A. Davis.

Jonsson, H., Josephsson, S., & Kielhofner, G. (2001). Narratives and experience in an occupational transition: A longitudinal study of the retirement process. *American Journal of Occupational Therapy, 55,* 424–432.

Kielhofner, G., & Forsyth, G. (2001). Measurement properties of a client self-report for treatment planning and documenting therapy outcomes. *Scandinavian Journal of Occupational Therapy, 8,* 131–139.

Kielhofner, G., Mallinson, T., Forsyth, K., & Lai, J. (2001). Psychometric properties of the second version of the Occupational Performance History Interview (OPHI–II). *American Journal of Occupational Therapy, 55,* 260–267.

2002

Kielhofner, G. (2002, June). *Keynote address: Challenges and directions for the future of occupational therapy.* Presentation at the World Federation of Occupational Therapy, Stockholm, Sweden.

Kielhofner, G. (2002). *A model of human occupation: Theory and application.* (3rd ed.). Baltimore: Williams & Wilkins.

Kielhofner, G., Forsyth, K., & Baron, K. (in press). Development for a client self-report for treatment planning and documenting therapy outcomes. *Scandinavian Journal of Occupational Therapy.*

References

Baron, K. B. (1991). The use of play in child psychiatry: Reframing the therapeutic environment. *Occupational Therapy in Mental Health, 11,* 37–56.

Barrett, L., Beer, D., & Kielhofner, G. (1999). The importance of volitional narrative in treatment: An ethnographic case study in a work program. *Work: A Journal of Prevention, Assessment & Rehabilitation, 12*(1), 79–82.

Barris, R., Kielhofner, G., Burch-Martin, R., Gelinas, I., Klement, M., & Schultz, B. (1986). Occupational function and dysfunction in three groups of adolescents. *Occupational Therapy Journal of Research, 6,* 301–317.

Barris, R., Kielhofner, G., & Watts, J. (1983). *Psychosocial occupational therapy: Practice in a pluralistic arena.* Laurel, MD: RAM Associates.

Blakeney, A. B. (1985). Adolescent development: An application to the model human occupation. In F. S. Cromwell (Ed.), *Occupational therapy and adolescents with disability* (pp. 19–40). New York: Haworth Press.

Borell, L., Gustavsson, A., Sandman, P., & Kielhofner, G. (1994). Occupational programming in a day hospital for patients with dementia. *Occupational Therapy Journal of Research, 14,* 4.

Borell, L., Sandman, P., & Kielhofner, G. (1991). Clinical decision making in Alzheimer's disease. *Occupational Therapy in Mental Health, 11,* 111–124.

Burton, J. E. (1989a). The model of human occupation and occupational therapy practice with elderly patients: Part 1. Characteristics of aging. *British Journal of Occupational Therapy, 52,* 215–218.

Burton, J. E. (1989b). The model of human occupation and occupational therapy practice with elderly patients: Part 2. Application. *British Journal of Occupational Therapy, 52,* 219–221.

Chen, C., Neufeld, P. S., Feely, C. A., & Skinner, C. S. (1999). Factors influencing compliance with home exercise programs among patients with upper extremity impairment. *American Journal of Occupational Therapy, 53*(2), 171–180.

Curtin, C. (1991). Psychosocial intervention with an adolescent with diabetes using the model of human occupation. *Occupational Therapy in Mental Health, 11,* 23–36.

DeForest, D., Watts, J. H., & Madigan, M. J. (1991). Resonation in the model of human occupation: A pilot study. *Occupational Therapy in Mental Health, 11,* 57–71.

Elliott, M. S., & Barris, R. (1987). Occupational role performance and life satisfaction in elderly persons. *Occupational Therapy Journal of Research, 7,* 215–224.

Forsyth, K., Lai, J., & Kielhofner, G. (1999). The Assessment of Communication and Interaction Skills (ACIS): Measurement properties. *British Journal of Occupational Therapy, 62,* 69–74.

Forsyth, K., Salamy, M., Simon, S., & Kielhofner, G. (1998). *A user's guide to the Assessment of Communication and Interaction Skills (Version 4.0) ACIS.* Chicago: Model of Human Occupation Clearinghouse.

Fossey, E. (1996). Using the Occupational Performance History Interview (OPHI): Therapists' reflections. *British Journal of Occupational Therapy, 59*(5) 223–228.

Gregory, M. (1983). Occupational behavior and life satisfaction among retirees. *American Journal of Occupational Therapy, 37,* 548–553.

Grogan, G. (1991a). Anger management: A perspective for occupational therapy (Part 1). *Occupational Therapy in Mental Health, 11,* 135–148.

Grogan, G. (1991b). Anger management: Clinical applications for occupational therapy (Part 2). *Occupational Therapy in Mental Health, 11,* 149–171.

Gusich, R. L. (1984). Occupational therapy for chronic pain: A clinical application of the model of human occupation. *Occupational Therapy in Mental Health, 4,* 59–74.

Gusich, R. L., & Silverman, A. L. (1991). Basava Day Clinic: The model of human occupation as applied to psychiatric day hospitalization. *Occupational Therapy in Mental Health, 11,* 113–134.

Haglund, L., Karlsson, G., Kielhofner, G., & Lai, J. (1997). Validity of the Swedish version of the Worker Role Interview. *Scandinavian Journal of Occupational Therapy, 4,* 23–29.

Helfrich, C., & Kielhofner, G. (1994). Volitional narratives and the meaning of occupational therapy. *American Journal of Occupational Therapy, 48,* 319–326.

Helfrich, C., Kielhofner, G., & Mattingly, C. (1994). Volition as narrative: Understanding motivation in chronic illness. *American Journal of Occupational Therapy, 48,* 311–317.

Henry, A., & Mallinson, T. (1999). The Occupational Performance History Interview. In B. J. Hemphill-Pearson (Ed.), *Assessments in occupational therapy mental health: An integrative approach* (pp. 59–70). Thorofare, NJ: Charles B. Slack.

Jonsson, H., Josephsson, S., & Kielhofner, G. (2001). Narratives and experience in an occupational transition: A longitudinal study of the retirement process. *American Journal of Occupational Therapy, 55,* 424–432.

Jonsson, H., Kielhofner, G., & Borell, L. (1997). Anticipating retirement: The formation of narratives concerning an occupational transition. *American Journal of Occupational Therapy, 51,* 49–56.

Khoo, S. W., & Renwick, R. M. (1989). A model of human occupation perspective on the mental health of immigrant women in Canada. *Occupational Therapy in Mental Health, 9,* 31–49.

Kielhofner, G. (1975). *The evolution of knowledge in occupational therapy: Understanding adaptation of the chronically disabled.* Unpublished master's thesis, University of Southern California, Los Angeles.

Kielhofner, G. (1977). Temporal adaptation: A conceptual framework for occupational therapy. *American Journal of Occupational Therapy, 31,* 235–242.

Kielhofner, G. (1980a). *Evaluating deinstitutionalization: An ethnographic study of social policy.* Unpublished doctoral dissertation, University of Southern California, Los Angeles.

Kielhofner, G. (1980b). A model of human occupation: Part two. Ontogenesis from the perspective of temporal adaptation. *American Journal of Occupational Therapy, 34,* 657–663.

Kielhofner, G. (1980c). A model of human occupation: Part three. Benign and vicious cycles. *American Journal of Occupational Therapy, 34,* 731–737.

Kielhofner, G. (1982a). Qualitative research: Part one. Paradigmatic grounds and issues of reliability and validity. *Occupational Therapy Journal of Research, 2,* 67–79.

Kielhofner, G. (1982b). Qualitative research: Part two. Methodological approaches and relevance to occupational therapy. *Occupational Therapy Journal of Research, 2,* 150–164.

Kielhofner, G. (Ed.). (1983). *Health through occupation: Theory and practice in occupational therapy.* Philadelphia: F.A. Davis.

Kielhofner, G. (Ed.). (1985). *A model of human occupation: Theory and application.* Baltimore: Williams & Wilkins.

Kielhofner, G. (1992). *Conceptual foundations of occupational therapy.* Philadelphia: F.A. Davis.

Kielhofner, G. (1993). Functional assessment: Toward a dialectical view of person–environment relations. *American Journal of Occupational Therapy, 47,* 248–251.

Kielhofner, G. (1995a). A meditation on the use of hands. *Scandinavian Journal of Occupational Therapy, 2,* 153–166.

Kielhofner, G. (1995b). *A model of human occupation: Theory and application* (2nd ed.). Baltimore: Williams & Wilkins.

Kielhofner, G. (1997). *Conceptual foundations of occupational therapy* (2nd ed.). Philadelphia: F.A. Davis.

Kielhofner, G. (2002a, June). *Keynote address: Challenges and directions for the future of occupational therapy.* Presentation at the World Federation of Occupational Therapy, Stockholm, Sweden.

Kielhofner, G. (2002b). *A model of human occupation: Theory and application* (3rd ed.). Baltimore: Williams & Wilkins.

Kielhofner, G., & Brinson, M. (1989). Development and evaluation of an aftercare program for young chronic psychiatrically disabled adults. *Occupational Therapy in Mental Health, 9,* 1–25.

Kielhofner, G., & Burke, J. P. (1977). Occupational therapy after 60 years: An account of changing identity and knowledge. *American Journal of Occupational Therapy, 31,* 675–689.

Kielhofner, G., & Burke, J. P. (1980). A model of human occupation: Part one. Conceptual framework and content. *American Journal of Occupational Therapy, 34,* 572–581.

Kielhofner, G., & Burke, J. P. (1985). Components and determinants of human occupation. In G. Kielhofner (Ed.), *A model of human occupation: Theory and application* (pp. 12–41). Baltimore: Williams and Wilkins.

Kielhofner, G., Burke, J., & Igi, C. H. (1980). A model of human occupation. Part four. Assessment and intervention. *American Journal of Occupational Therapy, 34,* 777–788.

Kielhofner, G., & Forsyth, K. (1997). The model of human occupation: An overview of current concepts. *British Journal of Occupational Therapy, 60,* 103–110.

Kielhofner, G., & Mallinson, T. (1995). Gathering narrative data through interviews: Empirical observations and suggested guidelines. *Scandinavian Journal of Occupational Therapy, 2,* 63–68.

Kielhofner, G., Mallinson, T., Crawford, C., Nowak, M., Rigby, M., Henry, A., & Walens, D. (1998). *A user's manual for the Occupational Performance History Interview (Version 2.0) OPHI–II.* Chicago: Model of Human Occupation Clearinghouse.

Kielhofner, G., Mallinson, T., Forsyth, K., & Lai, J. (2001). Psychometric properties of the second version of the Occupational Performance History Interview (OPHI–II). *American Journal of Occupational Therapy, 55,* 260–267.

Knapp, J. (1983). *A study of leisure values and life satisfaction among retirees.* Richmond: Virginia Commonwealth University.

Lai, J., Haglund, L., & Kielhofner, G. (1999). The Occupational Case Analysis Interview and Rating Scale: An examination of construct validity. *Scandinavian Journal of Caring Science, 13,* 267–273.

Lancaster, J. & Mitchell, M. (1991). Occupational therapy treatment goals, objectives, and activities for improving low self-esteem in adolescents with behavioral disorders. *Occupational Therapy in Mental Health, 11,* 3–22.

Lederer, J., Kielhofner, G., & Watts, J. (1985). Values, personal causation and skills of delinquents and non-delinquents. *Occupational Therapy in Mental Health, 5,* 59–77.

Lynch, K. B., & Bridle, M. J. (1993). Construct validity of the Occupational Performance History Interview. *Occupational Therapy Journal of Research, 13,* 231–240.

Lyons, M. (1983). *Employment and personal adjustment of mentally retarded persons: Towards an emic perspective of the relationship.* Richmond: Virginia Commonwealth University.

Mallinson, T., Kielhofner, G., & Mattingly, C. (1996). Metaphor and meaning in a clinical interview. *American Journal of Occupational Therapy, 50,* 338–346.

Mallinson, T., Mahaffey, L., & Kielhofner, G. (1998). The Occupational Performance History Interview: Evidence for three underlying constructs of occupational adaptation. *Canadian Journal of Occupational Therapy, 65,* 219–228.

Mattingly, C., & Fleming, M. H. (1994). *Clinical reasoning: Forms of inquiry in a therapeutic practice.* Philadelphia: F.A. Davis.

Model of Human Occupation Products (2002). *Occupational Circumstances Analysis Interview and Rating Scale.* (Available from American Occupational Therapy Association, 4720 Montgomery Lane, P.O. Box 31220, Bethesda, MD 20824-1220)

Munoz, J. P., Lawlor, M., & Kielhofner, G. (1993). Use of the model of human occupation: A survey of therapists in psychiatric practice. *Occupational Therapy Journal of Research, 13,* 117–139.

Nelson, D. L. (1988). Occupation: Form and performance. *American Journal of Occupational Therapy, 42,* 633–641.

Nelson, D. L. (1994). *Occupational form, occupational performance, and therapeutic occupation.* Rockville, MD: American Occupational Therapy Association.

Neville-Jan, A., Bradley, M., Bunn, C., & Gheri, B. (1991). The model of human occupation and individuals with co-dependency problems. *Occupational Therapy in Mental Health, 11,* 73–97.

Oakley, F. (1987). Clinical application of the model of human application in dementia of the Alzheimer's type. *Occupational Therapy in Mental Health, 7,* 37–50.

Pizzi, M. (1990). The model of human occupation with adults with HIV infection and AIDS. *American Journal of Occupational Therapy, 44,* 257–264.

Portney, L. G. & Watkins, L. G. (2000). *Foundations of clinical research: Application to practice.* Upper Saddle River, NJ: Prentice Hall Health.

Reilly, M. (1962). Occupational therapy can be one of the great ideas of 20th century medicine. *American Journal of Occupational Therapy, 16,* 1–9.

Reilly, M. (1974). *Play as exploratory learning.* Beverly Hills: Sage.

Rogers, J. C., & Kielhofner, G. (1985). Treatment planning. In G. Kielhofner (Ed.), *A model of human occupation: Theory and application.* Baltimore: Williams & Wilkins.

Rust, K., Barris, R., & Hooper, F. (1987). Use of the model of human occupation to predict women's exercise behavior. *Occupational Therapy Journal of Research, 7,* 23–35.

Salz, C. (1983). A theoretical approach to the treatment of work difficulties in borderline personalities. *Occupational Therapy in Mental Health, 3,* 33–46.

Scaffa, M. E. (1981). *Temporal adaptation and alcoholism*. Richmond: Virginia Commonwealth University.

Scaffa, M. E. (1991). Alcoholism: An occupational behavior perspective. *Occupational Therapy in Mental Health, 11,* 99–111.

Schaaf, R. C., & Mulrooney, L. L. (1989). Occupational therapy in early intervention: A family-centered approach. *American Journal of Occupational Therapy, 43,* 745–754.

Sepiol, J. M., & Froehlich, J. (1990). Use of the role checklist with the patient with multiple personality disorder. *American Journal of Occupational Therapy, 44,* 1008–1012.

Sholle-Martin, S. (1987). Application of the model of human occupation: Assessment in child and adolescent psychiatry. *Occupational Therapy in Mental Health, 7,* 3–22.

Sholle-Martin, S., & Alessi, N. E. (1990). Formulating a role for occupational therapy in child psychiatry: A clinical application. *American Journal of Occupational Therapy, 44,* 871–882.

Smith, N., Kielhofner, G., & Watts, J. (1986). The relationships between volition, activity pattern, and life satisfaction in the elderly. *American Journal of Occupational Therapy, 40,* 278–283.

Smyntek, L., Barris, R., & Kielhofner, G. (1985). The model of human occupation applied to psychosocially functional and dysfunctional adolescents. *Occupational Therapy in Mental Health, 5,* 21–40.

Tigges, K. N., & Sherman, L. M. (1983). The treatment of the hospice patient: From occupational history to occupational role. *American Journal of Occupational Therapy, 37,* 235–238.

Velozo, C., Kielhofner, G., & Fisher, G. (1998). *A user's guide to Worker Role Interview (Version 9.0) WRI*. Chicago: Model of Human Occupation Clearinghouse.

Velozo, C. A., Kielhofner, G., Gern, A., Lin, F., Azhar, F., Lai, J., & Fisher, G. (1999). Worker Role Interview: Toward validation of a psychosocial work-related measure. *Journal of Occupational Rehabilitation, 9,* 153–168.

Velozo, C. A., Kielhofner, G., & Lai, J. (1998). The use of Rasch analysis to produce scale-free measurement of functional ability. *American Journal of Occupational Therapy, 53,* 83–90.

Wieringa, N., & McColl, M. (1987). Implications of the model of human occupation for intervention with native Canadians. In F. S. Cromwell (Ed.), *Sociocultural implications in treatment planning in occupational therapy* (pp. 73–91). New York: Haworth Press.

Claudia Allen

8

Mary V. Donahue

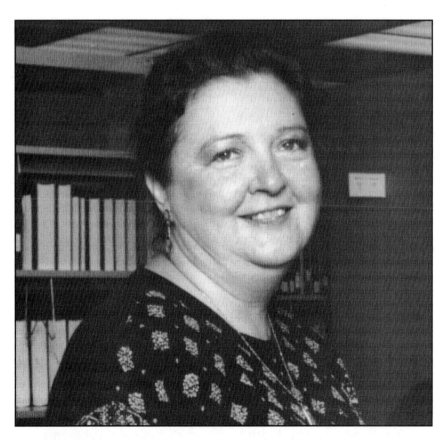

Therapeutic activities preserve the disabled person's dignity and personal identity. (C. Allen, 1989–1990 poster, compiled from Allen, 1985)

Therapeutic activity compensates for disability by utilizing remaining capabilities to accomplish desirable activities with satisfactory results. (Allen, 1987, p. 574)

In her work, Claudia Allen has focused on managing and adapting the activities and environments appropriate for the cognitive abilities of persons affected by a variety of cognitive disabilities. She has devised a hierarchy of cognitive levels, assessments to determine these levels, and environmental adaptations and structures to match these levels. Allen's theoretical framework is designed for individuals with chronic cognitive conditions such as schizophrenia and dementia. The therapeutic goal is to structure the environment and task to meet each individual's cognitive level.

Biographical Sketch

Childhood

Claudia Allen was born in Oregon in 1941 and grew up on a farm, where working with her hands, canning harvests, feeding animals, and making crafts were part of everyday life. During the long summers, she often borrowed a dozen books at a time from the library. She also developed a talent for getting close to animals that helped her become a keen observer of behavior. Being quiet, waiting, and being patient are traits that she carries with her from relating to farm animals, and that help her in working with people with disabilities who are unable to express their needs. Allen perceives that cognitive levels can be observed across a continuum of animal species (C. Allen, personal communication, May 16, 1992).

Allen had a grandmother who was an artist. One afternoon a week during the summers was devoted to learning pastel painting, embroidery, and other handwork under her grandmother's tutelage. Influenced by her father, who would have liked her to become a doctor, Allen thought for some time about becoming a dentist. Her interest in arts, crafts, and science made it logical that occupational therapy (OT) would later appeal to her.

Education

Allen received a traditional public school education with a college preparatory track in high school. Because she realized she needed to work on her writing skills, she selected every writing class she could attend. At a class reunion, one teacher was amazed to learn that Allen had become an author. Allen and her high school sweetheart kept in contact during college, and in 1963, the year she graduated, they married.

During her freshman year at the University of Oregon, Allen realized that dentistry did not appeal to her. A dormitory friend named Mary Foto told Allen about occupational therapy. Allen was intrigued by this field that clearly integrated art and science. She transferred to the OT program at San Jose State.

Professional Career

Allen began her OT career at Widner Memorial School, where she learned about Ayres's theories while working with children who had polio. Together with a physical therapist, she used Marianne Frostig's materials in a summer program designed to give 5-year-olds a head start for kindergarten. In an un–air-conditioned music room, they took the heavy leg braces off the children, put the children on mats, turned them around, used scooter boards, and had them crawl along strings on the floor. Without a formal design, they had fortuitously provided an environment for a comparison study, finding that the children who had received therapy achieved better kindergarten starting points than those who had not received therapy.

Allen reported how difficult it was to work at Widner because during the fall and spring sessions occupational therapists were only permitted to do pencil-and-paper work with the children in brief half-hour sessions. Meanwhile, the student population was shifting from children who had polio to children with cerebral palsy. The teachers and therapists had to adjust from teaching children who could keep up to expected educational norms, to teaching children with predictable falling-off points every 3 years, from 1st through 9th grades. During her time at Widner, Allen visited Penthurst State Hospital, an acknowledged "snake pit," where some of the Widner children had gone to live:

It was shocking and demoralizing to think that all of that effort had gone toward preparing the students for that, and that society was not really well equipped to deal with people with mental disorders. I think that had a very profound impression on me: no matter what anybody did, the special ed teachers, the OT's, PT's and speech pathologists could not help the students pass certain hurdles. So I think I got a real sense early on of what limitations there are that one can't overcome. (C. Allen, personal communication, May 16, 1992)

In the1960s, at a time when psychiatry still held out much hope for patients with mental illness, Allen took a position at Eastern Pennsylvania Psychiatric Institute (EPPI). There she worked in a uniquely stimulating intellectual environment. Each medical school in Philadelphia had its own ward in this hospital, so that a variety of frames of reference were being practiced. Many heated disagreements occurred in that accepting and nonrestrictive environment. Allen greatly enjoyed this exchange of theories and the interaction of unique personalities and lifestyles. There was also an extensive library at EPPI, with a helpful librarian. At the time, Allen assumed that all psychiatric patients and therapists enjoyed such a therapeutic and educational environment.

After several years at EPPI, Allen "decided that I really didn't know what I was doing . . . and . . . that I needed to go to graduate school" (C. Allen, personal communication, May 16, 1992). She entered the master's program at New York University (NYU), where she studied with Gail Fidler, Anne Mosey, and Sue Fine. EPPI paid for her tuition, fees, and books, in addition to giving her a full salary with the agreement that she return to work for a year after graduation.

Professional Challenges

Upon returning to EPPI, Allen found that what she had learned at NYU and during her residency with the higher level socioeconomic populations at New York State Psychiatric Institute did not apply to the average person with schizophrenia in a state hospital. While pondering this dilemma, she remembered that when she had first arrived at EPPI, it had struck her that many of the behaviors she observed were the same for people with schizophrenia as for children with cerebral palsy or mental retardation. The inability to follow more than one direction at a time was something both populations had in common (C. Allen, personal communication, May 16, 1992).

Meanwhile, Allen's husband, a psychiatrist, shared with her Philip May's research comparing four different treatment approaches for psychiatric patients. May's findings indicated the order of efficacy of treatment to be (a) psychotherapy plus medication, (b) medication alone, (c) electroconvulsive therapy alone, and (d) milieu therapy, of which OT was a part. Allen remembers being shocked and frightened at the implication that some of the things occupational therapists claimed to do were not valid. This study made it appear that "medication was really 'doing it,' and that the rest of the therapies were 'icing on the cake,' and that we had better define our roles" (C. Allen, personal communication, May 16, 1992).

Allen was concerned not only for the patients but also for the education of the OT students she was expected to mentor and supervise as part of the EPPI mission. This concern mobilized her to read extensively, covering every study she could obtain concerning psychopharmaceuticals and neurology, from Woodroff, Goodwin, and Guze's *Psychiatric Diagnosis* (1973) to the *Diagnostic and Statistical Manual of Mental Disorders–Third Edition–Revised* (American Psychiatric Association, 1987). While becoming immersed in this literature, she remained aware that psychotropic drugs are not cure-alls (C. Allen, personal communication, May 16, 1992).

In 1973, Allen moved to California to serve as chief of occupational therapy at Los Angeles County/University of Southern California (USC) Medical Center. She accepted a teaching position in the Department of Occupational Therapy at USC in 1975. Mary Reilly, still a dominant force at USC in 1975, perceived Allen as a foreigner with a master's degree from NYU. Allen raised questions and was something of an irritant on the scene. She recalls, however, being positively influenced by exposure to systems theory and by the emphasis on social roles in the department at USC (C. Allen, personal communications, May 16, 1992).

More recently, while Allen had been developing treatment goals, writing books, developing Medicare regulations and guidelines (Allen, Foto, Sperling, & Wilson, 1989), and writing on documentation, the USC department was developing its focus on occupational science. When asked about being in a department where emphasis historically was on occupational behavior and systems theory and now is on occupational science, Allen stated that it is difficult on all faculty: "Pure science and clinical practice operate within different value systems, and we all struggled with the conflicts that emerge" (C. Allen, personal communication, September 28, 1992).

In 1992, Allen's dual clinical and academic position included the title of chief of Occupational Therapy in Psychiatry at the Los Angeles County/USC Medical Center and instructor of Clinical Psychiatry and Behavioral Science at USC University Hospital. At that time, she was also a medical reviewer for allied health for Blue Cross of California. Her husband was then chief of a psychiatric unit at University Hospital and was also on the faculty at USC. Claudia has two daughters, one an occupational therapist (C. Allen, personal communication, August 24, 1992).

Assessments, Modules, Conferences, Books, and Videotapes

In the early 1990s, Claudia Allen, Cathy Earhart, and Tina Blue formed a partnership with S&S Crafts to produce the Allen Diagnostic Module (ADM) to market to occupational therapists a tool that assist clients in efforts to consolidate therapeutic gains and would make progress toward higher cognitive level skills. These standardized craft kits are designed to provide uniform assessment and growth opportunities for persons with cognitive or mental health impairments. The Allen Cognitive Level Test Manual was also published by S&S Worldwide (Allen, 1990).

To assist in expanding her work, in the 1990s, Claudia Allen established an office for Allen Conferences in Ormond Beach, Florida, headed by Jim Bertrand. In addition to arranging for conferences, Allen Conferences has published four books for therapists' use: *How To Use the Allen's Cognitive Levels in Daily Practice* (Allen, 1999), *Structures of the Cognitive Performance Modes* (Allen & Bertrand, 1999), *Starting an Allen's Cognitive Level Program in a Geriatric Facility* (Bertrand, 1997b), and *Understanding Cognitive Performance Modes* (Allen, Earhart, & Blue, 1995). The company has also produced teaching and training videotapes on the ACL Screen, Allen's theory, and the ADM

Placemat Project, and two tapes for training for interrater reliability. Information is available for Allen Cognitive Level products on the Web site for Allen Conferences, Inc. (http://www.allen-cognitive-levels.com/videos.htm).

Theory Overview and Development

Although Allen is aware that occupational therapists working with chronic cognitive disabilities need to alter their perspective from changing the person to managing the activities and environment, she is sensitive to the fact that "making these enormous shifts can be very tough" (C. Allen, personal communication, May 16, 1992). She traced the process of her own changing world view.

> When we got the first edition of Woodroff, Goodwin and Guze's *Psychiatric Diagnosis* (1973) out of St. Louis, which collected all of the research studies that became the precursor for DSM-III—whoa, this is an entirely different ballgame! I think it's still difficult to turn ourselves around because we have got to get rid of the Cartesian split [or dichotomy between "psychotic" and "organic/neurological" disorders], and adopt a very different world view, adopt a very different understanding of the mind. And you just don't do that quickly. I have done that three times: I started out with a psychoanalytic view with Fidler and Mosey, went into a Piagetian view with assimilation and accommodation, which didn't work, and have now gone to a much more neuroscience, DNA kind of view. (C. Allen, personal communication, May 16, 1992)

In summarizing her early influences and mentors, Allen includes Ruth Weimer, Gail Fidler, Anne Mosey, Mary Kay Bailey, and Betty Tiffany (C. Allen, personal communication, August 24, 1992). It is clear, however, that Allen is an original thinker.

Allen has a position of prominence in occupational therapy. She is a charter member of the Fellows of the American Occupational Therapy Association (FAOTA) and was the Eleanor Clarke Slagle Lecturer in 1987. She was a keynote speaker representing the United States at the World Federation of Occupational Therapists meeting in 1988 in Australia. Although Allen's name is associated with the cognitive levels she developed, she would have preferred that the title for her conceptual structure be the Functional Cognitive Levels instead of the Allen Cognitive Levels. Allen dislikes the notion of being considered a guru-type individual, and would prefer that the emphasis for her system be on the concept that is intrinsic to the type of cognitive process important to occupational therapists—that is, functional intelligence (C. Allen, personal communication, January 30, 2001).

Theoretical Concepts

Neurobiological Bases of Cognitive Disability

Allen has long been concerned about the Cartesian split or dichotomy between "organic" and "functional" disorders that has separated neurological medicine from psychiatry (Allen, 1985). She stated that OT practice began by delivering services to psychiatric patients at a time when empirical study of the brain was "thought to be impossible because the brain is so complex," but that neurobiological factors can no longer be excluded from occupational therapy models (Allen, 1982, p. 731). The first chapter of her first book, *Occupational Therapy for Psychiatric Diseases* (1985), remarkable for the time, was titled "Neuroscience Views of Routine Task Behavior." In it she argued that "a functional model of an emotional response to a task demand, based on a general description of total brain organization, is required for therapists to attain a holistic picture of an individual" (p. 182).

According to Allen, the evidence amassing in the literature of the 1960s to 1990s on psychopharmaceutical responses and the neurobiological bases of psychosocial disorders shows that the cause of psychiatric disorders cannot rest on psychodynamic explanations. In response to such evidence, Allen shifted in her view of cognitive disabilities from a psychoanalytic and then a Piagetian orientation to a neurological emphasis on Piagetian-based cognitive levels (Allen, 1987, 1988a; Allen et al., 1992). Her definition of cognitive disability as "a restriction in voluntary motor action originating in the physical or chemical structures of the brain and producing observable limitations in routine task behavior" speaks to her view of neurobiology as foundational to an understanding of the cognitive impairment underlying a cognitive disability (Allen, 1985, p. 31). Her definition, as well as statements such as "a cognitive disability is caused by a biologic defect" (Allen, 1985, p. 24), originally stirred up a great deal of controversy because they stood in sharp contrast to analytic perspectives that emphasized psychosocial causes of mental illness. However, both this perspective and Allen's cognitive levels are now widely accepted.

In 1998, Allen took another look at Piaget's work, finding that the dynamic process of organizing and refining her cognitive concepts had remained parallel to the iterations of cognitive structuralism of Piaget's outlook as a dynamic process (C. Allen, personal communication, January 30, 2001). Allen was pleased that her perspective remains within structural psychology—that is, the analysis of structure or content of conscious mental states by using introspective methods. Despite many modifications in Piaget's original conceptual cognitive-level labels as translated into Allen's OT-oriented cognitive-level labels, Allen believes that she has remained true to the spirit of Piaget's theoretical organization of intellectual abilities.

Cognitive Levels

Allen (1985) explained that she had examined the five cognitive developmental levels of Piaget—the sensorimotor, preconceptual, intuitive, concrete operational, and formal operational phases—so as to describe the cognitive disabilities manifested by the behaviors or voluntary motor actions of patients treated in occupational therapy. Allen attempted to correlate each of Piaget's abstract cognitive levels with its external manifestations in behavioral function. Thus, her schema represents an "occupational" or action-oriented interpretation of Piaget's cognitive levels.

Allen commented that she cannot follow Piaget too closely: "If one assumes that the Piagetian hierarchy is only partially correct in describing the functional behavior of adults with mental disorders, then one must be prepared to look beyond the realm of the Piagetian hierarchy" (Allen, 1985, p. 328). Consequently, she revised her first formulations by winnowing the denotations and connotations of the labels to represent the indications of intelligence that she had observed. Her original schema recognized six distinct functional cognitive levels: automatic actions, postural actions, manual actions, goal-directed activities, exploratory actions, and planned actions (Allen, 1985, 1988a, 2000; Allen et al., 1992). These concepts provide an ordinal scale of observable behaviors, thus enabling the development of a calibrated hierarchy of adequate specificity for measuring cognitive functions.

Levels 1 and 2, automatic actions and postural actions, most closely resemble Piaget's sensorimotor cognitive level; Level 3, manual actions, resembles Piaget's preconceptual level; and Level 4, goal-directed activities, resembles Piaget's level of intuitive thought. Levels 5 and 6, exploratory actions and planned actions, may be viewed as representing Piaget's concrete and formal operational levels, respectively. In the current formulation, Allen has changed the title of the fifth level from exploratory actions to independent learning because the former term was considered too abstract. The term *exploratory actions* may not have connoted an achievement of a cognitive skill, but rather aimless wanderings of exploration (C. Allen, 1999; Allen, personal communication, January 30, 2001).

Allen (1999) modified the schema of cognitive levels of function in two additional ways. One change is the provision of more easily understood descriptors within the schema to condense the seven earlier descriptors of sensory cues, motor actions, conscious awareness, purpose, experience, process, and time. The descriptors for the six cognitive levels are now delineated across "Abilities," "Attention Toward," and "Thinking About." The vocabulary of the new explanations is more direct and clearer than previous language (Allen, 1999).

Allen's other change was to split Level 1 into two parts, creating a lower level called Level 0, which is a coma state. In this state of being unconscious, the patient shows no response to stimulus and no capacity for arousal. Allen states that she added this level for the sake of neurologists. Table 8.1 shows Allen's conceptual configuration, including these more recent changes (Bertrand, 1997b).

Functional Information Processing System or Performance Modes

In delineating subdivisions of the original Allen Cognitive Levels, Allen divided each of Levels 1 through 5 into five categories of performance modes to provide specificity in standards of per-

Table 8.1
Cognitive Levels

| | Descriptors | | |
Cognitive Level	Abilities	Pays Attention To	Thinking About
Level 0: Coma	Generalized reflexive actions	Unconscious: lack of response to stimuli; autonomic flexion/extension; opening mouth	No thoughts; startle reactions
Level 1: Automatic Actions	Protective reflexes Locating strong stimuli Sustaining life	Five senses	Survival
Level 2: Postural Actions	Overcoming the effects of gravity Body movements: sit, stand, walk, range of motion, push Avoid barriers	Trunk balance Movements of extremities Large external objects Cues to barriers	Proprioceptive cues Stability, falls Safety, comfort
Level 3: Manual Actions	Handling objects Repetitive actions Follows cues to next step	Gross hand coordination Finger opposition Perceptual categories of size, shape, row Sustains actions	Feeling, moving, and identifying objects Cause and effect on objects
Level 4: Goal-Directed Activities	Goes to next step Self-care alone Complies with directions	Figure–ground perception Striking visual cues Old effects of actions Errors, samples Possessions	"What's next?" "Is this right?" "This is mine/yours." "I've done this before."

(continues)

Table 8.1 *Continued.*

		Descriptors
Level 5: Independent Learning (originally called Exploratory Actions)	New exploratory actions Fine motor adjustments Talking and working Impulsiveness (Individuals at Level 5.4 and below do not recognize their illness)	Discovery of new effects and remembers Surface properties: sheens and texture Spatial properties: assembly, part-whole, tiny part Feelings of self and personal rights	"How can I make this faster, easier, better?" "What's in it for me" "It's not my fault." "I wonder what they meant by that?"
Level 6: Planned Actions	Stopping to think Seeking more information Checking clock or schedule Considering needs of others Organizing and prioritizing activities	Symbolic, abstract cues: time, gravity, evaporation Hypothetical risks as anticipated hazards Social expectations and personal obligations Greater good	"What would happen if . . . ?" "What do you think of this?" "What are my options?" "How can I help you?"

Note Adapted from *Occupational Therapy Treatment Goals for the Physically and Cognitively Disabled*, by C. K. Allen, C. A. Earhart, and T. Blue, 1992, Rockville, MD: American Occupational Therapy Association.

formance that can be used to accurately evaluate cognitive disability levels (Allen, 1985, 1987; Allen et al., 1992). She created performance modes both for the sake of patients and to develop interdisciplinary credibility for observations in occupational therapy. In recent years, Allen clarified the descriptions of the performance modes, making them more occupational therapy oriented by gearing them toward activities of daily living (ADLs), and renamed this performance mode structure the Functional Information Processing System (FIPS; Allen & Bertrand, 1999) The outline of this processing system is provided in Table 8.2.

Persons capable of automatic action only (Level 1) are able to respond in a sensory manner to stimuli with movement of body parts while lying in bed, but are unable to maintain postural actions of sitting or walking. Individuals who have the ability of postural actions (Level 2) can sit, stand, and walk, but at the lower Level 2 stages may not know where they are going. Later, they may walk to an identified location and use grab bars and railings for support. People with the capacity for manual actions (Level 3) initially can grasp and move their hands when objects are placed within reach. With higher Level 3 processes, they can distinguish between objects, sustain actions on objects, note the effects of their actions on objects, and recognize when an activity is completed.

Individuals capable of goal-directed activities (Level 4) have the cognitive ability to sequence steps independently through the parts of a simple, routine short-term task. These individuals can complete a simple goal, scan the environment, and attempt to memorize new skill steps. To learn a total activity pattern or to build a habit, they may rely on memory of steps practiced through months of repetition (Allen et al., 1992). People with the capacity for independent learning (Level 5) have the mental ability to discover improved effects of actions and to remember details of actions. At this level, the individual engages in self-directed learning. In an effort to relate to others and to learn through them, the individual considers social standards and consults with other people. Learning by doing through a process of trial and error includes the advantage of adaptability and the disadvantage of time-consuming or costly mistakes. People capable of planned actions (Level 6) have the intellectual capacity to anticipate results and to select courses of action that are projected as desirable. Covert thought processes may be revealed

Table 8.2
Functional Information Processing System: Procedural Memory[a]

Cognitive Levels	Performance Modes
Level 1: Automatic Actions	1.0 Withdraws from stimuli 1.2 Responds to stimuli 1.4 Locates stimuli 1.6 Moves in bed 1.8 Raises body parts
Level 2: Postural Actions	2.0 Overcomes gravity 2.2 Stands and uses righting reactions 2.4 Walks 2.6 Walks to an identified location 2.8 Uses railings and grab bars for support
Level 3: Manual Actions	3.0 Grasps objects 3.2 Distinguishes between objects 3.4 Sustains actions on objects 3.6 Notes effects of actions on objects 3.8 Uses all objects and senses completion of an activity
Level 4: Goal-Directed Activities	4.0 Sequences self through steps of an activity 4.2 Differentiates between parts of an activity 4.4 Completes a goal 4.6 Scans the environment 4.8 Memorizes new steps
Level 5: Independent	5.0 Learns to improve effects of action Learning 5.2 Improves the fine details of actions 5.4 Engages in self-directed learning 5.6 Considers social standards 5.8 Consults with other people
Level 6: Planned actions	6.0 Plans actions

[a] Formerly termed "Modes of Performance Within the Cognitive Levels."

Note. Adapted from *Structures of the Cognitive Performance Modes,* by C. K. Allen and J. Bertrand (Eds.), 1999, Ormond Beach, FL: Allen Conferences.

by pauses to stop and think before acting, by information gathering as preparation for action, or by requests to deliberate on alternatives before making a decision (Allen, 2000; Allen et al., 1992).

As an example of progress through the performance modes within a cognitive level, Allen mentioned that some individuals experience a rapid decline in cognitive ability following stroke, and in natural recovery may ascend through the mode levels quickly (C. Allen, personal communication, January 30, 2001). For others, however, movement through the levels can be slow or nonexistent.

Allen also provided an extended example of what may be performed at each level of the FIPS schema for a single task of food preparation. For the three lower performance levels, eating is usually the activity that is done best. At Level 3.8, an individual may be trained to make a simple sandwich. At Level 4.4, some persons with disabilities can prepare simple, well-learned dishes; follow a fixed diet; and shop for routine items, but they go to the store repeatedly to purchase immediate needs only. At Level 5.2, people may be expected to know how to shop, wash, prepare, cook, and store food properly, with awareness of spoilage problems and ability to check quality of produce. However, due to lack of higher independent learning skills achieved at the upper end of Level 5, they may impulsively change a shopping list and fail to follow dietary precautions in their meandering, exploratory style (Allen, 2000; Allen et al., 1992).

Allen believes that at Levels 1 through 5, humans share sensorimotor processes with other species, but that the cognitive abilities of Level 6 are uniquely human. Many of the activities of everyday life are done at lower levels of cognition because it is human nature to conserve energy when doing routine tasks. Also, when people are fatigued or lack motivation, they are content to operate at lower levels, on automatic pilot. However, the intellectual competence of the individual without a cognitive disability includes the capacity to function at Level 6 when the need or desire arises (Allen et al., 1992; Katz, 1998).

Cognitive Levels 4 and 5 are perplexing to therapists wishing to determine whether lack of motivation or inability is the cause of the individual's lack of participation or effort. Allen admits that motivational explanations cannot always be eliminated. For that reason, when assessing cognitive levels, the therapist should permit the patient to choose the activity (Allen, 1985, 1988a; Allen et al., 1992). Also, because about 20% of the nondisabled population may operate for the most part at Level 5, it is not always possible to determine whether the Level 5 performance of a person with a disability is a temporary or usual mode of function (C. Allen, personal communication, May 16, 1992). This observation needs to be studied empirically.

Allen has expanded most of her earlier troublesome definitions to the point of universality of conceptualization. For example, Allen's earlier definition of cognitive disability seemed to omit an important element. Allen (1985) stated that "a cognitive disability is a restriction in voluntary motor action originating in the physical or chemical structures of the brain and producing observable limitations in routine task behavior" (p. 31). Allen's adoption in 1992 of an ICIDH (International Classification of Impairments, Disabilities and Handicaps; World Health Organization [WHO], 1980) distinction between *disability* (concerned with global, functional limitations) and *impairment* (existing at the organ level) has helped to resolve some of the lack of clarity in the original statement (Allen et al., 1992, p. 345).

Working and Procedural Memory

Basic to the understanding of the FIPS are the two types of memory, working and procedural. Allen has described working memory as an active system of recall of functional skill elements that can dynamically select subskills needed for a new task (C. Allen, personal communication, January 30, 2001). Working memory operates sequentially and is found on the left side of the brain. By contrast, procedural memory is the hardwired recall of specific steps of an activity that has been performed so frequently that the process is routine in nature. Procedural memory operates instantaneously. A person can use procedural memory to drive a car home from work through a usual route. However, if that simple routine is broken by stopping at a store for an errand, working memory needs to be employed for the dynamic adjustment to the typical procedure (Allen, 1999).

In OT assessment for return to the community, if the individual is evaluated for ADLs at home, the test merely taps into procedural memory of familiar functional steps in a familiar setting. If working memory is to be tested, a dynamic task needs to be selected. Allen maintains that crafts are needed in OT to evaluate working memory for its capacity to problem-solve and to follow steps in a new sequence unfamiliar to the individual

(C. Allen, personal communication, January 30, 2001). In occupational therapy, if only ADLs are tested, the capacity of the individual for dynamic, working memory required for new tasks during reentry into the community remains unknown.

Figure 8.1 presents the differences between the information processing of working memory and that of procedural memory. The upper portion of the figure shows the relationships of cues,

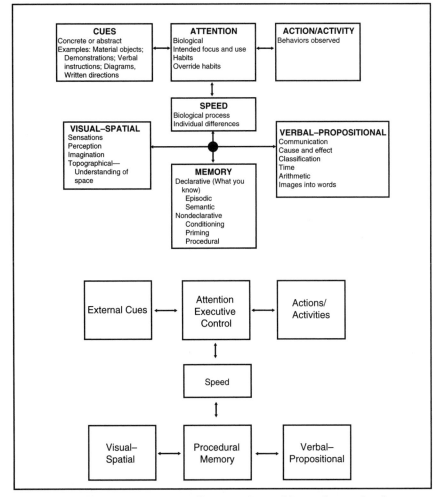

Figure 8.1. Information processing diagrams for working and procedural memory. *Note:* From *How to Use Allen's Cognitive Levels in Daily Practice* (p. 10), by C. K. Allen, 1999, Ormond Beach, FL: Allen Conferences. Reprinted with permission from Allen Conferences, Inc., 385 Coquina Avenue, Ormond Beach, FL 32174.

attention, speed, visual–spatial abilities, and verbal input as elements of processing of information for memory functions. In this model, the elements are depicted as separate entities. By contrast, in the lower portion of the figure, the elements that play a role in procedural memory are more closely integrated. In procedural memory, the brain requires fewer conscious steps to undertake functions that are repeatedly used (Allen, 1999). In both models, actions and activities are the observable behaviors of the inferred mental processes of the rest of the models.

Assessment of Cognitive Levels

Initially Allen began assessment of patients through clinical observation to develop face validity for the cognitive levels. She insisted that occupational therapists should never abandon the strengths of their own clinical observation skills no matter how technical or stratified the format of formal assessments they use (C. Allen, personal communication, May 16, 1992).

Allen and her OT colleagues have developed numerous methods for evaluation of the cognitive levels. The first was the Allen Cognitive Levels (ACL; Allen, 1988a), a craft-oriented leather-lacing task that incorporates three levels of difficulty in forming stitches. It has been used clinically since 1973 for evaluative purposes, and is now produced by S&S Worldwide. The ACL has three versions: the original, the expanded (ACL–E), and the problem-solving ACL (ACL–PS). In addition, the Large ACL (LACL) was developed by Kathy Kehrberg (1992) for use in geriatric assessment. Allen emphasizes that users always need to check patients for visual impairment before beginning screening with the ACL. In Josman and Katz's (1991) ACL–PS, the therapist permits much Level 5 independent learning behavior before instructing the patient in the stitches and provides an opportunity for the patient to correct a deliberate error in the stitches. Allen (1990) saw the conceptual value of this addition, which removed the ceiling effect of the earlier ACL, and she incorporated this improvement in 1990, renaming the test the ACL–90. The ACL–90 incorporates several steps of problem solving to provide challenges for individuals with higher cognitive levels, and the test has additional discriminatory power through a refinement of intervals within the test (Allen et al., 1992). "The range of scores is 3.0 to 5.8, which seems to be more logically related to what leather lacing can measure" (Allen et al., 1992, p. 33).

Allen now considers the ACL to be a quick screening tool (Allen et al., 1992; C. Allen, personal communication, May 16, 1992) and has added the name "Screen" to the title (ACLS). She believes that a therapist should begin an assessment with an interview to determine the individual's functional history, then screen with the ACLS, and finally use the comprehensive Routine Task Inventory (RTI; Allen et al., 1992), which aims at analyzing a basic and broad spectrum of independent living activities. Allen also encourages clinicians to develop their own assessment for activities that they constantly use in certain groups by calibrating them through the hierarchies of the performance modes of the cognitive levels (see Table 8.2).

> [The ACLS] is so fast to administer, and so easy, that it goes into research designs very well. But it is still this fast little thing. The real power is in the RTI, not in the ACLS. The real power is not in the leather lacing; it's in the activities of daily living pattern of performance, and people don't get that. They get hung up on this test. And maybe it's just an evolutionary process. Maybe it takes a year of administering the test before you get a Gestalt of what the performance modes are really all about. We now feel more comfortable with our clinical observation scores than with our ACLS scores, and if there is a disparity, we take our clinical score over the ACLS score. I keep telling people that they've got to get to that point. They can't stay wedded to that one little thing, [the leather lacing]. So the ACLS is the best documented and the best investigated, but ... I want people to get to where they trust their own judgment, and their own ability to assess from observing performance, because the natural performance is our ace in the hole. (C. Allen, personal communication, April 16, 1992)

Allen now recommends using the RTI in addition to the ACLS to provide a comprehensive evaluation battery that can serve as an indicator of goals to be addressed with the client through discussion, problem solving, training, or drilling. Because cognitive disabilities, which are often hidden, can have a more pervasive impact than obvious physical disabilities, Allen has argued that the instrument used to assess cognitive problems needs to be detailed and hierarchical in its calibrations in order to provide a well-documented, comprehensive picture of the person (Allen et al., 1992). The RTI, with its multiple levels of distinctions of cognitive and behavioral indicators, provides this specificity for the ADL area. Table 8.3 outlines the four major kinds of disability that are analyzed through the RTI: self-awareness disability, sit-

Table 8.3
Activities Analyzed on the Routine Task Inventory
to Assess Behavior Disabilities

10. Self-awareness disability	12. Occupational role disability
.0 Grooming	.0 Planning/doing major role activities
.1 Dressing	.1 Planning/doing spare-time activities
.2 Bathing	.2 Pacing and timing activities
.3 Walking/exercising	.3 Exerting effort
.4 Feeding	.4 Judging results
.5 Toileting	.5 Speaking
.6 Taking medications	.6 Following safety precautions
.7 Using adaptive equipment	.7 Responding to emergencies
.8 Other	.8 Other
.9 Unspecified	.9 Unspecified
11. Situational awareness disability	13. Social role disability
.0 Housekeeping	.0 Communicating meaning
.1 Preparing/obtaining goods	.1 Following instructions
.2 Spending money	.2 Contributing to family activities
.3 Shopping	.3 Caring for dependents
.4 Doing laundry	.4 Cooperating with others
.5 Traveling	.5 Supervising independent people
.6 Telephoning	.6 Keeping informed
.7 Adjusting to change	.7 Engaging in good citizenship
.8 Other	.8 Other
.9 Unspecified	.9 Unspecified

Note. The numbers 10 to 13 are based on the World Health Organization's (1980) ICIDH format and include activities that "are apt to be most important to most people" and "are apt to be affected by cognitive disability" (Allen, Kehrberg, & Burns, 1992). From "Evaluation Instruments," by C. K. Allen, K. Kehrberg, and T. Burns, in *Occupational Therapy Treatment Goals for the Physically and Cognitively Disabled* (p. 36), by C. K. Allen, C. A. Earhart, and T. Blue, 1992, Rockville, MD: American Occupational Therapy Association. Copyright 1992 by the American Occupational Therapy Association. Reprinted with permission.

uational awareness disability, occupational role disability, and social role disability (Allen et al., 1992, p. 36). Allen uses the ICIDH (WHO, 1980) definitions of these disabilities: "Self-awareness disability is a mental disturbance in the ability to meet the natural demands of one's body"; "situational awareness disability is a mental disturbance of the capacity to register and understand relationships between objects and persons within the context of daily living"; "occupational role disability is a mental disturbance of the ability to organize and participate in routine activities connected with the occupation of time, not only confined to the performance of work"; and "social role disability is a mental disturbance in the ability to meet social expectations when interacting with other people" (Allen et al., 1992, p. 349).

Allen et al. (1992) describe each of the four disability areas and their activities in detail. Within each area, they list eight basic ADLs essential for discrimination of safety and independence. In *Occupational Therapy Treatment Goals for the Physically and Cognitively Disabled,* Allen et al. (1992, p. 40) wrote, "This book is designed to give you feedback about the accuracy of your activity analysis so that you can confidently analyze any activity that is important to your patient." Extended examples detailed in Chapter 6 of the book include the activities of sanding, staining, gluing, polishing/cleaning, cutting, sewing, measuring, and mixing ingredients, all of which are calibrated through the levels of the performance modes for each activity.

Allen describes the difficulties in delineating the evaluation of human cognitive levels and in developing a schema of performance modes for cognitive assessment.

Things are pretty clear all though level four, but level five is a serious concern, and we really don't understand the difference between [difficulties in] problem-solving at level five when that's a disability or when it's normal [for that individual]. And we're having tremendous trouble with level six because the hierarchy from motor behavior and through symbolism as Piaget delineated it simply doesn't work. So we don't have a view of a hierarchy of normal learning that is really working. We have to develop our own.

The surprising thing is that we have some very bright left-hemisphere dominant people who score 5.2 or 5.4 on the ACLS, and function that way with their hands, my husband being one, who is very good conceptually, but becomes a level five on me routinely. There are some people who just don't problem-solve with their hands. . . . Perhaps the capacities of the left-dominant abstract thing became level 6, and may be hemispheric. . . . All of that stuff is fouled up between 5.4 and whatever goes into level 6. We just stopped at 6.0 in this last book. It just got too confusing. (C. Allen, personal communication, April 16, 1992)

Application to Occupational Therapy

Practical Application of Theory by Allen

In 1985, Allen discussed the question, "Can occupational therapy services change the cognitive level?" She gave a negative answer, admitting that this was a shocking reply (Allen, 1985, p. 31). Occupational therapists, she stated, needed "to switch from trying to change the patient to changing the activity" (Allen, 1985, p. 27). In 1992, Allen commented on the general inability of patients with cognitive impairments to move beyond their cognitive level, even with intensive training.

It was very frustrating for me because clearly the thing to do is . . . to try to move a person to the next level. If we had a learning theory that worked, we could do it. But we can't seem to do it. We can't seem to make it work. Even with the new book, with 52 modes of performance, we just can't do it.

For example, if the patient is performing cognitively at a Level 4.4 in the performance modes,

every time you give them a 4.6 cue, they ignore it. They don't know what to do with it, or they reject it, or they just don't see it. And we still come up against these brick walls. I think it goes back to having no good theory about learning. Maybe it's in the DNA, in that genetic stuff, and if the DNA is all fouled up, you just can't go on. (C. Allen, personal communication, August 24, 1992)

Instead of trying to change the patient, "change is made by getting the patient to do everything that he or she would like to do within his or her range of ability" (Allen et al., 1992, p. 23). The occupational therapist first identifies the patient's range of ability by assessing the individual's cognitive level, then selects and modifies tasks to bring them within that range. Allen (1985) emphasized that the tasks selected should appeal to the patient and in fact be pleasant.

Occupational Therapy as Compensatory Intervention

Allen's approach to treatment of patients with cognitive disabilities is in keeping with her broader views on OT treatment in general as she expressed them in her 1987 Eleanor Clarke Slagle Lecture, "Activity: Occupational Therapy's Treatment Method." In this lecture, Allen stated that "therapeutic activity compensates for disability by utilizing remaining capabilities to accomplish desirable activities with satisfactory results" (1987, p. 574). She emphasized the emotional satisfactions of successful activity and the occupational therapist's role of helping the patient to obtain or regain these satisfactions. She pointed out, for example, that "activity actualizes a person's strengths" and that " . . . people with spinal cord injuries who are the most productive do not express their loss in physical terms; the greatest loss is expressed as a loss in activity" (1987, p. 573). Although activity is valued by everyone, it "is especially important to disabled people because their opportunity to engage in successful activity is limited" (1987, p. 574).

Functional Safety

Allen has asserted that "safety in doing ordinary activities is the primary treatment goal" (Allen et al., 1992, p. 339) in working with patients who have any type of cognitive disability. She refers to the cognitive levels as a functional safety scale because lack of attention to cues is the principal problem of patients with cognitive disabilities.

When a patient is discharged, "the expected outcome is a recommendation of the least restrictive environment that the patient can function in safely" (Allen et al., 1992, p. 20). The Allen Cognitive Levels have proven useful for making this determination. Allen indicates, for example, that a person who stabilizes at Level 3.5 most likely needs 24-hour supervision. A patient remitting at Level 4.5 does not need such supervision but has deficits that prevent "efficient and error-free performance of high level ADLs" (Allen et al., 1992, p. 49).

Allen pointed out that the safety of the patient with a cognitive disability is a legal issue in which occupational therapists are necessarily involved.

> What is the difference between looking at a person in the simulated environment versus the real environment? . . . How much can you predict in those carefully controlled situations as to what patients are going to do in an uncontrolled environment where a lot of out of the ordinary things happen? It's not going to be an either or kind of thing, but a weighted, multiregression analysis kind of prediction. We really need to go into that kind of depth to really understand what we are doing when we get into these legal questions. . . . We have to prepare ourselves for that. Ultimately is it "child" custody or not? Where do we draw the line, and what factors determine where we draw the line? Really tough questions. (C. Allen, personal communication, May 16, 1992)

Allen continues to stress that the assessment and intervention for safety issues is essential not only for people with cognitive information processing deficits, but also for occupational therapists. Each of the 25 performance mode levels in her book, *Understanding Cognitive Performance Modes* (Allen, Earhart & Blue, 1995), has a one- to two-page analysis of the safety problems for people at each level in the ADL categories of moving, bathroom, dressing, eating, housekeeping, and physical disabilities. These issues overlap from one level to another, but are outlined in such great detail that they could be shared with family members to highlight the therapist's concerns for the safety of the patient and the family. Support people frequently need confirmation of their own unstated concerns about the prevention of accidental fires, falls, and "wanderings."

Allen has turned the spotlight onto issues of functional safety that occur when individuals have cognitive limitations of focus, concentration, and directionality; are unable to learn new tasks; or have difficulty sequencing steps in tasks. In considering the need for adaptation, change of environment, or supervision to accommodate safety issues for a patient, an occupational therapist needs to act as an environmental and safety consultant.

Legal Definitions of Function

Allen credited *Black's Law Dictionary* (1979) and the ICIDH (WHO, 1980) as sources that helped her to define such terms as *competence, capacity, reasonable care, negligence, reasonable thought, prudent and diligent behavior, incapacitated status,* and *custody* (Allen et al., 1992). "Our patients are mostly involuntary. We are faced with those kinds of legal questions [regarding competency] daily" (C. Allen, personal communication, May 16, 1992). Allen also has distinguished between *impairment* and *disability, recovery* and *remediation,* and *environmental compensations* and *social assistance* by drawing on official health definitions put forth in the ICIDH (WHO, 1980) and in the *International Classification of Diseases* (Karaffa, 1992).

Third-Party Payer Definitions of Function

From the beginning, Allen's work has been guided by practical considerations. Her schema of cognitive levels and performance modes and her construction of the RTI were to a great extent responses to the dilemma of writing satisfactory progress notes for Blue Cross and Medicaid. She sought to remedy classifications that were too broad in scope to detect the distinctions of varying cognitive disability levels or the small refinements therapists made to accommodate patients' disabilities. To make the subtle changes in patients visible to the insurer, Allen broke apart each of the six cognitive levels into multiple performance modes (as shown in Table 8.2). She then incorporated these distinctions into the RTI to make assessments of functioning as highly calibrated as possible.

The need to justify OT services to third-party payers also has contributed to Allen's emphasis on safety as the primary goal in treating individuals with cognitive disabilities.

> The way to get out of being boxed in by Medicare for the self-care activities, to look at a broader view of the activities that people are going to do, is to emphasize safety. That's our key to getting paid if we are looking at the quality of life—a very practical approach. (C. Allen, personal communication, April 16, 1992)

Clinical Observations

Allen is also practical in another way. Her publications are filled with down-to-earth guidelines for clinical assessment, task analysis and accommodation, and preparation for the environment to which persons with cognitive disabilities are returning. Her books use graded case examples to teach OT students and practitioners how to incorporate her concepts, propositions, and philosophy into their practice. Through leading questions, she enables the reader to ferret out pertinent facts within the cases for evaluation and provides direction for possible change or accommodation.

Application of Theory by Occupational Therapists

Practitioners in cognitive and psychosocial OT tend to refer conversationally and frequently to the Allen Cognitive Levels by number when describing a person's cognitive functional ability. This practice has been in common usage in oral clinical descriptions since about 1985, even by therapists in settings not formally using the ACLS (personal communications with New York area occupational therapists, 1985 to present). The Allen Cognitive Levels (Allen, 1985, 1987, 1988a, 1988b, 1999, 2000; Allen et al., 1992, 1995) are popular among therapists because they are user friendly in terms of evaluating and citing numeric level names as representative of the cognitive gradations of functional behavioral abilities that remain intact in individuals. Among occupational therapists working in mental health, the statement that a person is "operating at Level 4" needs little or no explanation.

Allen's work is taught in OT departments in colleges, universities, and clinics across the country. Allen also has provided workshops and created videotapes instructing people in the use of her tools and system through Allen Conferences (http://www.allen-cognitive-levels.com).

Theory Validation and Research

Early critiques of Allen's work focused on her apparently iconoclastic position of a neurological base for psychiatric disorders, her skepticism about patients' abilities to change their cognitive levels, and the definitions of some of her concepts. Her early ideas were based on her work with people with schizophrenia and other chronic disorders. Most of these earlier problems that occupational therapists had with Allen's views have now been resolved. In some instances, Allen has shifted to a new position through development of her perceptions and assessment tools. She has expanded the cognitive levels with the performance modes so that patients and therapists can clearly perceive the small, incremental steps through which patients have been treated by cognitive drilling, training, learning, problem solving, and goal setting.

In his 1992 text, *Conceptual Foundations of Occupational Therapy,* Kielhofner focused his discussion of Allen's cognitive disabilities model on concerns voiced about her earlier work: the concern that occupational therapists must not inadvertently limit patients' opportunities to learn; insistence that research must be done to support or refute Allen's claim that learning does not occur within Levels 1 through 4; and the need for research into issues of motivation and its effect on performance. In that Kielhofner and Allen published their 1992 texts almost simultaneously, Kielhofner was likely unaware that Allen had gradually developed her model to include these issues. Kielhofner noted Allen's concern for motivation, dating as far back as 1985, in her emphasis on the patient's selection of desirable activities. He did have a point, with which Allen would no doubt agree, that lack of change in patients may be partially attributable to the paucity of resources for patients in the current health care delivery system (Kielhofner, 1992). Kielhofner called for further research comparing the relative importance of motivational factors with cognitive functional factors as contributors to the rehabilitation process.

An example of the application of the Allen Cognitive Levels by one occupational therapist was described by Bertrand (1997a):

> After the cognitive level is determined, the manual, *Understanding Cognitive Performance Modes,* outlines each mode by description, tells the percentage of cognitive and physical assistance needed and the amount of supervision the patient will require to be safe. For example, a patient who is at Level 4.2 will require 38% (or Moderate) cognitive assistance. This person needs 24-hour supervision to remove dangerous objects outside of the visual field and to solve problems arising from minor changes in the environment.

This degree of specificity in treatment intervention is typical of therapists applying the Allen levels and performance modes to the patient's daily life.

Cheatum (1994) reported that occupational therapists at the Veterans Administration Medical Center in Wilkes-Barre, Pennsylvania, were asked by the Surgery Department to administer the Allen Cognitive Levels preoperatively to 26 patients about to undergo hip replacement surgery. Following surgery, the patients were given the following simple precautions:

1. Don't bend the hip more than 90 degrees.

2. Don't cross the operated leg over the other leg.

3. Don't turn the operated leg inward (pigeon-toed).

Despite these simple instructions, patients with lower scores on the ACL had a higher incidence of dislocation. Cheatum reported the following results:

1. Persons with a score of 4.4 ($n = 5$ out of 26) or lower had a 100% chance of dislocation.

2. Persons with a score of 4.7 to 5.0 ($n = 4$ out of 26) had a 44% chance of dislocation.

3. Persons with a score of 5.2 or better ($n = 17$ out of 26) had no dislocation.

These results occurred even though occupational therapists provided persons in the lowest level group with verbal cues, written materials, and videotapes of behaviors. This is an excellent illustration of cognitive problems overriding postsurgical intervention (Cheatum, 1994), as well as of research on cognition relevant to physical disability practice.

Reliability and Validity Studies

Numerous studies of reliability and validity have been carried out by occupational therapists using Allen's instruments, including the Allen Cognitive Levels (ACL; Allen, 1988a), Routine Task Inventory (RTI; Heimann, Allen & Yerxa, 1989), Cognitive Performance Test (Burns, 1992), and Functional Information

Performance System (FIPS; Allen et al., 1992). These studies are described in this section.

Allen Cognitive Level

The ACL has been found to have good test–retest and interrater reliability. In 1978, Moore tested the original ACL leather-lacing task and found a high level of interrater reliability ($r = .99$) of five pairs of occupational therapists with 32 participants. These therapists had extensive experience administering the ACL test for several years. Newman (1987) found good interrater reliability ($r = .95$) and good test–retest reliability ($r = .75$) of the ACL–Extended (ACL–E), the version featuring a lengthened score sheet with more numerous graded intervals and developed for use with populations in whom little cognitive change is expected. Concurrent validity with the ACL varied but was generally supported. Allen's (1985) investigations of concurrent validity showed moderate and low correlations between the ACL and the Brief Psychiatric Rating Scale ($r = .53$) and between the ACL and the Block Design subtest of the Wechsler Adult Intelligence Scale (WAIS) ($r = .46$) in hospitalized patients. In 50 nondisabled persons, Allen (1985) found moderate correlations between the ACL and the Hollingshead Two-Factor Index of Social Position subtests of education ($r = .50$), occupation ($r = .53$), and social position ($r = .51$). Katz (1979) found a low correlation between the ACL and the WAIS Block Design subtest ($r = .45$) in people with depression; however, Mayer (1988) found a good correlation ($r = .72$) between the ACL and WAIS Block Design and Object Assembly subtests in people with psychosis, and a moderate correlation ($r = .55$) of the ACL and the WAIS Performance IQ. In children with emotional disturbance, the ACL was not predictive of scores on the Visual Motor Integration (VMI) or the Perceptual Memory Task (Shapiro, 1992).

Discriminate validity of the ACL has also been addressed. In Moore's (1978) study, the validity of the ACL for placing patients in an OT group was supported, and she found a good correlation ($r = .76$) between six therapists ratings of the patients for general clinical group levels and patients' performance levels on the ACL.

The ACL has been used to assess patients with schizophrenia, depression, and dementia and to compare them to normal controls. Figure 8.2 shows comparison of ACL scores among

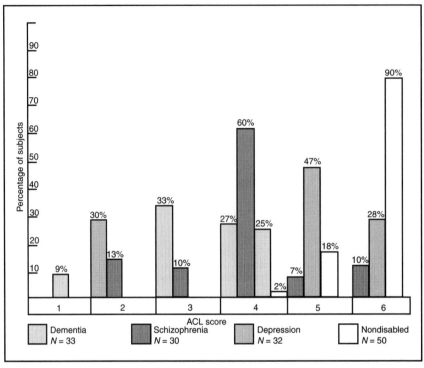

Figure 8.2. Frequency distribution of scores on the Allen Cognitive Level test (ACL). *Note.* From *Occupational Therapy for Psychiatric Diseases: Measurement and Management of Cognitive Disabilities* (p. 369), by C. K. Allen, 1985, Boston: Little, Brown. Copyright 1985. Reprinted with permission.

these four groups. The partially overlapping histograms are found in the position relative to each other that most clinicians would expect, giving the results clinical or face validity. The majority of patients with dementia were in Levels 1 to 4. Patients with schizophrenia ranged from Levels 2 to 6, with over half of this diagnostic group in Level 4. Average scores of patients with depression fell in Levels 4 to 6, with about 50% in Level 5. Nondisabled individuals ranged from Levels 4 to 6, with 80% ranking in Level 6 (Allen, 1985, p. 369). Thus, it can be seen that certain known psychiatric groups are associated with specific levels of functional cognitive performance, providing "known group" or discriminant validity. Table 8.4 (Allen, 1988), which illustrates the overlapping levels of various diagnoses dependent on

Table 8.4
Diagnoses Associated with Cognitive Disability Levels

Cognitive Level	Diagnoses
Level 1: Automatic Actions	Organic brain syndrome Severe dementia Recent traumatic brain injury Cardiovascular accidents Occasional psychiaric disorder
Level 2: Postural Actions	Dementia Cardiovascular accidents Traumatic brain injury Severely psychotic disorders
Level 3: Manual Actions	Dementia Traumatic brain injury Cardiovascular accidents Developmental disabilities Acute manic episodes Acute schizophrenic episodes
Level 4: Goal-Directed Activities	Mild dementia Traumatic brain injury Cardiovascular accidents Developmental disabilities HIV/AIDS Acute manic episodes Acute depressive episodes
Level 5: Independent Learning	Affective disorders in remission Good-prognosis schizophrenic disorders Personality disorders Early-onset dementia Usual level of function for about 20% of persons with no distressing disability or symptamology
Level 6: Planned Actions	Affective disorders in full remission Good-prognosis schizophrenic disorders Acute brain syndromes, cleared Usual level of function for most "normal" persons

Note. From "Cognitive Disabilities," by C. K. Allen, 1888, in *Mental Health Focus* (pp. 3-28 to 3-32), by S. Robinson (Ed.), Rockville, MD: American Occupational Therapy Association. Copyright 1988 by American Occupational Therapy Association. Reprinted with permission.

the degree of severity of cognitive deficit, includes diagnoses that are graphed in Figure 8.2.

Allen has openly invited occupational therapists to test the validity and reliability of the ACLS through additional studies. In 1988, Katz, Josman, and Steinmetz reported from Israel that in a study of 20 psychiatric adolescent patients and matched healthy controls, a significant difference was found in cognitive levels of the two groups ($p < .01$). None of the controls scored under Level 5 on the ACL and half of them scored at Level 6. By contrast, the patients had a wide range of cognitive skills, with 25% below Level 5, 50% at Level 5, and 25% at Level 6 (Katz et al., 1988). Again, the cognitive performance levels of function of known groups, such as the control groups, provide discriminant validity for the ACLS. In a comparison of the ACLS results with another cognitive measure, the Class Inclusion subtest of the Riska Object Classification (ROC) Test, "All subjects in the control group fully understood class inclusion relations, compared with only 60% of the patients" (Katz et al., 1988, p. 35).

In their 1992 book, Allen et al. acknowledged that some diagnostic groups of patients, such as those with affective disorders or good-prognosis schizophrenia, may experience a remission, thus changing cognitive levels. Other more chronic patients can solidify gains within a cognitive level through training and drilling, and thus move upward through the performance modes. Although some patients, such as those with dementia, may manifest a decline in cognitive level as part of the natural progression of their disease, others can be stabilized through a reasonably stimulating activity program to maintain their cognitive level.

In Allen et al.'s 1992 text, Tina Blue set up a comparison of the Allen Cognitive Levels with the Rancho Cognitive Levels, which also builds a bridge across physical and mental assessments of cognitive losses, thus testing concurrent validity (C. Allen, personal communication, August 24, 1992). Blue matched the Rancho levels of No Response, Generalized Response, and Localized Response with Allen's Level 1, Automatic Actions; the Rancho Confused–Agitated and Confused–Inappropriate levels with Allen's Levels 2 and 3, Postural Actions and Manual Actions; the Rancho Confused–Appropriate and Automatic–Appropriate levels with Allen's Level 4, Goal-Directed Activities; and the Rancho Purposeful–Appropriate level with Allen's Level 5, Independent

Learning. This comparison provides a clinical clarification and face validity of the two systems from divergent parts of the field of OT that are reconverging in the cognitive domain. Allen's cognitive levels seem more useful due to their greater clarity, simplicity, and ease of recall based on their correspondence to Piaget's well-known, though abstract, cognitive levels.

Allen (1998) developed a table that compares the ACLS with a number of other evaluation tools in addition to the Rancho Cognitive Levels. These include Medicare Cognitive and Physical Assessments (Medicare Guidelines: HCFA Publication 13-3), Rancho Head Trauma (Ranchos Los Amigos Professional Staff Association, 1986), Global Deterioration Scale (Reisberg, Ferris, Leon, & Cook, 1988), Function Improvement Measure ADL and Eat (Hamilton, Granger, Sherwin, et al., 1987), Global Assessment Scale (American Psychiatric Association, 1980), and Global Assessment of Function Scale (American Psychiatric Association, 1994). It is suggested that the reader look into Allen's (1998) source for complete references and information.

Routine Task Inventory

Heying (1983) and Heimann (1985; Heimann et al., 1989) did studies using the Routing Task Inventory (RTI). For example, examining the RTI in a study of 41 patients with Alzheimer's disease, Heimann et al. (1989) found good interrater reliability ($r = .98$) and test–retest reliability ($r = .91$), with an internal consistency alpha coefficient of .94. Good test–retest reliability ($r = .99$) for the RTI was also reported in a population with senile dementia (Wilson, Allen, McCormack, & Burton, 1989).

Concurrent validity of the RTI and the ACL was supported in several studies. In persons with senile dementia, correlations were moderate between the RTI and the ACL ($r = .56$) and between the RTI and the Mini-Mental Status Exam ($r = .61$) (Wilson et al., 1989). Secrest, Wood, and Tapp (2000) examined the concurrent validity of the ACLS and the RTI in a study of 33 men with schizophrenia. The ACLS was found to be significantly correlated with community function as measured by the RTI ($r = .67$). In a study on discharge planning, community living, and cognition with 40 adult psychiatric patients, McAnanama, Rogosin-Rose, Scott, Joffe, and Kelner (1999) found the highest correlation between the ACLS and the RTI–2 (Routine Task

Inventory–Second Edition) for the Instrumental Scale ($r = .97$) and for the Physical Scale ($r = .81$). Because the RTI shares a common theoretical base with the ACLS in measuring and predicting task performance, the relationship between the ACL and the RTI is not surprising.

Cognitive Performance Test

In 1985, Theresa Burns began developing the Cognitive Performance Test (CPT) to provide a standardized ADL assessment for functional levels manifested in Alzheimer's disease based on Allen's cognitive levels of processing information. Burns selected six of the RTI tasks: Dress, Shop, Toast, Telephone, Wash, and Travel. Studies of reliability and validity of the CPT have been carried out at the Minneapolis Veterans Administration Medical Center's Geriatric Research, Education and Clinical Center. External validity for 77 patients was measured in contrast to the Mini-Mental Status Examination ($r = .67$) and two caregiver's measures, Instrumental Activities of Daily Living ($r = .64$) and the Physical Self-Maintenance Scale ($r = .49$). Interrater reliability for 18 patients at 4 weeks was .91, and test–retest reliability for 36 patients at 4 weeks was .89 (Burns, 1992, pp. 46–50). Burns's analysis of IADLs within the CPT is similar to Earhart's Analysis of Activities (Allen et al., 1992) based on Allen's modes of performance.

Reliability and Validity of ACL, RTI, and CPT Summarized

Three tables are provided in this chapter to summarize the results of the validity and reliability studies that have been performed on the Allen Cognitive Level Screen (Allen, 1998) and the Routine Task Inventory (Allen, 1998). As shown in Table 8.5, the results of most of the reliability studies done for both the ACLS and the RTI have been high, ranging from .89 to .99, with one exception (.75) in the case of a test–retest study for people with schizophrenia (Newman, 1987).

Two tables of validity studies have been organized, one comparing the ACLS with other related assessment tools, and one comparing ACLS scores of "known groups." The first, Table 8.6, compares ACLS with six evaluation tools: the Wechsler Adult Intelligence Scale, the Bay Area Functional Performance Evaluation, the Riska Object Classification, the Mini-Mental Status

Table 8.5
Studies of Reliability of Three of Allen's Assessment Tools

Study	Diagnosis	n	Type of Reliability	r	p
Allen Cognitive Levels Screen (ACLS)					
Moore (1978)	Schizophrenia (inpatient)	32	Interrater	.99	
Newman (1987)	Schizophrenia	21	Interrater	.95	.01
	Schizophrenia	22	Test–Retest	.75	.01
Partida (1992)	Psychiatric illness	4	Interrater	1.00	
Howell (1993)	Depression	20	Interrater	.91	< .0001
Penny, Musser, & North (1995)	Psychiatric illness	8	Interrater	.98	
Studies of Reliability of the Allen Routine Task Inventory (RTI)					
Heimann (1985)	Psychiatric illness (outpatients)		Interrater	.99	< .001
			Test–Retest	.99	< .0001
Heimann, Allen, & Yerxa (1989)	Cognitive disabilities		Interrater	.99	
			Test–Retest	.91	
			Alpha	.94	
Wilson (1985)	Dementia		Test–Retest	.99	< .0001
Studies of Reliability of the Cognitive Performance Task (CPT)					
Burns (1992)	Alzheimer's disease	18	Interrater	.91	
		36	Test–Retest	.89	

Table 8.6

Studies of Validity of the Allen Cognitive Levels Screen (ACLS)
Through Comparison with Other Related Assessment Tools

Study	Diagnosis or Population	n	Validity Comparison	r	p
Katz (1979)	Depression		Wechsler Adult Intelligence Scale (WAIS) Block Design	.45	< .001
Wilson (1985)	Senile dementia		Riska Object Classification	.66	< .001
Wilson (1985)	Senile dementia		Mini-Mental Status Exam	.90	< .001
Newman (1987)	Schizophrenia		Bay Area Functional Performance Evaluation	.63	.01
Mayer (1988)	Psychiatric inpatients	40	WAIS Block Design and Object Assembly	.729	< .0001
			WAIS Performance IQ	.55	< .0003
Katz, Josman, & Steinmetz (1988)	Adolescent psychiatric patients	20	Class Inclusion of Riska Object Classification		< .0001
Heimann, Allen, & Yerxa (1989)	Psychiatric diagnoses	20	Routine Task Inventory	.64	< .001
Wilson, Allen, McCormack, & Burton (1989)	Senile dementia	20	Mini-Mental Status Exam	.61	
			Routine Task Inventory	.56	.01
Kehrberg (1992)	Senile dementia		Large Leather Lacing	.95	.001
McAnanama, Rogosin-Rose, Scott, Joffe, & Kelner (1999)	Psychiatric inpatients	40	ACLS at discharge and ACLS 28 days postdischarge	.72	.01
Secrest, Wood, & Tapp (2000)	Schizophrenia	31	Routine Task Inventory	.67	< .01
			Wisconsin Card Sort Categories	.57	< .01

Note. Missing values were not reported.

Exam, the Wisconsin Card Sort, the RTI, and the Large Leather Lacing (Allen, 1998). Correlations range from .45 to .95; the fact that no two tools are exactly alike in the factors they examine may account for some moderate-level correlations. This table does not include studies with modest results (Shapiro, 1992) which compared the ACLS with tools assessing vocabulary, IQ, and some social skills, or which would not necessarily be expected to correlate highly with the ACLS (David & Riley, 1990; Gokey, 1986; Penny, Musser, & North, 1995).

Table 8.7 lists studies of the ACLS that compared identified groups on specific factors. Known comparison groups include people without disability, specific age groups, and sheltered workshop controls to be compared with people with dementia, schizophrenia, and mixed psychiatric diagnoses, and adolescents with psychiatric diagnosis. The reader is referred to the original sources of these studies for more complete information.

Performance Modes or Functional Information Performance System

Since Allen has developed the modes of performance within the cognitive levels (Allen, et al., 1992), or the FIPS" (Allen & Bertrand, 1999), she has called for testing of these levels, which appear to have conceptual or face validity. "The task that needs to be done right away is establishing the interrater reliability of the modes of performance" (Allen et al., 1992, p. 101). Allen's goal in achieving reliability is to develop sufficient agreement in perception of the performance modes so that average therapists score the modes in the same way. As Allen has indicated, an accurate sequencing of the performance modes in cognitive development steps is essential. She has pointed out that Rasch analysis tools "hold promise for being able to investigate the validity of the sequence as well as the distances between the modes" (Allen et al., 1992, p. 102).

Future Directions

The theory underling the Allen Cognitive Levels is a dynamic system. It is responsive to input not only from Allen herself, but from others who use her constructs and concepts. It is a vital

Table 8.7

Studies of Validity of the Allen Cognitive Levels Screen (ACLS) Through Comparison of Identified Groups with Specific Factors

Study	Diagnosis or Population	n	Comparison Groups	Specific Factors	F or z	p
Williams (1981)	No disability		Identified group social levels	In education, social, and occupational status		
Katz, Josman, & Steinmetz (1988)	Adolescents with psychiatric diagnosis	49	Controls ($n = 29$)	In age, sex, education, and place of residence		
Josman & Katz (1991)	Adolescents with psychiatric diagnosis	49	Controls ($n = 29$)	In age, sex, education, and place of residence		
Kaeser (1992)	Dementia		Identified cognitive levels	Levels of ability in tiling	$F(1,14)$	<.001
Breeding (1993)	Normal 6- to 9-year-olds	84	Four age groups			
Raweh (1996)	Schizophrenia (2 groups)		ACL Treatment group; Sheltered workshop controls	Improvement for Treatment group	$z = 2.52$	<.01
McAnanama, Rogosin-Rose, Scott, Joffe, & Kelner (1999)	Psychiatric diagnosis ($M = 4.72$ cognitive level)	16	Nonpsychotic group ($n = 24$) ($M = 5.02$ cognitive level)	Means of scores of ACLS at discharge; post-discharge; RTI Total, Instrumental, and Physical		

structure used by clinicians in an organic rather than static manner, both formally and informally. This theory attracts clinicians to use Allen's assessments both as evaluations and as tools to plan treatment. It also attracts researchers to examine its validity, reliability, efficacy, and predictability. For these reasons, it likely will continue to be used in the future.

Because Allen focuses on issues of safety, as she has highlighted in *Structures of the Cognitive Performance Modes* (Allen & Bertrand, 1999), her theory has applicability for future health and social systems of care. Through the delineations of the performance modes, or the FIPS, issues of safety (e.g., in the home around stairs, in the community in terms of directionality in finding new or old locations, and on the highway with slower reflexes behind the wheel) will become more prominent as the population ages. Therapists' competence to evaluate the cognitive level of clients living at home will become paramount.

Because of the efficiency of the ACLS and the RTI, these tools have been helpful in assessment of patients with a brief length of stay and limited coverage for hospitalizations. In locations where the population has a greater length of treatment time, the ACLS is also efficacious because of the detail provided in the structure of the cognitive performance modes.

Numerous studies have examined people with psychosocial problems using the ACLS. However, based on the success of the ACLS in predicting surgical recovery as an intervention in hip rehabilitation, perhaps more studies should be done on using the ACLS with preoperational patients with other physical disabilities. In addition, further outcome studies using a standardized instrument such as the ACLS will strengthen the credibility of the field of OT. In some clinics, staff who administer assessment tools are being retained while others who merely treat clients are being let go. Use of OT assessment tools provides a unique service that occupational therapists can offer the public.

Recently Allen has reiterated the rationale for the use of crafts in OT to tap into the ability of the individual's working memory, which is needed to follow the new steps of an unfamiliar task. By contrast, Allen points out that the steps of a well-established activity of daily living merely require procedural memory. Allen has standardized certain crafts so as to evaluate the cognitive level of the individual accurately. Allen is unique in the field in that she has made these crafts commercially available for ease of use by busy therapists (C. Allen, personal communication, January 30, 2001).

In their recent books, Allen and her colleagues provide well-organized details for evaluation and treatment of cognitive disabilities (Allen, 1999; Allen & Bertrand, 1999; Allen et al., 1995; Bertrand, 1997e). This degree of detail is both a strength and a weakness of Allen's work. Although some therapists and family members need this type of concrete explanation, this amount of specificity may be a hindrance for others more advanced in rehabilitation. Also, adhering to the detailed steps might stifle beginning therapists' creativity and independent learning in designing activities for and with the patient.

Allen (1988a) remarked in summing up the presentation of her work, "The history of this frame of reference has only just begun" (p. 24). The years that have passed since the first edition of this chapter in 1993 have been productive for Claudia Allen. In addition, the clinical use of the ACLS, the RTI, and her cognitive schema of functional levels and performance modes and research into these systems has become more widespread.

Placed in perspective of the totality of Allen's work, the issues for which she is criticized are of minor concern. Allen is to be admired not only for her expansion of Piaget's ideas into the functional realm of voluntary motor actions, but also for her further refinement of providing performance modes to solve both conceptual and clinically pragmatic problems. Allen has opened a door of opportunities to empirical research in the psychosocial area of OT. She has enabled occupational therapists to understand what many have been doing intuitively in placing patients into cognitive levels. She has provided the field with an organized schema that has clinical and concurrent validity. She has established a model that lends itself to development of the realms of higher planning and problem solving. She has been open to suggestions and modifications by colleagues and researchers. She has even welcomed the consideration of a combination of the model of human occupation with cognitive disability theory (Allen, 1988b, pp. ix, x), thus bringing disparate elements of the field of OT into greater integration.

Cognitive disability theory can help therapists understand human cognitive levels in general. Piaget examined the mistakes his children made in order to get a glimpse of their covert and overt cognitive processes within sequential levels of thought. Likewise, Allen's work enables occupational therapists to examine varying cognitive process performance modes through levels of disability in voluntary motor actions of their patients so as to better comprehend normal adult problem solving, independent learning, and planned cognitions. In two of her books, Allen (1985; Allen et al., 1992) has presented a holistic approach to occupational therapy. She has categorized the primary health problems treated by occupational therapists across traditional subspecialties as cognitive or noncognitive disabilities, regardless of the boundaries of typical areas of practice.

Bibliography

1982

Allen, C. K. (1982). Independence through activity: The practice of occupational therapy. *American Journal of Occupational Therapy, 36,* 731–739.

Allen, C. K., & Mendel, W. M. (1982). Chronic illness and staff burnout: Revised expectations for change in the supportive-care model. *International Journal of Partial Hospitalization, 1,* 191–201.

1985

Allen, C. K. (1985). *Occupational therapy for psychiatric diseases: Measurement and management of cognitive disabilities.* Boston: Little, Brown.

1987

Allen, C. K. (1987). Activity: Occupational therapy's treatment method. 1987 Eleanor Clarke Slagle lecture. *American Journal of Occupational Therapy, 41,* 563–575.

Allen, C. K., & Allen, R. E. (1987). Cognitive disabilities: Measuring the social consequences of mental disorders. *Journal of Clinical Psychiatry, 48,* 185–191.

1988

Allen, C. K. (1988). Cognitive disabilities. In S. Robinson (Ed.), *Mental health focus: Skills for assessment and treatment.* (pp. 18–33). Rockville, MD: American Occupational Therapy Association.

Allen, C. K. (1988). Preface. The development of standardized clinical evaluations in mental health. *Occupational Therapy in Mental Health, 8,* ix–x.

Allen, C. K. (1988). Occupational therapy: Functional assessment of the severity of mental disorders. *Hospital and Community Psychiatry, 39,* 140–142.

1989

Allen, C. K. (1989). Psychiatry. In T. Malone (Ed.), *Physical and occupational therapy: Drug implications for practice* (pp. 207–228). Philadelphia: Lippincott.

Allen, C. K. (1989). Treatment plans in cognitive rehabilitation. *Occupational Therapy Practice, 1,* 1–8.

Allen, C. K., Foto, M., Sperling, T. M., & Wilson, D. (1989). Outpatient occupational therapy: Medicare part B guidelines (DHHS Transmittal No. 565). In *Health insurance manual.* Baltimore: Health Care Financing Administration.

Heimann, N. E., Allen, C. K., & Yerxa, E. J. (1989). The Routine Task Inventory: A tool for describing the functional behavior of the cognitively disabled. *Occupational Therapy Practice, 1,* 67–74.

Wilson, D. S., Allen, C. K., McCormack, G., & Burton, G. (1989). Cognitive disability and routine task behaviors in a community based population with senile dementia. *Occupational Therapy Practice, 1,* 58–66.

1990

Allen, C. K. (1990). Development of a research tradition. *Mental Health Special Interest Section Newsletter, 13*(2), 1–3.

1991

Allen, C. K. (1991). *Change within the Allen Cognitive Level 3, 4 and 5.* Paper presented at the annual conference of the American Occupational Therapy Association, Houston.

Allen, C. K. (1991). Cognitive disability and reimbursement for rehabilitation and psychiatry. *Journal of Insurance Medicine, 23,* 245–247.

Allen, C. K. (1991). Some thoughts about rehabilitation and case management: An insurer's viewpoint. *Journal of Insurance Medicine, 22*(4), 217–218.

1992

Allen, C. K. (1992). Cognitive disabilities. In N. Katz (Ed.), *Cognitive rehabilitation: Models for intervention and occupational therapy.* Boston: Andover Medical.

Allen, C. K., Earhart, C. A., & Blue, T. (1992). *Occupational therapy treatment goals for the physically and cognitively disabled.* Rockville, MD: American Occupational Therapy Association.

1993

Allen, C. K., & Robertson, S. C. (1993). *A study guide of occupational therapy treatment goals for the physically and cognitively disabled.* Rockville, MD: American Occupational Therapy Association.

Earhart, C. A., & Allen, C. K. (1993). *Allen Diagnostic Module instruction manual.* Colchester, CT: S&S Worldwide.

1994

Allen, C. K. (1994). Creating a need-satisfying, safe environment: Management and maintenance approaches. In C. B. Royeen (Ed.), *AOTA self study series: Cognitive rehabilitation.* Rockville, MD: American Occupational Therapy Association.

1995

Allen, C. K., Earhart, C. A., & Blue, T. (1995). *Understanding cognitive performance modes.* Ormond Beach, FL: Allen Conferences.

1996

Allen, C. K. (1996). *Allen Cognitive Level test manual.* Colchester, CT: S&S Worldwide.

1998

Allen, C. K. (1998). Cognitive disabilities model. In N. Katz (Ed.), *Cognition and occupation in rehabilitation: Cognitive models for intervention in occupational therapy* (pp. 225–280). Bethesda, MD: American Occupational Therapy Association.

1999

Allen, C. K. (1999). *How to use the Allen's Cognitive Levels in daily practice.* Ormond Beach, FL: Allen Conferences.

Allen, C. K., & Bertrand, J. (Eds.) (1999). *Structures of the cognitive performance modes.* Ormond Beach, FL: Allen Conferences.

Assessments

1988

Earhart, C. A., & Allen, C. K. (1988). *Cognitive disabilities: Expanded activity analysis.* Colchester, CT: S&S Worldwide.

1990

Allen, C. K. (1990). *Allen Cognitive Level Test manual.* Colchester, CT: S&S Worldwide.

1991

Josman, N., & Katz, N. (1991). Allen Cognitive Level Test Problem-Solving (ACL–PS) test. *American Journal of Occupational Therapy, 45,* 331–338.

1992

Allen, C. K., Kehrberg, K., & Burns, T. (1992). Evaluation instruments. In C. K. Allen, C. A. Earhart, & T. Blue (Eds.), *Occupational therapy treatment goals for the physically and cognitively disabled* (pp. 31–84). Rockville, MD: American Occupational Therapy Association.

1993

Kehrberg, K. (1993). *Large Cognitive Level Test.* Minneapolis: VA Medical Center's Geriatric Research, Education, and Clinical Center.

2000

Allen, C. K. (2000). *Cognitive levels 0 and 0.8.* (Available from Ivelisse Lazzarini, Edward and Margaret Doisey School of Allied Health Professions, St. Louis University, St. Louis, MO, 63103)

References

Allen, C. K. (1982) Independence through activity: The practice of occupational therapy. *American Journal of Occupational Therapy, 36,* 731–739.

Allen, C. K. (1985). *Occupational therapy for psychiatric diseases: Measurement and management of cognitive disabilities.* Boston: Little, Brown.

Allen, C. K. (1987). Activity: Occupational therapy's treatment method. 1987 Eleanor Clark Slagle Lecture. *American Journal of Occupational Therapy, 41,* 563–575.

Allen, C. K. (1988a). Cognitive disabilities. In S. Robinson (Ed.), *Mental health focus: Skills for assessment and treatment* (pp. 18–33). Rockville, MD: American Occupational Therapy Association.

Allen, C. K. (1988b). Preface. The development of standardized clinical evaluations in mental health. *Occupational Therapy in Mental Health, 8,* ix-x.

Allen, C. K. (1990). *Allen Cognitive Level test manual.* Colchester, CT: S&S Worldwide.

Allen, C. K. (1998). Cognitive disabilities model. In N. Katz (Ed.), *Cognition and occupation in rehabilitation: Cognitive models for intervention in occupational therapy* (pp. 225–280). Bethesda, MD: American Occupational Therapy Association.

Allen, C. K. (1999). *How to use the Allen's Cognitive Levels in daily practice.* Ormond Beach, FL, Allen Conferences.

Allen, C. K. (2000) *Cognitive levels 0 and 0.8.* Retrieved October 12, 2000, from www.allen-cognitive-levels.com/level0_1.htm

Allen, C. K., & Bertrand, J. (Eds.) (1999). *Structures of the cognitive performance modes.* Ormond Beach, FL: Allen Conferences.

Allen C. K., Earhart, C. A., & Blue, T. (1992). *Occupational therapy treatment goals for the physically and cognitively disabled.* Rockville, MD: American Occupational Therapy Association.

Allen, C. K., Earhart, C. A., & Blue, T. (1995). *Understanding cognitive performance modes.* Ormond Beach, FL: Allen Conferences.

Allen, C. K., Foto, M., Sperling, T. M., & Wilson, D. (1989). Outpatient occupational therapy: Medicare part B guidelines (DHHS Transmittal No. 565). In *Health insurance manual.* Baltimore: Health Care Financing Administration.

Allen, C. K., Kehrberg, K., & Burns, T. (1992). Evaluation instruments. In C. K. Allen, C. A. Earhart, & T. Blue (Eds.), *Occupational therapy treatment goals for the physically and cognitively disabled* (pp. 32–84). Rockville, MD: American Occupational Therapy Association.

American Psychiatric Association (1987). *Diagnostic and statistical manual of mental disorders–Third edition.* Washington, DC: Author.

American Psychiatric Association (1994). *Diagnostic and statistical manual of mental disorders–Fourth edition.* Washington, DC: Author.

Bertrand, C. (1997a). *Interdisciplinary benefits of the Allen's Cognitive Levels in geriatric rehabilitation.* Paper presented at the meeting of the National Geriatric Rehabilitation Conference, Boston.

Bertrand, C. (1997b). *Starting an Allen's cognitive level program in a geriatric facility.* Ormond Beach, FL: Allen Conferences.

Black's Law Dictionary (5th ed.) (1979). St. Paul, MN: Western.

Breeding, C. J. (1993). *Performance of six to nine year old children without disability for the Allen Cognitive Level Test, Expanded Version.* Unpublished master's thesis, University of Southern California, Los Angeles.

Burns, T. (1992). Part III: The Cognitive Performance Test: An approach to cognitive level assessment in Alzheimer's disease. In C. K. Allen, C. A. Earhart, & T. Blue (Eds.), *Occupational therapy treatment goals for the physically and cognitively disabled* (pp. 46–50). Rockville, MD: American Occupational Therapy Association.

Cheatum, L. S. (1994). Utilization of the Allen Cognitive Levels in predicting outcoming of hip replacements. *Physical Medicine and Rehabilitation Service Newsletter.* Retrieved from http://www.allen-cognitive-levels.com/old.htm

David, S. K., & Riley, W. T. (1990). The relationship of the Allen Cognitive Level test to cognitive abilities and psychopathology. *American Journal of Occupational Therapy, 44,* 493–497.

Gokey, M. A. (1986). *The relationship between cognitive level and daily functioning in persons with chronic schizophrenia.* Unpublished master's thesis, San Jose State University, San Jose, CA.

Heimann, N. E. (1985). *Investigation of the reliability and validity of the Routine Task Inventory: A tool for describing the functional behavior of the cognitive disabled.* Unpublished master's thesis, University of Southern California, Los Angeles.

Heimann, N. E., Allen, C. K., & Yerxa, E. J. (1989). The Routine Task Inventory: A tool for describing the functional behavior of the cognitively disabled. *Occupational Therapy Practice, 1,* 67–74.

Heying, L. M. (1983). *Cognitive disabilities and activities of daily living in persons with senile dementia.* Unpublished master's thesis, University of Southern California, Los Angeles.

Howell, F. F. (1993). *The Allen Cognitive Level test–1990: Reliability studies with the depressed population.* Unpublished master's thesis, University of Florida, Gainsville.

Josman, N., & Katz, N. (1991). Problem-solving version of the Allen Cogntive Level (ACL) Test. *American Journal of Occupational Therapy, 45,* 331–338.

Kaeser, D. S. (1992). *Cognitive disability theory as a basis for activity analysis for elderly persons with dementia.* Unpublished master's thesis, Western Michigan University, Kalamazoo.

Karaffa, M. C. (1992). *International classification of diseases* (4th ed.). Los Angeles: Practive management Information Corp.

Katz, N. (1979). *An Occupational therapy study of cognition in asult inpatients with depression.* Unpublished master's thesis, University of Southern California, Los Angeles.

Katz, N. (Ed.) (1998). *Cognition and occupation in rehabilitation: Cognitive models for intervention in occupational therapy.* Bethesda, MD: American Occupational Therapy Association.

Katz, N., Josman, N., & Steinmetz, N. (1988). Relationship between cognitive disability theory and the model of human occupation in the assessment of psychiatric and nonpsychiatric adolescents. *Occupational Therapy in Mental Health, 8,* 31–43.

Kehrberg, K. L. (1992). Part II: The Large ACL. In C. K. Allen, C. A. Earhart, & T. Blue (Eds.). *Occupational therapy treatment goals for the physically and cognitively disabled.* Bethesda, MD: American Occupational Therapy Association.

Kielhofner, G. (1992). *Conceptual foundations of occupational therapy.* Philadelphia: F.A. Davis.

Mayer, M. A. (1988). Analysis of information processing and cognitive disability theory. *American Journal of Occupational Therapy, 42,* 176–183.

McAnanama, E. P., Rogosin-Rose, M.L., Scott, E. A., Joffe, R. T., & Kelner, M. (1999). Discharge planning in mental health: The relevance of cognition and community living. *American Journal of Occupational Therapy, 53,* 129–135.

Moore, D. S. (1978). *An occupational therapy evaluation of sensorimotor cognition: Initial reliability, validity, and descriptive data for hospitalized schizophrenic adults.* Unpublished master's thesis, University of Southern California, Los Angeles.

Newman, M. (1987). *Cognitive disability and functional performance in individuals with chronic schizophrenic disorders.* Unpublished master's thesis, University of Southern California, Los Angeles.

Partida, A. (1992). *Reliability and validity of two alternate versions of the Allen Cognitive Level test among adults with mental illness.* Unpublished master's thesis, University of Southern California, Los Angeles.

Penny, N. H., Musser, K. L., & North, C. T. (1995). The Allen Cognitive Level test and social competence in adult psychiatric patients. *American Journal of Occupational Therapy, 49,* 420–427.

Raweh, D. (1996). *Treatment effectiveness of the cognitive disabilities theory of Allen with adult schizophrenic outpatients: A primary study.* Unpublished master's thesis, Hebrew University of Jerusalem, Israel.

Secrest, L. Wood, A. E., & Tapp, A. (2000). A comparison of the Allen Cognitive Level test and the Wisconsin Card Sorting Test in adults with schizophrenia. *American Journal of Occupational Therapy, 54,* 129–133.

Shapiro, M. E. (1992). Application of the Allen Cognitive Level test in assessing cognitive level functioning of emotionally disturbed boys. *American Journal of Occupational Therapy, 4*(6), 514–518.

Williams, L. R. (1981). *Development and initial test of an occupational therapy object-classification test*. Unpublished master's thesis, University of Southern California, Los Angeles.

Wilson, D. S. (1985). *Cognitive disability and routine task behaviors in a community based population with senile dementia*. Unpublished master's thesis, San Jose State University, San Jose, CA.

Wilson, D. S., Allen, C. K., McCormack, G., & Burton, G. (1989). Cognitive disability and routine task behaviors in a community based population with senile dementia. *Occupational Therapy Practice, 1*, 55–66.

Woodroff, W. A., Goodwin, D. W., & Guze, S. B. (1973). *Psychiatric diagnosis*. New York: Oxford University Press.

World Health Organization. (1980). *International classification of impairments, disabilities and handicaps*. Geneva, Switzerland: Author.

Occupation-Based and Occupation-Centered Perspectives

9

Ferol Menks Ludwig

> *To serve mankind well requires that we discover much more knowledge about people as agents, in their own environments, engaged in daily occupations. . . . To learn what we need to know requires that we accept the challenge of becoming ardent students of life's daily activities, grappling courageously with the ambiguity and complexity of occupation, the occupational human, and the contexts in which occupation takes place.*
> (Yerxa, 1998a, p. 418)

We added this chapter to this edition of our book in order to present an overview of the many developments in occupation-based and occupation-centered theories and practice models that are currently influencing occupational therapy (OT) practice nationally and internationally. Occupation has been called the basis and core of the OT profession; however, throughout the field's history, professionals have struggled with their commitment to it, their ability to articulate its value, and their efforts to expand theories and integrate them into practice. Many exciting occupation-based and occupation-centered theories and conceptual frameworks have recently been posited and are being researched and applied to practice. To reflect this current diversity and richness, this chapter differs from the preceding ones in that one particular theorist is not selected for in-depth discussion. Instead, some of the major occupation-based and occupation-centered contemporary theoretical developments are described in an overview that is intended to provide the reader with a schema or framework in which to conceptualize these concepts.

The organization for this chapter is as follows: First, the sociohistorical background of the theory of occupation-based and occupation-centered practice is presented. Next, contemporary theoretical concepts and major premises are discussed. Third, application to OT practice is presented, which is followed by theory validation and research. The chapter finishes with a section on conclusions and one on future directions.

Due to space limitations, this chapter by no means covers all of the work and contributions made in occupation-based and occupation-centered practice. Nor does it attempt to discuss specific theories and research in depth. Although I am unable to recognize everyone who is contributing to occupation-based and occupation-centered theory and practice within the confines of this chapter, I hope that I have provided a useful overview and conceptual framework that will help readers to better organize, understand, integrate, develop, and apply findings and knowledge in this area. The reference list will direct the reader to some outstanding works, which in turn will lead to more references in a stimulating journey of discovery.

In this chapter, I refer to occupation-based and occupation-centered practice. Words can have significant nuances that reflect subtle, but significant differences. *Occupation-based* means that the approach relies on occupational constructs but does not necessarily use occupation as ends and means. Occupation-centered implies a more integrated use of occupation as both ends and means. However, the definitions may vary with authors.

Background of Theory of Occupation-Based and Occupation-Centered Practice

Political and social reform marked the 19th and beginning of the 20th centuries in Western Europe and the United States. The confluence of diverse social movements—arts and crafts movement, settlement movement, and resurrection of the moral treatment movement within the mental hygiene movement—pragmatism, and scientific engineering influenced the creation of occupational therapy. OT's founders were concerned with the relationship between occupation and health and dysfunction and with the therapeutic value of occupation. The adverse effects of industrialization, mechanization, and urban living led to the end of cottage industries, and people became consumers more than producers of whole goods. Social theorists, architects, and designers started the arts and crafts movement in Victorian Britain. Arts and crafts societies spread through Western Europe and the United States "to provide an alternative code to the harshness of late nineteenth-century industrialism, to foster spiritual harmony through the work process and to change that very process and its works" (Cumming & Kaplan, 1991, p. 9). These societies encouraged individualism, creation of handmade products instead of machine uniformity, and reappraisal of design materials. They created a new aesthetic value in contrast to the strict design morality of early Victorian Britain. The arts and crafts movement provided a foundation for early occupational therapists to value processes that produced individually well-made objects and to apply these to practice with populations with chronic disabilities. They viewed idleness as a negative state of being.

Jane Addams at Hull House Settlement in Chicago led the settlement movement, and Eleanor Clark Slagle, who became one of the first occupational therapists, studied and worked with her. This movement, involving primarily women in social activism, sought to lessen the devastating effects of poverty, industrialization, and cultural alienation of immigrants. The settlement movement believed in the power of creative activities to address some of these problems and had a strong influence on the development of OT (Quiroga, 1995).

The mental hygiene movement had many proponents among the founders of OT, such as Julia Lathrop and Adolph Meyer. Meyer, a physician who was associated with Hull House, was also a pragmatist and associate of John Dewey, an educator and psychologist. Dewey, a leading pragmatist along with William James, wrote and taught extensively about the importance of doing, especially in education. Occupational therapy also has its roots in the conceptual themes that arose from the functionalist school of psychology and the pragmatist school of philosophy. The concept that one learned by doing had a moral tone in that character was formed and expressed by what one did (Dewey,

1922; James, 1892/1985; Peirce, 1957). Both pragmatism and occupational therapy posit the relationship between the productive use of time and the need to organize daily activities for health and well-being. Thus, occupations were used to enable persons to adapt to environmental demands through direct experience. The early founders built upon the basic premises of pragmatism and functionalism and skillfully wove these into the treatment programs they established. They used occupation to alter habit patterns and ways of thinking to develop "decent habits of living" (Slagle & Robeson, 1941). It was primarily through the work of Meyer and Slagle that occupational therapy was based on the proposition that there was health-maintaining and health-generating potential in one's balanced and purposeful use of time. (See Chapter 1 for more discussion of early ideas and writings concerning occupation.)

Frank and Lillian Gilbreth (F. B. Gilbreth & Gilbreth, 1920; L. Gilbreth, 1927) and Cristine Frederick (1913) promoted techniques aimed to make persons more efficient on the job and in the home, which reflected societal values of efficiency and productivity. This influence is seen in OT's view of occupation and emphasis on productive occupation as the outcome for which patients are prepared in therapy as they learn to perform occupations effectively according to principles of scientific engineering. This emphasis differed from that of the arts and crafts movement, in which the worth of the occupation was related to the quality and purposefulness of the end product, not to its earning power or production efficiency and uniformity. Scientific engineering regarded the individual as an extension of the machine, whereas the arts and crafts movement emphasized individual workmanship, quality craftsmanship, a way of life, and moral aesthetic. The term *activity analysis* was developed by Frank Gilbreth (1911), an engineer, to refer to the process of the systematic study of jobs, workers' movements, and adapting activity to be more efficient. Thus, methods originally used in time and motion studies of jobs were applied to vocational retraining and a wider variety of occupations such as therapeutic crafts and "reeducation of the crippled soldier" (F. B. Gilbreth & Gilbreth, 1920). Activity analysis in occupational therapy was initially used in physical dysfunction, especially during World Wars I and II in military hospitals (L. M. Gilbreth, 1943). This emphasis on efficiency and productivity aligned with a gradual shift in occupational therapy toward a focus on medical outcomes and away from the earlier sociohistorical, humanitarian social reform movements (Creighton, 1992).

Changes in health and social care, as well as the wars, influenced the context in which occupation-based practice developed. Theory development and practice became increasingly reductionistic as it allied with medical and scientific models that focused on remediating discrete areas of physical and mental dysfunction (Kielhofner & Burke, 1977; Madigan & Parent, 1985). Peloquin (1989; 1996) wrote,

> Moral treatment's decline relates closely to a lack of inspired and committed leadership willing to articulate and redefine the efficacy of occupation in the face of medical and societal challenges. The desire to embrace the most current trend of scientific thought led to the abandonment of moral treatment in spite of its established efficacy. The failure to identify and address the social and institutional changes that had gradually made the practice and success of moral treatment virtually impossible led to the erroneous conclusion that occupation was not an effective intervention. (p. 46)

Friedland (1998) presented an interesting argument that as occupational therapy became a part of rehabilitation, its core values "eroded" (p. 373), and this has contributed to the field's identity problems. "It is as though the core concept of occupation as a means of promoting health and well-being was somehow elusive and, in not being well enough articulated, became dissipated" (p. 374). OT professionals lost sight of the concept that it was engagement in occupation that could have a transformative therapeutic effect. Instead, graded activity was aimed at improving range of motion and strength in isolated and reductionistic practice of remedial exercises. The medical model offered more status.

Friedland (1998) made a strong point when she stated,

> As occupational therapists continued to compete in the reductionistic environment of medicine, we found that our qualifications were generally not as good as others who could fix broken parts. And although *no one else* could do what we did, no one, including ourselves, seemed to value that. No one, including

> ourselves, seemed to notice that we had abdicated our role in
> developing and maintaining health and well-being through oc-
> cupation in order to join the ranks of the reductionists. (p. 378)

Friedland (1998) and Yerxa (1992) stated that the results of this alignment with the medical model led occupational therapists to become more like physical therapists and to compete with them.

Theorists such as Fidler (see Chapter 2) and Reilly (see Chapter 6) fueled the recommitment to assumptions about humans and occupation that initially infused the practice of occupation. Kielhofner with Burke (see Chapter 7) further expanded theory that focused on occupation and context. Currently, the profession is grappling with its definition and focusing again on occupation-based and occupation-centered practice. This is primarily as a result of changes in health care delivery and reimbursement, dissatisfaction with current non-occupation-based modalities being used, recognition by other professions and consumers of the importance of occupation to health and wellness, and advances in education that have led to more doctoral-level theorists and researchers. Occupation-based practice has been broadened beyond the founding concepts and use of arts and crafts as a cure.

Occupation-based and occupation-centered practices are important foci of the profession as a whole, as indicated in the following paragraphs:

The American Occupational Therapy Association (AOTA), published the *AOTA Self-Study Series—The Practice of the Future: Putting Occupation Back Into Therapy* (Royeen, 1994), which focused on models that used an occupation-based approach.

The May 1998 special issue of the *American Journal of Occupational Therapy* was devoted to occupation-centered practice and education. This was followed in June 1998 with another issue focused on occupation-centered research. Wendy Wood served as guest editor for both issues (Wood, 1998a, 1998b).

Beginning with the winter 2002 issue, the board of the American Occupational Therapy Foundation (AOTF) changed the name of *Occupational Therapy Journal of Research* (OTJR) to *OTJR: Occupation, Participation, and Health*. The reasons for this change were to advance the understanding of the role that occupation plays in facilitating participation and enhancing health; to emphasize to the public the profession's commitment to the study of occupation, participation, and health; and to foster interdisciplinary dialogue with contributions from disciplines such as psychology, economics, anthropology, sociology, geography, rehabilitation science, nursing, and social work (Baum, 2001).

The AOTF is targeting occupation-based practice in a major project and has also sponsored and secured grants for two multidisciplinary scholarly symposia on habit. A third one is in the planning stages. The AOTF published the presentations from the conferences in the *Occupational Therapy Journal of Research (AOTF,* 2000, *AOTA,* 2002b).

Occupational science has evolved as an academic discipline dedicated to the scholarly inquiry of occupation and the human as an occupational being. Results of these inquiries are facilitating occupational therapy's articulation of basic concepts, beliefs, theory development, and practice. For example, Jackson, Carlson, Mandel, Zemke, and Clark (1998) describe the development and implementation of a preventive OT program for independent living, healthy elderly adults. They describe the integration of OT methods into a program based on research and theory generated from occupational science. This program, Lifestyle Redesign, was the basis of the landmark largest OT outcome study. The results were published as the lead article in an issue of the *Journal of the American Medical Association* (Clark et al., 1997). Through their involvement in Lifestyle Redesign, these older adults were enabled to fashion patterns of occupations that improved their health, well-being, and life satisfaction.

> This study demonstrated not only the empirical value of an innovative occupation-centered program for an at-risk population, but also notable progress has been made on a puzzle plaguing occupational therapy since its inception: that of discerning characteristics of inconsequential activity programs from those that are substantial in impact. (Wood, 1998a, p. 323)

▶ An increasing number of OT curricula are including an occupation-centered or occupation-based focus, and some programs are adding occupational science in addition to occupational therapy to their departmental names.

Contemporary Theoretical Concepts and Major Premises

The theoretical base of occupation-based and occupation-centered treatment is wide and relies on theories from many diverse fields. I cover three major areas in this section. The first, contextual relevance, relates to the power of occupation in that quality of life for a person is influenced by the performance of occupations within his or her naturally lived contexts. Thus, occupation is most powerful when it occurs naturally and is not decontextualized. The second refers to the power of occupation as a therapeutic agent and its relationship to health and well-being. Third, the study of the human as an occupational being relies on theories that address human functioning and motivation, as well as those that have occupation as their focus.

Contextual Relevance

The importance of the relationship among context, occupation, and the person has become officially recognized in occupational therapy. AOTA (1994, p. 1047) expanded the third edition of its Uniform Terminology to "reflect current practice and to incorporate contextual aspects of performance. Performance Areas, Performance Components, and Performance Contexts are the parameters of occupational therapy's domain of concern." These areas dynamically interact with each other and do not operate in isolation. Performance contexts are composed of temporal (chronological, developmental, life cycle, and disability status) and environmental (physical, social, and cultural) contexts

> The occupational therapist views function at a level which considers the dynamic transactional relationship of persons, occupations, and environments, and assumes an inseparability of contexts, temporal factors, and physical and psychological phenomena. Canadian occupational therapists label the outcome of this relationship *occupational performance* while their colleagues in the United States often use the term *function*. (Law et al., 1997, p. 74)

Thus, OT intervention focuses on the person, the context, and the occupation in a dynamic manner that acknowledges this inseparability.

Because AOTA's Commission on Practice recognized that the practice environment and core constructs had changed considerably since the 1994 revision of AOTA's Uniform Terminology, the group developed the "Occupational Therapy Practice Framework: Domain and Process" (AOTA, 2002a). This official document even more strongly commits and articulates OT's focus on occupation and daily life activities. It outlines dynamic evaluation and intervention processes that focus on the use of occupation as both means and an end. The document emphasizes that "engagement in occupation to support participation in context is the focus and targeted end objective of occupational therapy intervention" (p. 611). Likewise, engagement in occupation naturally facilitates participation within context. Context also influences performance, and this must be integrated into practice. On the international level, the World Health Organization (WHO; 2001) calls for rehabilitation professionals to use broader models that include environment as it facilitates or creates barriers to participation.

Occupation-centered theories, models of practice, and frames of reference explain how humans influence their contexts through occupation and the way in which environments influence humans and occupation. Work, play, self-care, and leisure are dependent on successful interactions among the person, occupation or task, and relevant contextual factors. The following subsections examine some contemporary theoretical frameworks that include environmental, temporal, and lifespan dimensions of context.

Environment as Context

Environment is one of the contexts in which occupation occurs and affects the performance, purpose, and meaning of occupation. Environment refers to the physical, social, and cultural milieu that exists outside of the person that has the potential to influence him or her. Political, economic, and institutional environments also need to be included (Law, Cooper, et al., 1996). Some theories speak of environment in more bounded terms, such as the immediate physical and sociocultural milieu surrounding the person, whereas others take a more ecological and global view. A paradigm shift has occurred in the profession from an emphasis on the internal properties of the person or the disorder within the person to an emphasis on the important dynamic relationship of the environment to development, health, and well-being (Baum & Baptiste, 2002; Letts, Rigby, & Stewart, 2003). Occupation-based practice theories and practice models focus on the dynamic and complex relationships between individuals or communities and their environments and occupations. They view the person's need for occupation as central to the treatment process, with activity or participation as the outcome.

All of the occupation-centered and occupation-based models recognize the influence of the environment on occupational performance; however, they differ in how inclusive their concepts of environment are. The sociocultural environment is a very important aspect of environmental context. Some theories deal with sociocultural issues more explicitly than others. Generally, occupation-centered and occupation-based theories consider the sociocultural environmental context to be extremely relevant because the meaning of occupation is strongly influenced by culture. This premise has pervaded the OT literature from its roots through current times.

Berger and Luckman (1966) wrote about the "social construction of reality" as the process through which meaning is made and shared in social groups. For example, preparing a meal can have many realities or meanings: In one social group it may signify nurturing and giving, whereas in another it may be considered as menial work. Gelya Frank (1994) described the many different meanings of the ordinary daily activity of self-care and discussed how society stigmatized those who deviated from its norms. If people are what they do, then it follows that their identity and self-worth are also socially constructed. Historical times, socioeconomics, and politics are some additional facets of the sociocultural environment that have contextual relevance. Social supports and liabilities are important contextual aspects as well. The contextual relevance of the sociocultural environment to occupation and meaning making, identity, and self-worth is a very rich area that uses many theories from sociology and anthropology in particular and reflects a conceptual shift to a more social view of health.

Person–Activity–Environment Fit Occupation-based and occupation-centered theories are based on the fundamental concept of person–activity–environment fit, which refers to the match among the skills and capabilities of the person, demands of the occupation, and environmental demands and resources (Letts et al., 2003). This type of theory involves concepts and assumptions about the person, the environment, and the occupation as well as the dynamic nature of their interrelationships. Theories about the influence of the environment on human behavior come from many disciplines, including behavioral science, environmental psychology, architecture, urban studies, social science, geography, and occupational therapy.

Environment in OT models is seen as a facilitator or enabler of occupational performance, but it can also present heavy demands that limit or prevent occupational performance. The environment can be altered by adapting or modifying it to improve occupational performance. The idea that the environment rather than the person can be changed to improve occupational performance demonstrates a paradigm shift, especially from medical models.

Holm, Rogers, and Stone (1998) developed their person-task-environment transaction model as an adaptation of Lawton's (1982) environmental competence model. Lawton described behavior (B) as a function (f) of a person's capabilities (P) and environmental demands (E). He stated this in formula form to demonstrate the dynamics of each variable. Thus, if one's capabilities decrease, the influence of the environment on behavior increases, and vice versa. Holm et al. (1998) similarly theorized that task performance (behavior) is dependent on the fit between the capabilities of the person and the demands that the environment places on those capabilities; however, they also emphasized the role of nonhuman environmental factors, such as assistive devices (ATD) and adaptations or objects in the environment (OE), to help equalize the relationship between the person's capabilities and the environmental demands. Holm et al. (p. 473) gave this in formula form as:

$$B = f\,[(P + ATD) \times OE \times SE].$$

In words, this means behavior is a function of the person's capability with an assistive device times the objects in the environment and the structural environment (SE). For example, the behavior might be sewing a hem. Sewing a hem (B) is then a function (f) of the person's ability to see. Let us say that Ms. Jones's eyesight is impaired. Her ability to mend the hem can be improved by environmental compensations such as increased lighting, a needle threader, and eyeglasses. At the other extreme, a person with excellent eyesight can work in a more demanding environment with fewer compensations. Thus, as impairment increases, so does dependence on the environmental conditions and enhancements (Holm et al., 1998).

Law et al. (1997) reviewed 10 theoretical models from environment-behavior studies that offer "key theoretical ideas that underpin occupational therapy practice" (p. 72). These authors provide an excellent discussion of these models, which in turn impart a basis for emerging models of practice that emphasize occupational performance and person–environment fit. Each model addresses conceptualizations about the person, the environment, the relationship between them, and the outcome or adaptive relationship or outcome that results (see Table 9.1). "Most of the theoretical models are complementary and vary only in focus or emphasis rather than in conceptualization. Potentially all can be of use to occupational therapy practice" (p. 76). These theoretical models, however, are not from OT practice.

After they presented the 10 theoretical backgrounds listed in Table 9.1, Law et al. (1997) reviewed six contemporary and emerging occupational models of practice that focus on person-environment-occupation relationships and their implications for practice. These are derived in part from the 10 theoretical backgrounds. Again, Law et al. (1997) provided an excellent overview and critique of each of these models.

Overviews of the major theoretical constructs and premises of these six models are presented in the following subsections. Letts et al. (2003) provide more information on these models in their chapter titled "Environment and Occupational Performance: Theoretical Considerations."

Person–Environment–Occupational Performance Model. Christiansen and Baum's (1991, 1997) person–environment–occupational performance model (see Table 9.2) views occupational performance as an open and complex system that is composed of

(*text continues on p. 389*)

Table 9.1

Key Elements of Person-Environment Model

Theorist	How is the person conceptualized?	How is the environment conceived?	Person-Environment Interaction (adaptation)	OT application
Baker and Intagliata	Individual: • physical status • mental status • needs • knowledge • beliefs and attitudes	• the individual's perceived or experienced environment and the actual environment	The individual responds as: • an active participant or • and instinctive responder	• focus on client perceptions of environments and quality of life • clients with mental health problems
Bronfenbrenner	Individual: • as a social agent seeks and creates meaning in the social environment	• social and cultural milieu of the individual	Interdependence: • change in one domain on social environment effects change in another domain	• emphasis on client's social environment (e.g., family interventions); pediatric practice, social development
Bandura	Individual: • six basic cognitive capacities	• the individual's perceptions of the environment are key	Perceived self-efficacy: • person's perceptions of his or her ability to be successful in an activity in a particular environment	• focus on environmental perceptions • encourages consultation with clients
Gibson and Gibson	Individual: • as a developing, curious, motivated learner • task oriented • perception	• the context or surroundings of the individual • supportive or constraining (affordance)	Interdependence: • personal activities matched to affordable of environment	• child development in the context of his or her surroundings *(continues)*

Table 9.1 *Continued.*

Theorist	How is the person conceptualized?	How is the environment conceived?	Person–Environment Interaction (adaptation)	OT application
Mandala of Health	Community: • distinctive needs of community • social policy	• biological • physical • cultural • economic	• social and political implications of health • need to change environment not people	• community health • advocacy
Kahana	Individual: • needs • preferences	• the social characteristics of the residential setting	Congruence: • the well-being and function of the individual • individual choice of environment	• discharge planning, particularly with older adults • social environments
Kaplan	Individual: • the internal organization of including information about the environment	Individual: • opportunities • choices	Temporal flexibility: • to each experience one brings memories of past experiences which affect perception and anticipation	• general practice • psychiatric environments
Lawton	Individual: • the person possesses a set of abilities which constitute competence	Environmental press: • the forces in the environment in terms of their demand characteristics	Two possible responses: • adaptive behavior whether + or – • affective response	• gerontology and frail individuals

Table 9.1 *Continued.*

Theorist	How is the person conceptualized?	How is the environment conceived?	Person–Environment Interaction (adaptation)	OT application
Moos	Group of persons: • residing in an institutional setting • sociodemographics • self-concept • health factors • functional abilities	Environmental system consisting of: • physical factors • policy factors • suprapersonal factors • social climate factors	• stability and change within the institution for well-being of residents and staff	• assessing institutions and sheltered-care environments
Weisman	Employees	Physical setting. • properties • components Organizations: • policy • objective	Congruence: • manipulation of the physical environment to ensure that the policies and objectives of the organization are met	• work environments

Note. From "Theoretical Contexts for the Practice of Occupational Therapy," by M. Law et al., 1997, in *Occupational Therapy: Enabling Function and Well-Being* (2nd ed., pp. 77–78), by C. Christiansen and C. Baum (Eds.), Thorofare, NJ: SLACK. Copyright 1997 by SLACK, Inc. Reprinted with permission.

Table 9.2
Person–Environment–Occupational Performance Model

Developers:	C. Christiansen and C. Baum
Origin:	Developed to emphasize a view of performance as an interaction between a person and his or her environment
Population:	All ages
Theoretical Foundations:	• General systems theory • Occupational Therapy theorists (Howe and Briggs, Kielhofner and Burke, Reilly, Reed) • Environmental theories • Neurobehavioral theories • Psychological theories (personality, motivation, values, agency)
Concepts and Assumptions:	• Performance results from complex interactions between person and the environments in which he or she carries out tasks • Developmental state influences performance • Performance is facilitated by intrinsic enablers (in person), environmental factors and meaning of occupation • Occupational therapy intervention can facilitate a person's adaptation when he or she encounters problems in performance • A personal sense of competence influences performance
Client/Therapist Relationship:	Active patient involvement is important; therapist as "teacher–facilitator"
Expected Outcome:	Competence, occupational performance Development of "life performance skills" Improved health and well-being
Assessment:	Assess person's "assets, deficits" Pay attention to person's environment(s) Could be formal, standardized, observation, interview Outcomes should focus on well-being

Intervention:	• Uses a problem–asset–oriented model
	• Produces as client/family centered plan
	• Should be unique to each person and be driven by client goals
	• Intervention principles:
	  1. Uses occupation as a therapeutic medium
	  2. Uses compensatory adaptive strategies to overcome intrinsic factors (psychological, cognitive, physiological, neurobehavioral)

(continues)

Table 9.2 *Continued.*

Intervention:	3. Modifies physical environment within cultural parameters
	4. Develops social networks
	5. Works to remove barriers that limit occupational performance
	6. Educates the client, family, and others (e.g., employers) in strategies to optimize performance, promote health, and prevent secondary conditions

Note. From "Theoretical Contexts for the Practice of Occupational Therapy," by M. Law et al., 1997, in *Occupational Therapy: Enabling Function and Well-Being* (2nd ed., p. 87), by C. Christiansen and C. Baum (Eds.), Thorofare, NJ: SLACK. Copyright 1997 by SLACK, Inc. Reprinted with permission.

the person, environment, and occupation. Many intrinsic and extrinsic factors influence occupational performance and are considered in planning treatment. Intrinsic factors are those within the person such as psychological, physiological, and neurobehavioral influences. Motivation, experience, beliefs, abilities, and skills are intrinsic enablers of performance. Extrinsic factors include interpersonal, societal, cultural, and physical environmental factors. This model relies heavily upon principles of client-centered practice, as does the person–environment–occupation model (discussed later). One of the fundamental theoretical constructs of this model is that people naturally are motivated to explore and demonstrate mastery in their environment. This mastery is a measure of how successfully they have adapted to or met the challenges of daily living by using their personal, social, and material resources. Another basic premise is that people develop their self-identity through their meaningful occupations and find fulfillment.

This model is an emerging one that has not been widely tested. Law et al. (1997) commented that the strength of this model is its focus on the complexity of relationships among person, environment, and occupation that result in occupational performance. "It presents the viewpoint that in order to understand performance, we must consider the characteristics of individuals, the unique environments in which they function, and the nature and meaning of the actions, tasks, and roles to the person" (Cristiansen & Baum, 1997, p. 48). These elements are dynamically related with each changing and influencing the other two

(Stewart et al., 2003). This framework provides a conceptual model to view and study human behavior in terms of integrating knowledge about impairments that limit performance; environments that support performance; and the person's needs, preferences, adaptive strategies, values, and goals.

Ecology of Human Performance Model (EHP). EHP, proposed by OT faculty at the University of Kansas (see Table 9.3), focuses on the interactive, dynamic influence of context on the person and performance. Human performance is therefore a transactional process through which person, context, and performance affect each other. Each transaction affects a future performance range and options because the person, the context, or available performance range may be altered by the experience. Different variables may be more salient at one time than others. The match between these variables is the essential performance issue. Although theoretical bases are provided by both environmental psychology and occupational therapy, EHP defines person, task, performance, and context using AOTA's (1994) terminology and describes possible interactions among these four components. There is interdependence between the person's capabilities and the demands of the task and surrounding environment. EHP identifies five approaches to intervention incorporating all four components; these are establish or restore, alter, adapt, prevent, and create (Dunn, Brown, & McGuigan, 1994; Dunn, McClain, Brown, & Youngstrom, 1998). EHP aims to facilitate occupational performance and involves collaboration among the person, family, and occupational therapist (Dunn, McClain, Brown, & Youngstrom, 2003). Additional work is needed to apply the theoretical constructs to practice.

Model of Human Occupation (MOHO). Barris (1982) organized environmental dimensions into a conceptual framework, which was expanded with subsequent work by Barris, Kielhofner, Levine, and Neville (1985). MOHO (Kielhofner, 1995, 2002) is currently the most developed and researched model (see Table 9.4). (See Chapter 7 for more about this model.) MOHO uses a systems approach that incorporates environmental influences. The more recent version (Kielhofner, 1995) has expanded the concept of environmental influences. Environmental demands

Table 9.3
Ecology of Human Performance Model

Developers:	W. Dunn and Occupational Therapy Faculty at University of Kansas
Origin:	Developed in response to the lack of consideration for complexities for context in occupational therapy
Population:	All ages
Theoretical Foundations:	• Environmental psychology • Occupational Therapy theorists (Kiernat, Barris, Howe and Briggs, Spencer)
Concepts and Assumptions:	• Ecology (the interaction between person and environment) affects human behavior and performance • Performance cannot be understood outside of context • Context/environment includes physical, temporal, social, and cultural elements, and is considered to be broader than environment as it also includes the phenomenological experience of the person • Relationships exist between the key variables of person, context, tasks, and performance • Environmental cues and features are used by a person to support performance of tasks
Client/Therapist Relationship:	Collaborative
Expected Outcome:	Performance of tasks Changes in context are used to support performance
Assessment:	Incorporate consideration of context Now, contextually relevant assessment tools are needed
Intervention:	Five alternatives described: 1. Establish/restore (remediate) person's skills/abilities 2. Alter the actual context in which persons perform 3. Adapt contextual features and/or task demands to support performance in context 4. Prevent the occurrence or evolution of maladaptive performance 5. Create circumstances which promote more adaptable or complex performance in context

for performance are associated with available people and objects and strongly influence the establishment of roles, habits, and skills.

Competence involves the ability to effectively interact with a wider range of environments. This model, like Holm et al.'s (1998),

Table 9.4
A Model of Human Occupation

Developer:	Gary Kielhofner
Origin:	Influenced from original occupational behavior work at University of Southern California and Gary Kielhofner's master's thesis, which was refined/elaborated upon with Janice Burke & Cynthia Heard Igi for 1980 publication. Roan Barris and Anne Neville-Jan, together with many others, contributed to the first edition textbook. Twenty-two people contributed to the second edition
Population:	All ages
Theoretical Foundations:	• Occupational Therapy theorists (Reilly, Shannon, Nelson) • Systems theory; Cultural theory; Role theory • Environmental theories (Gibson, Lawton) • Personality theorists (Seligman, Allport, Maslow)
Concepts and Assumptions:	• Human occupation: "doing culturally meaningful work, play, or daily living tasks in the stream of time and in the contexts of one's physical and social world" (Kielhofner, 1995, p. 3) • Change is a function of changes in the internal organization (e.g., growth, increased strength, skill acquisition) or new environmental conditions • Human system is a dynamic, changing, open system comprised of three subsystems: volition, habituation, mind-brain-body performance • These systems arrange themselves according to the demands of the situation in which they are performing; each contributes different but complimentary function to the operation of the whole system • Environment influences occupational behavior • Occupational performance: "meaningful sequences of action in which a person completes an occupational form" (Kielhofner, 1995, p. 113) using motor, process, communication, and interpretation skills

(continues)

Table 9.4 *Continued.*

Concepts and Assumptions (*continues*)	• Occupational dysfunction:
	  • Disability results in breakdown of life's meaning or unable to place self in a "personal narrative" with possibilities and hope, loss/restrictions of habits and role
	
	  • Dysfunction occurs when people don't use their capacities In reasonable way to respond to reasonable societal expectations and when behavior negatively affects integrity of human system

Client/Therapist Relationship:	Not explored in detail other than notation that data gathering is to be interactive.
Expected Outcome:	Develop a theory of the circumstances of the individual patient based on interview, structured assessments, and situated means. Enable an adaptive process and minimize the impact of impairments
Assessment:	Assessment process is interactive with client, analytical, and asks questions in three framework areas: Human System's Organization—clients' assets & liabilities; Environmental Influences—how it affords or presses occupational behavior; and Systems Dynamics—examine skills demonstrated when engaged in occupations in their environment

Intervention:	Principles of Program Development:
	1. Promoting self-organization
	2. Using occupational forms as a context for change
	3. Using the environment as the context for assembling occupations
	4. Intervening across a functional continuum
	  • Goal is to support change or reorganization
	  • Asserts the primary tool which therapists have at their disposal is to change the relevant environment to support or precipitate a change in the human system
	  • Therapy focuses on replacing roles and uses meaningful occupational forms to produce changes in skills

Note. From "Theoretical Contexts for the Practice of Occupational Therapy," by M. Law et al., 1997, in *Occupational Therapy: Enabling Function and Well-Being* (2nd ed., pp. 91–92), by C. Christiansen and C. Baum (Eds.), Thorofare, NJ: SLACK. Copyright 1997 by SLACK, Inc. Reprinted with permission.

addresses the concept of environmental demands or press. Thus, the environment can influence performance by its demands or press and by opportunities for performance. The physical environment is composed of natural and constructed environments and objects. The social environment involves social groupings and rule-bound socially constructed action sequences. These social and behavioral environments create occupational behavior settings, which refer to meaningful contexts for occupational performance.

MOHO clarifies environmental characteristics and their influence on persons. The model also includes a wider range of contextual factors such as temporal and lifespan. However, one has to learn terminology that seems specific to the model. "Differences between task, activities, occupation, occupational forms, and their relationship with the environment are at times unclear. The model would benefit from further development of how persons create and shape their occupations and their environments" (Law et al., 1997, p. 90). MOHO is not as comprehensive in the area of environmental context as some of the other models, such as the person–environment–occupation and the person–environment–occupational performance models. (See Chapter 7 for more information on MOHO.)

Person–Environment–Occupation Model. The person–environment–occupation model emanated from work begun by six occupational therapists who created The Environment Research Group at McMaster University in 1991. "After conducting reviews of the literature in occupational therapy, and more broadly, we focused on reviewing environmental assessment measures and in developing a model of practice" (Letts et al., 2003, p. xv). The group has been productive in developing this model and conducting research that focuses on persons and their occupations within their daily natural environments (Law et al., 1996, 1997; Stewart et al. 2003; Strong et al., 1999).

The person–environment–occupation model is perhaps the model that best reflects the dynamic interplay or "transactional relationship" among the person, context, and occupation in a client-centered approach to practice (Law et al., 1997, p. 92). It is similar to the EHP framework in that it also separates the concept of occupation from the performance of the occupation. It highlights the consequences to occupational performance when there is any change in the person, the environment, or the occupation, which is a strength of the model along with its highly and dynamically transactional interrelationships. (See Table 9.5.)

Table 9.5
The Person–Environment–Occupation Model:
A Transactive Approach to Occupational Performance

Developers:	M. Law, B. Cooper, S. Strong, D. Stewart, R. Rigby, L. Letts
Origin:	Developed as part of an environmental research program in the School of Rehabilitation Science, McMaster University
Population:	All ages
Theoretical Foundations:	• Canadian Guidelines for Occupational Therapy • Environmental theorists (Lawton and Nahemow) • Theory of "flow" (Csikszentmihalyi)
Concepts and Assumptions:	• The *person* is a unique being who assumes a variety of roles simultaneously. These roles are dynamic, varying across time and context in their importance, duration, and significance. • Environment us defined broadly including cultural, socioeconomic, institutional, physical, and social considerations of the environment. • Occupation is defined as groups of self-directed, functional tasks and activities in which a person engages over the lifespan. Time patterns and rhythms characterize the occupational routines of individuals over a day, a week, or longer. • Occupational Performance is the outcome of the transaction of the person, environment, and occupation. It is defined as the dynamic experience of a person engaged in purposeful activities and tasks within an environment. Over a lifetime individuals are constantly renegotiating their view of self and their roles as they ascribe meaning to occupation and the environment around them. • The model assumes that its three major components (person, environment, occupation) interact continually across time and space in ways that increase or diminish their congruence. The outcome of greater compatibility is therefore represented as more optimal occupational performance

(continues)

Table 9.5 *Continued.*

Client/Therapist Relationship:	Interdependent partnership to address occupational performance issue defined by the client
Expected Outcome:	Improved fit between person, occupation, and environment will result in optimal occupational performance
Assessment:	The client, together with the therapist, identifies the client's occupational strengths and issues/problems in occupational performance. This can be done using a semi-structured interview (e.g., Canadian Occupational performance Measure), or standardized assessment (e.g., Occupational Performance History Interview). Assessment of performance components, environmental conditions, and occupation helps to determine the focus and level of intervention
Intervention:	Interventions can target the person, occupation and the environment, offering multiple avenues for eliciting change. The goal is to facilitate changes which result in improved occupational performance

Note. From "Theoretical Contexts for the Practice of Occupational Therapy," by M. Law et al., 1997, in *Occupational Therapy: Enabling Function and Well-Being* (2nd ed., p. 93), by C. Christiansen and C. Baum (Eds.), Thorofare, NJ: SLACK. Copyright 1997 by SLACK, Inc. Reprinted with permission.

Behavior and context are inseparable. "The strength of the model is its focus on the transactional relationship between the person, occupation, and environment" (Law et al., 1997, p. 92) which is called occupational performance. It also includes temporal features of routines from a daily basis to lifespan development perspectives. Thus, it is more comprehensive in its inclusion of components of contextual relevance.

Occupational Adaptation (OA). The OA frame of reference is guided by a conceptual model that is based on core OT premises about occupation and adaptation. "One of the most important features of the occupational adaptation perspective is the integration of the constructs of occupation and adaptation into a single interactive concept" (Schkade & Schultz, 1992, p. 829). Many theories discuss both occupation and adaptation, but OA is unique in the way that it proposes that these two concepts are not separate, but rather comprise an interactive process that explains the adaptation process as it is experienced throughout the lifespan. Schultz and Schkade (1992, 1997) have provided with an extensive overview of the literature on adaptation, as well as a therapeutic frame of reference that can be used to facilitate individual adaptation.

OA describes an internal adaptation process that occurs through engagement in occupation and for successful occupational engagement. Occupations have the following three characteristics: (a) active involvement of the person, (b) meaning to the person, and (c) a tangible or intangible product such as a tasty meal or a solution to a mental problem. OA has influenced practice, education, and research. Although a comprehensive perspective on adaptation has been often identified in the OT literature, it has not been broadly and systematically organized and developed into specific frameworks for practice. Schultz and Schkade (1992) assert that promoting internal adaptation has been and will always be an integral part of OT. The success of person–environment transactions depends on the quality and nature of the individual's adaptive processes.

OA describes (a) a normal developmental process that leads to competence in occupational functioning, (b) processes though which OT outcomes occur, and (c) holistic processes. Schkade and Schultz (1992) carefully laid out the assumptions and theoretical background of OA. (See Table 9.6.)

OA is a frame of reference for practice, education, and research. One of OA's strengths is that it uses a developmental, as well as environmental, context. This frame of reference focuses on the person's experience in relevant occupational contexts using meaningful occupations to influence his or her internal adaptation process. This inner adaptation process is the goal of intervention, which leads to efficacious responses to environmental demands. Dysfunction occurs when disability, handicapping conditions, and stressful life events disrupt the adaptation process. Intervention focuses on maximizing the individual's internal adaptation process, which in turn will improve occupational performance (Schkade & Schultz, 1993; Schultz & Schkade, 2003). Environment plays an important role in the adaptive process and in evaluating the outcome.

Table 9.6
Occupational Adaptation Model

Developers:	J. Schkade and S. Schultz
Origin:	Concept for occupational adaptation was selected by Texas Woman's University as a focus for research
Population:	All ages
Theoretical Foundations:	• Occupational therapy theorists (Reed, Kielhofner, Nelson) • General Systems theory
Concepts and Assumptions:	• Integrates constructs of occupational and adaptation into a single interactive construct • Occupation provides the means by which people adapt • Occupational adaptation is a normative process that is most pronounced in periods of transition • Person is made up of three systems: sensorimotor, cognitive, and psychosocial, as well as underlying subsystems • Occupational environments are those that call for an occupational response—they are contexts in which occupations occur (work, play, leisure, self-maintenance) • Occupations are activities characterized by three properties: active participation, meaning, and a product that is the output of the process • Adaptation is a change in the functional state of the person • Occupational adaptation is both a state (of competency in occupational functioning) and a process
Client/Therapist Relationship:	Interdependent/collaborative—Therapist functions as an agent of the patient's occupational environment, and the patient functions as the agent of his or her unique person systems
Expected Outcome:	• Improvement in the person's internal occupational adaptation process (self-initiation, generalization, and mastery) • Occupational adaptation as a state of competency in occupational functioning
Assessment:	• Identify the sources of dysfunction in the occupational adaptation process • Data gathering about the patient's occupational environments, role expectations, effect of presenting problem on the person's systems

(continues)

Table 9.6 *Continued.*

Intervention:	<ul><li>Focus in on the patient's internal adaptation process and the use of meaningful occupations</li><li>Directed at improving the patient's internal ability to generate, evaluation, and integrate adaptive responses in which relative mastery is experienced</li><li>The occupational environment is an important as the patient's condition</li><li>Activities, tasks, methods, and techniques must be centered on occupational activity that promotes satisfaction</li></ul>

Note. From "Theoretical Contexts for the Practice of Occupational Therapy," by M. Law et al., 1997, in *Occupational Therapy: Enabling Function and Well-Being* (2nd ed., p. 95), by C. Christiansen and C. Baum (Eds.), Thorofare, NJ: SLACK. Copyright 1997 by SLACK, Inc. Reprinted with permission.

Contemporary Task-Oriented Approach. The contemporary task-oriented approach uses motor theories for intervention while incorporating environmental influences on performance. (See Table 9.7.) Occupation is considered as part of the environment (Bass Haugen & Mathiowetz, 1995; Mathiowetz & Bass Haugen, 1994). Thus, some of the complexity of the interaction between occupation and environment is lost. This approach uses motor theories that have been developed and tested mainly on people without disabilities. Therefore, the validity of generalizing this approach to populations with disabilities remains to be determined (Law et al., 1997).

Additional Contexts

Other contextual components that some of the theories and models incorporate are ecological, temporal, developmental, lifespan, and disability status. Ecological models vary in scope and complexity, ranging from a systems approach to less complex and less multidirectional dynamics. Few occupation-centered perspectives are unidirectional. The consensus among models seems to lie in their reflecting a transactive process. The emphasis on the various components and how they work are some areas of difference. Thus, occupational performance is a result of transactions among the capabilities of the person; the demands of the task or occupation; and the demands of the physical,

Table 9.7
Contemporary Task-Oriented Approach

Developers:	Virgil Mathiowetz and Julie Bass Haugen
Origin:	Developed to emphasize that occupational therapy should focus on occupational performance and use contemporary motor theories as a basis for intervention
Population:	All ages, although primarily tested with adults
Theoretical Foundations:	• Systems model of motor control • Motor learning theory • Developmental theories
Concepts and Assumptions:	• Motor behavior is facilitated and organized through performance of functional tasks • Performance of functional tasks is influenced by personal characteristics and the performance context • Personal characteristics and environmental factors are organized in a hierarchical fashion; control parameters which are personal characteristics or environmental factors are important in hindering or enabling performance • Use of motor learning strategies to practice a functional task will enhance the development of skilled performance
Client/Therapist Relationship:	Collaborative
Expected Outcome:	Improvement in task performance and role performance
Assessment:	• Assess functional tasks required to be performed by the person • Determine personal characteristics and environmental factors which are hindering performance • No specific recommendations about outcome measures
Intervention:	• Use and active learning approach • Client is an active participant in therapy intervention • Describe seven intervention principles: 　1. Client identifies tasks of interest and importance 　2. Client is encouraged to actively experiment with movements to achieve task performance 　3. Therapist performs and analysis of client's movement strategies

(continues)

Table 9.7 *Continued.*

4. Important personal characteristics and environmental factors which are hindering performance are changed

5. Outcome in terms of improved task performance is recorded

6. Further intervention can focus on developing more efficient movement strategies

7. Motor learning principles such as varying practice are used to enhance learning

Note. From "Theoretical Contexts for the Practice of Occupational Therapy," by M. Law et al., 1997, in *Occupational Therapy: Enabling Function and Well-Being* (2nd ed., p. 97), by C. Christiansen and C. Baum (Eds.), Thorofare, NJ, SLACK. Copyright 1997 by SLACK, Inc. Reprinted with permission.

social, cultural, temporal, and lifespan contexts in which the occupation or task takes place. Clients are not viewed as passive in their environment. They both act on and are affected by the environment. These models are similar to biopsychosocial models in that intervention or change can be focused on one or more of the following: the person, the occupation, and the environment. For example, when a therapist cannot change the patient by remediating her eyesight, the therapist can change the environment by providing a reader, books on tape, more light, and needle threaders. If a cognitive task is too difficult for the person's capabilities, the occupation or task can be altered.

The temporal contextual aspect relates to the experience of actions and occupations in time. Meyer (1922) emphasized the importance of balance among work, rest, play, and sleep. Shannon (1977) reiterated this importance in relation to adaptation and occupational role. Kielhofner (1977) stated that the context of time is important and the way in which one uses and organizes time is one of the best measures of adaptiveness. Christiansen (1996) presented a highly informative, scholarly review of three perspectives of the concept of balance in occupation. His analysis of the literature found evidence to support the premise that daily patterns of time use are influenced by "sociocultural patterns, psychological dispositions, physiological rhythms, and physical and mental capacities" (p. 447). He found less conclusive evidence on activity patterns and well-being. Further research is needed to demonstrate that balance of occupations is beneficial to health and well-being. The study of ritual, routine, and habit are interesting areas of exploration and discovery (Crepeau, 1995; Ludwig, 1997, 1998; Zemke, 1995). Developmental, lifespan, and disability contexts are discussed further in relation to their applicable models.

The Human as an Occupational Being

A powerful and fundamental concept of occupational science is the conceptualization that people are occupational beings who create meaning in their lives through the occupations in which they engage (Clark, 1997; Clark et al., 1991; Clark, Wood, & Larson, 1998; Wilcock, 1993, 1998; Yerxa et al., 1990). This concept goes further than positing that occupation has purpose; it also links meaning, occupation, well-being, and therapeutic change. A rich and exciting body of literature is emerging that presents various perspectives on the meanings that people derive and express through engagement in daily occupation and that is contributing to theory development. These theoretical frameworks are multidisciplinary and come from many fields in addition to occupational therapy and occupational science. The following sections present an overview of additional relevant theories and theoretical constructs that are reflected in contemporary occupation-centered and occupation-based theoretical frameworks. The sections are intrinsic motivation, occupation and identity, occupation and health and survival, and occupational science.

Intrinsic Motivation

Much of the earlier theoretical work and research on the human as an occupational being centered around theories of intrinsic motivation and biological need for occupation (Florey, 1969; White, 1971). Later Csikszentmihalyi (1990), a developmental psychologist, described intrinsic motivation for the experience of "flow," which occupational therapists related to in terms of providing "just the right challenge." A line of research in OT began with Kircher (1984), who hypothesized that performing a purposeful occupation would be more intrinsically motivating and persons would work longer and harder than for a rote or non-product-oriented one. Other studies followed (Rocker & Nelson, 1987; Steinbeck, 1986; Thibodeaux & Ludwig, 1988). Some researchers continue to explore variations of this hypothesis with various task enhancements (Murphy, Trombly, Tickle-Degnen, & Jacobs, 1999; Thomas, 1996; Thomas, Wyk, & Boyer, 1999; Yoder, Nelson, & Smith, 1989). Some researchers are now moving to examining the effects of contextual relevance on occupational performance under a similar research paradigm (Ferguson & Rice, 2001; Ma, Trombly, & Robinson-Podolski, 1999).

Occupation and Identity

Another perspective of the human as an occupational being centers around the relationship between occupation and identity. Christiansen (1999), in his Eleanor Clarke Slagle Lecture, asserted that people build and express their identities through engagement in occupations. He further "postulated that performance limitations and disfigurement that sometimes result from illness or injury have identity implications that should be recognized by occupational therapy practitioners" (p. 547). Helfrich, Kielhofner, and Mattingly (1994) wrote that people construct self-understanding and meaning through their volitional narratives. In the manual to the second edition of the Occupational Performance History Interview (OPHI-II), Kielhofner et al. (1998) identified the construct of occupational identity as the degree to which the individual has integrated and feels confident about his or her values, interests, and occupational roles. In these perspectives, identity is developed and expressed through occupation, and occupation is a means to experience life meaning. The Canadian model of occupational performance (Canadian Association of Occupational Therapists [CAOT], 1997) adds the concept of spirituality. These theoretical perspectives posit that "understanding people as occupational beings is to understand the core themes of their lives and the meanings they experience and express through occupation (i.e., why people do something, what they might do in the future, who they perceive they are becoming)" (Hocking, 2001, p. 464).

Occupation, Adaptation, Health, and Survival

In her Eleanor Clark Slagle Lecture, King (1978) argued the
need for a unifying comprehensive theory that addressed ordinary purposeful behavior. She proposed adaptation as a unifying
concept. "Perhaps it is time that some of our implicit assumptions about adaptation be made explicit. Only when these assumptions are articulated can their validity be examined
through research" (p. 431). She presented four features of the individual adaptation process: (a) It must be actively created by
the person, not imposed; (b) it is called forth by environmental
demands; (c) it is most efficiently organized at the subcortical
level, below level of consciousness, with conscious attention focused on tasks or objects; and (d) it is self-reinforcing and serves
as a stimulus for doing the next more complex challenge. Her
thesis was that "the essential purpose of occupational therapy is
to stimulate and guide the adaptive processes through which an
individual may best survive and develop" (p. 433). Ayres's (see
Chapter 5) theoretical concepts and writings heavily influenced
King's conceptualizations, especially in terms of theoretical constructs that posited that sensory input and motor output are the
essentials of individual adaptation. Thus, sensory integration is
adaptive development.

Schultz and Schkade (1997) consider adaptation to be a continuous thread throughout the profession. From their review of
literature, they delineated major concepts in the OT perspective
of adaptation and posed a paradigm of adaptation, which posits
that the role of OT is to facilitate the internal adaptation process
in clients to enhance occupational performance. Engagement in
tasks and occupations that are part of one's occupational roles
facilitates internal adaptation. The authors describe the relationship of this paradigm to their occupational adaptation
frame of reference discussed previously. Adaptation is posited to
be the mechanism by which person–environment transactions
are negotiated.

Occupation has been seen not only as essential to adaptation, but also to survival. Wilcock (1993) wrote that humans engage in occupation for many reasons, which she summarized as
aimed at meeting "immediate bodily needs of sustenance, self-
care, and shelter"; developing "skills, social structures, and technology aimed at safety and superiority over predators and the

environment"; and using personal capabilities (p. 20). This description is reminiscent of Maslow's (1954) hierarchy. Wilcock (1998) stated that "humans have occupational needs" (p. 11). Her major contribution has been to link occupation to health and survival. She takes the constructs of occupation and health and opens new vistas for OT by describing their potential impact on society and their broader global ecological effect and their relationship to OT and public health. Her work expands considerably on Reilly's (1962) often quoted hypothesis "that man through the use of his hands, as they are energized by mind and will, can influence the state of his own health" (p. 2). (See Chapter 6 for more about Reilly.)

Yerxa, a colleague of Mary Reilly's at the University of Southern California (USC), wrote, "One of the greatest challenges society faces today is understanding the relationship between engagement in occupation and health" (Yerxa et al., 1990, p. 1). She richly described the orchestration of a daily round of occupations. She stated, "To fully understand occupation it is necessary to comprehend the experience of engagement in it" (p. 9). This is also a major theme of Fidler (see Chapter 2 for more about Fidler's contributions). Yerxa also felt that the meaning of occupation could not be assessed from outside by observation. She wrote that occupation is highly individualized, is complex, and occurs in environmental and temporal contexts. She saw many purposes for occupation.

Occupational Science

Occupational science (OS) emerged out of the early 20th-century values, beliefs, and concepts of the founders of OT. Thus, it is based on the same sociohistorical context as the profession of OT described in Chapter 1 and in the beginning of this chapter. Occupational therapy is a profession, whereas occupational science is an academic discipline. What this means is that OS, as an academic discipline, is a "branch of knowledge or learning recognized by the university community as legitimate for scholarly investigation" (USC, 1989, p. 143). A profession offers service to the public by the application of a specialized base of knowledge and skills (Freidson, 1994).

Occupational science is a social science that is concerned with the study of the form, function, and meaning of human occupation. The concept of occupation is its central focus of study. Under the leadership of Yerxa at USC, a doctoral degree program in occupational science was established (Clark et al., 1991). Occupational science is not a single theory, frame of reference, or model. Yerxa et al. (1990) envisioned that the knowledge generated from occupational science could be applied to support the practice of occupational therapy. Although OS includes the study of the therapeutic uses of occupation in medical contexts, it also examines the centrality of occupation to health. This relationship of occupation to health is a crucial one in providing the linkage, evidence, and rationale for expanded practice in new settings and in health and wellness.

Occupational science can be expected to generate numerous theories about occupation that are likely to be applied to practice by OT practitioners in concert with other theories, models, or frames of reference that practitioners find useful. Its unique and primary contribution to OT will be to provide a corpus of knowledge sharply focused on the concept of occupation. This contribution can build professional unity by giving practitioners a more explicit and expansive sense of the complexity and power of human occupation employed to serve the public good (Clark et al., 1998, p. 13).

To be an occupational scientist requires that one be engaged in the scholarly study of occupation. Occupational scientists come from a variety of academic disciplines including occupational therapy; however, one does not need to be an occupational therapist to be an occupational scientist. The occupational therapist can become an occupational scientist through postprofessional education that enables him or her to have research skills and knowledge to pursue a scholarly study of occupation.

Occupational science is a relatively new multidisciplinary field of study that has received wide support internationally. In the United States, it was initially treated with some "diffidence, even conflict within the profession" (Wilcock, 1998, p. 203). Some of the reasons Wilcock listed for this reaction included (a) OS being considered just another theory in competition with OT; (b) OT being seen as fitting within OS; (c) therapists being very medically oriented and not recognizing any need for an occupational perspective; and (d) the desire for an embracing overall theory, or a view of the human in tightly fit boxes.

Occupational science, however, offers OT many things. Wilcock (1998) stated,

> If occupational science grows, there is no doubt that it will increase complexity of understanding because it will include many models, frames of reference, and theories, changing direction according to sociocultural change and advances in biological knowledge. Complexity will lead to heated debate between scientists . . . but collectively contribute to the science. (p. 203)

Mosey (1992, 1993) argued for the complete partition of OS from OT. Chapter 3 on Mosey provides more information about her position and her debate with the faculty from USC (Carlson & Dunlea, 1995; Clark et al., 1993) on this issue.

Application to Occupational Therapy Practice

Clinical practice is grounded in theoretical bases. This section examines how occupation-based and occupation-centered theories have been, and can be, linked to practice or intervention. Practice theories and frames of reference link theory and practice. Since the beginning of the profession, theories regarding the application of occupation to change have evolved. Recently, there has been a national and international recommitment to and resurgence of interest in occupation as OT's core or center. These occupation-based and occupation-centered approaches build upon theoretical constructs discussed in the previous section that relate occupation, the human as an occupational being, and context to therapeutic change, health, and well-being.

Contextual Relevance in Practice

Occupational therapy practitioners include performance contexts when determining feasibility and appropriateness of interventions (AOTA, 1994; Commission on Practice, AOTA, 2002).

New understandings and beliefs about the environment and person-environment relations are promoting the development of practice models that incorporate a social view of health and disability. As a result, we now acknowledge the importance of environmental factors in the lives of the people we work with, and we are changing our assessment and treatment practices to reflect this. (Letts et al., 2003, p. 13)

When using models that emphasize the individual, context, and occupation, it is important to understand that each model lends itself to somewhat different evaluation approaches. For example, models that emphasize the individual's perception of the environment might be better suited to self-report measures, whereas others might benefit from observational instruments (Law et al., 1997). Models that consider the individual, context, and occupation as inseparable and transactional might involve more complex and in-depth measures, such as the ethnographic interview (Gitlin, Corcoran, & Leinmiller-Eckhardt, 1995; Hasselkus, 1990; Spencer, Krefting, & Mattingly, 1993).

The six occupation-based and occupation-centered theoretical models reviewed earlier in this chapter have implications for practice. Law et al.'s (1997) matrix that presents each of these models in relation to a specific case in terms of client–therapist relationship, assessment, and intervention provides an excellent illustration of their applied use. In the following subsections, these six models are discussed in relation to intervention.

Person–Environment–Occupational Performance Model

The person–environment–occupational performance model provides a broad framework in which to organize information about the individual. Principles and guidelines for client-centered practice are essential processes of this model. Thus, assessment and treatment emphasize that the therapist collaborate with the client to plan intervention around occupational performance goals that the client has identified. For a therapeutic client–therapist relationship, the client should understand the breadth of the therapist's knowledge, skills, and resources, and the therapist needs to understand the client's knowledge and experience of his or her problem or condition. The primary focus is on the person's necessary and meaningful daily occupations that are limited as a result of health condition or disability (Christiansen & Baum, 1997).

Assessment and intervention strategies are not unique to this model, but it uses a wide variety of evaluations and approaches that further enable the person to develop his or her resources to perform occupations that are personally necessary and meaningful. Assessment is concerned with identifying the intrinsic and extrinsic factors that limit and support occupational performance. "Assessment data should include details about the individual assets as well as deficits and should always reflect the environmental context in which the individual typically performs the activities, tasks, and roles of daily living" (Christiansen & Baum, 1997, p. 64). Narrative reasoning, which involves understanding the client in terms of his or her life story, can be particularly effective in gaining the individual's perspective of the problem (Mattingly, 1998; Mattingly & Fleming, 1994).

"The goal of occupational therapy is to prevent, remediate, or reduce dysfunction that impairs or limits occupational performance of an individual" (Christiansen & Baum, 1997, p. 63). A wide variety of community, family, and other environmental resources may be used to facilitate improved occupational performance. Christiansen and Baum identified five major categories for strategies that address occupational performance: *modification of the physical environment, application of technical aids and devices, strategies for sensory and neuromotor remediation, occupation as therapeutic medium or means*, and *teaching or learning strategies*. The first two are environmental interventions, and the third is an intrinsic (within the person) intervention. The client selects strategies using an informed decision-making process.

Law et al. (1997) commented that the "occupational therapy process which accompanies the Person Environment Occupational model appears quite linear in its focus" (p. 86). Christiansen and Baum (1997), however, described the process as nonlinear because the therapist moves back and forth between elements to meet the patient's unique needs.

Ecology of Human Performance Model (EHP)

Therapeutic intervention involves a collaboration among the client, family, significant others, and the OT practitioner of the

EHP model. The intended outcome is to improve occupational performance by changing any combination of person, context, or task variables. For example, to establish or restore a person's abilities in context, the practitioner might use an intervention that targets having the person learn or relearn a skill or ability. Another intervention might be to alter the context or task so that the person can perform it with his or her current abilities. Also, interventions can be designed for a person who has no disability, impairment, or contextual factors that inhibit performance. In this situation, intervention is aimed at enriching contextual and task experiences that will enhance performance for the person in the natural contexts of life (Dunn et al., 1994).

EHP provides guidelines for inclusion of physical, temporal, and sociocultural contexts. It is generic and can be applied to everyday clinical practice. "This framework provides direction for the development of specific models of practice that recognize the interrelationship of the person and his or her context during task performance. It also recognizes the multifaceted nature of occupational therapy intervention" (Law et al., 1997, p. 89). However, little clinical evidence has been documented.

Model of Human Occupation

Regarding MOHO, Law et al. (1997) wrote, "Therapists find particularly useful the suggestions about how to apply the model in practice through case illustrations, review of potential assessments, a detailed theoretical question list, and an explicit sample of a program development project" (p. 90). Only a few suggested assessments focus on the environment, and most of those do so mainly on the presence or absence of supports and systems maintenance rather than "clearly articulating disabling environmental barriers" (p. 90). The OPHI-II, however, provides many occupation-centered constructs for assessment (Kielhofner et al., 1998; Kielhofner, Mallinson, Forsyth, & Lai, 2001).

Person–Environment–Occupation Model

The person–environment–occupation model reflects its Canadian roots in the Client-Centered Guidelines for the Practice of Occupational Therapy (CAOT, 1991). Occupational performance and context and the person are inseparable and highly transactive in nature (Law, Cooper, et al., 1996). Thus, intervention can enter in a variety of areas and target any combination of the person, occupation, and environment. Intervention seeks to identify important occupations to the client, and specific guidelines and examples are described for this model (CAOT, 1997; Strong et al., 1999). Assessments have been widely used and conceptually fit the model well. Letts et al. (1994) discussed person–environment assessments for OT. Researchers are developing an impressive body of literature supporting the use of the Canadian Occupational Performance Measure (Law et al., 1998) as an assessment tool and as an outcome measure (Carpenter, Baker, & Tyldesley, 2001; Sewell & Singh, 2001). Considerable testing of the model is occurring, particularly among Canadian and British therapists (Law, 1993a, 1993b, 1998; Rebeiro & Cook, 1999; Rebeiro, Day, Semeniuk, O'Brien, & Wilson, 2001). Letts et al. (2003) have provided therapists with theoretical background and a broad range of applications of contemporary theories that involve environment in OT practice to enable occupational performance. Examples focus on community, social groups, and individuals. Environmental features include physical, cultural, social, political, and technological features.

Occupational Adaptation (OA)

Occupational adaptation is identified as a frame of reference that was created to serve as a guide that spans across treatment settings and populations (Schkade & Schultz, 1992, 1993; Schultz & Schkade, 1992). This frame of reference is designed for clinical application that provides a theoretical foundation (as discussed previously), the method of intervention, the outcome of therapy, and the roles of the therapist and patient. Occupational adaptation is seen as both a state of occupational function and as a normative process in which competent occupational function develops. Schultz and Schkade and colleagues outline a practice model, which guides therapists to look holistically at the person's internal processes as well as the environment (Schkade & McClung, 2001; Schkade & Schultz, 1992; Schultz & Schkade, 1992). Adaptation processes are critical and have significant implications for prevention and remediation efforts.

Occupational adaptation is not so much a compendium of techniques, as it is a process of thinking and clinical reasoning to organize and guide the intervention process.

> The essential task of the practitioner is to acknowledge and facilitate the client as the agent of therapeutic change. The practitioner sets the stage for the client to progressively assume the agency role. This is critical in influencing the client's internal adaptation process. (Schkade & Schultz, 1993, p. 530)

Close client-centered collaboration between the client and the practitioner is crucial throughout the intervention process. Schultz and Schkade (1994) and Ford (1995) described this frame of reference in home health and provided good examples of how this process works.

The relationship between the therapist and patient and the assumptions can be somewhat vague and hard to translate into practice. Schkade and McClung wrote *Occupational Adaptation in Practice: Concepts and Cases* (2001, p. xi) "to make the occupational adaptation frame of reference more understandable and easier to use clinically." They have accomplished this by describing the theoretical ideas and illustrating them with case examples. Basic and applied research is being conducted because this framework was developed as a focus of research and for application to practice for the doctoral program at Texas Woman's University (Garrett & Schkade, 1995; Gibson & Schkade, 1997; Pasek & Schkade, 1996; Spencer et al., 1998). The model seems to work best in settings where the therapist has longer contact with the patient.

Contemporary Task-Oriented Approach

The contemporary task-oriented approach uses "top-down" approach to assessment and intervention. The major emphasis is on the performance of functional tasks. Personal characteristics, such as cognitive, psychosocial, and sensorimotor, and the physical, socioeconomic, and cultural environmental contexts are important factors affecting performance. Learning strategies based on motor learning theories that provide feedback of results from practice are used to help clients relearn tasks (Bass Haugen & Mathiowetz, 1995; Mathiowetz & Bass Haugen, 1994). Clear and detailed evaluation and intervention strategies are described (Law et al., 1997).

Summary

All six models conceptualize the importance of environment on occupational performance. All of them value occupation as a core concept, with occupational performance being a primary outcome. They vary in terms of whether they differentiate occupation from occupational performance, a differentiation that is most developed by the person–environment–occupation and person–environment–occupational performance models. Whether specific interventions are tied to measurement procedures, such as in the model of human occupation and the person–environment–occupation model, is another area of difference. In most of the models, the main focus on intervention is the person, whereas in the ecology of human performance and person–environment–occupation, and person–environment–occupational performance models, change can focus on any one or more of the person, occupation, and the environment. Law, Baum, and Baptiste (2002) edited *Occupation-Based Practice: Fostering Performance and Participation* to explore issues concerning preparing occupation-based treatment plans and practice.

Infusing Occupation into Practice

Under the leadership of Patricia Crist beginning in 1996, AOTA's Education Special Interest Section has initiated and conducted workshops on infusing occupation into practice. These workshops have been organized to (a) help to reduce the disconnection between occupation-based and occupation-centered theory and practice; (b) use theory and research in a real-life setting and application; (c) apply current and emerging theories in occupation-based and occupation-centered practice to actual persons in occupational therapy; (d) compare three theoretical views through a case study approach; and (e) further the dialogue on the practical application of approaches using occupation and the science of occupation (Crist, Royeen, & Schkade, 2000). Crist et al. (2000) stated, "The seamless integration of occupation into our professional core for occupational therapy is essential. The scientific study and application of occupation are tantamount to occupational therapy being fully recognized as a profession" (p. viii).

The following persons presented at the first workshop in 1996: Florence Clark on occupational science, Gary Kielhofner on the model of human occupation, and Sally Schultz on occupational adaptation. The following persons presented at the second workshop in 1999: Winnie Dunn on the ecology of human performance, Mary Law on the person–environment occupation model, and David Nelson on the conceptual framework of therapeutic occupation. At a third workshop in 2001, the following persons presented: Claudia Allen on the cognitive disabilities model, Beatrice Abreau on holistic rehabilitation using the quadraphonic approach, and Joan Toglia on the dynamic interactional approach to cognitive rehabilitation. Published proceedings from the first two workshops, in 1996 & 1999, present a case study approach in which theoretical information about occupation is infused into practice applications (Crist & Royeen, 1997; Crist et al., 2000). The 2000 edition includes comments by the six theorists from the first two workshops concerning continuing development of their approaches "through clinical and research questions" (Crist et al., 2000, p. vii). That edition is a "must read" for scholars, students, practitioners, and educators. The richness of the dialogue and the words of the six theorists highlight how their work integrates OT practice. All of these theories regard occupational performance or occupational behavior as the outcome of interactions between persons and their environments. Each postulates slightly different dynamics of those interactions. Comparative insights from the theorists themselves, case applications, and references are invaluable.

Integration and Synthesis of Theories, Frameworks, and Models

The most recent developments have been collaborations between some of these theorists to integrate and synthesize their theories, frameworks, and models to focus on comprehensive assessment and treatment of occupational performance. Law, Baum, and Dunn (2001) have edited and contributed several chapters to *Measuring Occupational Performance: Supporting Best Practice in Occupational Therapy*. This text provides background on measurement concepts and issues, along with a wide range of information that occupational therapists must consider when conducting assessments and utilizing measurement information for intervention. This book promotes an occupation-centered, evidence-based approach to measurement. Reviews of assessments are current and focus on all aspects of occupational performance and the environment. Reviews of both qualitative and quantitative assessment methods are included. Emerging trends in occupational performance assessment and their impact on the field of OT are also included. This work is an excellent resource for evidence-based practice, research, and health care policy.

In her foreword to Fearing and Clark's book, *Individuals in Context: A Practical Guide to Client-Centered Practice,* Law (2000) stated, "A significant challenge in occupational therapy practice today is to ensure that our services are client-centered, focused on occupation, and supported by research evidence" (p. xi). In that book, Fearing and Clark (2000) presented the occupational performance process model (see Figure 9.1), originally presented by

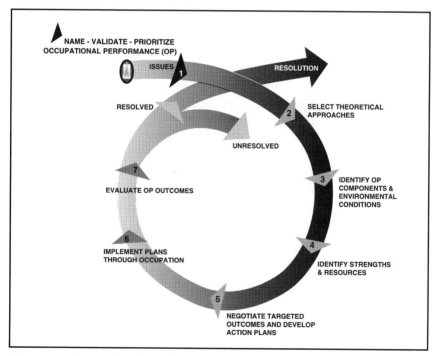

Figure 9.1. Occupational performance process model. OP = occupational performance. *Note.* From Occupational Performance Process Model," by V. Fearing, M. Law, and J. Clark, 1997, *Canadian Journal of Occupational Therapy, 64,* p. 11. Copyright 1997 by Canadian Association of Occupational Therapists. Reprinted with permission.

Fearing, Law, and Clark (1997), as a client-centered practice framework that is centered on occupation. In the foreword, Law referred to the model as a "compass" with OT practice as a "journey."

> The result of this journey will be the following: an evidence based occupational therapy practice grounded in theory and research, a client-centered practice that enhances client and therapist outcomes and satisfaction, a focus on enabling clients to perform their chosen occupations, and continual documentation of outcome and the quality of your practice. (Law, 2000, p. xi)

Occupation-Based and Occupation-Centered Assessment and Treatment

Assessment forms the basis from which occupational therapists determine the nature of their clients' occupational performance in terms of strengths, challenges, and priorities. This is the groundwork for intervention goals. In 1991, AOTA and AOTF convened the Symposium on Measurement and Assessment: Directions for the Future in Occupational Therapy, which resulted in the publication of a series of articles and recommendations in the *American Journal of Occupational Therapy* in March and April of 1993. These publications challenged occupational therapists to focus assessment processes and instruments on individualized meaningful occupation rather than the discrete components that underlie performance problems (Fisher & Short-DeGraff, 1993). Trombly (1993) stated that the usual approach to assessment, which she referred to as bottom-up, does not communicate to OT clients the relevance to daily-life occupations that occupational therapists have to offer. In other words, evaluations that do not focus on meaningful occupations that clients find problematic will not relay the purpose of OT to them and others, which will contribute to misunderstanding and displeasure with services. Clients need to understand the purpose of OT and its potential outcomes in order to participate fully in a client-centered approach.

Speakers at the symposium recommended a top-down assessment process, which they believed would result in improved communication about authentic OT and support occupation-centered intervention. The top-down approach begins by finding out what the person needs or wishes to do, the natural context in which he or she usually does these, and the person's current limitations to accomplishing them. The occupation-centered theories previously discussed are compatible with this approach. What is needed are psychometrically sound assessment tools that are congruent with the core concepts about occupation, contextual relevance, and the human as an occupational being.

The disadvantages of top-down approaches are that they may be task specific. Also, for interventions to be maximally effective, they must happen in the client's natural occupational context. It is essential in these frameworks for the practitioner to integrate the complexity of contextual factors that are impinging on occupational performance.

Interventions can use occupation as ends or as means, or as a top-down or bottom-up approach. Therapists who use a bottom-up approach focus evaluation and treatment on the client's generic task abilities and focus specifically on impairments, according to WHO's (2001) model and performance components of AOTA's (1999) Uniform Terminology. The rationale is that, with remediation, generic task abilities, such as postural control, arm strength, and bilateral coordination, will translate into gains in everyday occupational performance. In this approach the therapist focuses on discrete performance components without having to consider demands of the occupation or environment. Demands for real-life performance are begun after performance component abilities have been restored or plateaued.

Another problem with the assumptions of a bottom-up approach to assessment and intervention is that it is not supported by recent research testing the hypothesis that normalizing performance components will result in independent occupational performance (Fisher, 1992b; Mathiowetz, 1993). Further research has demonstrated that improvement in performance components does not automatically transfer into better occupational performance (Mathiowetz & Bass Haugen, 1994; Trombly, 1995).

Many occupation-centered theorists and practitioners find that a top-down approach to performance discrepancy is effective (Gray, 1998). The top-down approach begins at the highest level, the so-called top of occupational performance areas described by AOTA (1994). A basic assumption of this approach is that even though impairments cannot always be cured, performance in valued occupations can be improved by adaptations.

According to Trombly (1993), the main advantage of the top-down approach is that evaluation and intervention center on impaired role and task performances that are meaningful to clients. This focus imparts relevance of treatment to improving a client's ability to engage in meaningful occupations. Theoretically, this may be more motivating Thus, real-life performance, rather than being contrived, is both the medium and the outcome of treatment. Another strength of the top-down approach was described by Holm et al. (1998):

> When difficulties are encountered in doing tasks, we tend to seek the assistance of others, use a tool to help us, or try a different way of performing the task. These compensatory procedures foster task completion. Because the top-down approach enhances procedures that humans turn to naturally when problems are encountered, it is familiar to clients, hence, it is likely to be well accepted by them. (p. 480)

Holm et al. (1998) stated that another advantage of the top-down approach is that it facilitates the identification of impairments in the context of occupational performance and ascertains the relevance of the impairment in functional occupational performance. In the bottom-up approach, impairments may be evaluated in isolation and their effect on performance can only be inferred. Another advantage of the top-down approach is that it enables a more efficient and targeted evaluation of impairments directly affecting occupation-related performance and, therefore, more precisely directs interventions.

Hocking (2001) and Fisher (1992a, 1992b) expressed concern that occupational therapists who center evaluations exclusively on performance components risk focusing treatment on those components and therefore fail to "address critical occupational issues" (Hocking, 2001, p. 463). In addition, performance component-based assessments are not likely to disclose client's strengths, adaptive strategies, and environmental interactions and resources. Thus, abilities and impairments can be observed as they interact synergistically in the actual doing of contextually relevant real-life tasks.

As discussed earlier, several occupational therapists have developed occupation-centered assessments for practice, such as the Canadian Occupational Performance Measure (Law et al., 1998), the Occupational Performance History Interview (Kielhofner et al., 1998), application of ethnographic methods (Hasselkus, 1990; Spencer et al., 1993), and narrative (Clark, Ennevor, & Richardson, 1996; Helfrich et al., 1994). Coster (1998) presented an adaptation of the functional assessment model proposed by Trombly (1993) that is tailored for children. This is a useful model for organizing the occupation-centered assessment process with children. Law et al. (2001) have compiled a wide range of assessments that augment this framework. Occupation-centered assessments need to utilize frameworks that are organized around the field's understanding of occupation.

The Human as an Occupational Being

Occupational therapists are increasingly coming to agree that "evaluations that focus directly on occupation are most true to the basic concepts of occupational therapy. The complexities of implementing occupation-based assessments, however, have received little attention" (Hocking, 2001, p. 463). The field needs models that guide clinical reasoning. Hocking outlined three broad strategies to evaluate the use of available occupation-based instruments. She also agreed that therapists need to be trained to use a top-down approach. She expanded upon Trombly's (1993) ideas and proposed a hierarchical method (see Figure 9.2) that relies first on understanding clients as occupational beings who create meaning through their engagement in occupation. For example, Hocking (2001, p. 464) listed the following meaning-related questions that the therapist might ask:

How does this person describe himself or herself?

How does this person's occupation contribute to constructing or maintaining identity, to expressing and experiencing meaning, or to achieving his or her life purpose?

What are this person's occupational goals?

In what ways do the occupations this person finds problematic affect his or her identity or expression or experience of meaning?

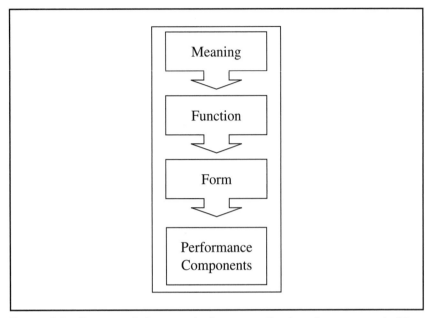

Figure 9.2. Conceptual framework for occupation-based assessment. *Note.* From "The Issue Is—Implementing Occupation-Based Assessment," by C. Hocking, 2001, *American Journal of Occupational Therapy, 55,* p. 464. Copyright 2001 by American Occupational Therapy Association. Reprinted with permission.

Because meaning is also socially constructed, it is important to know how the client's significant others and the sociocultural environment consider the client's occupational fit.

Function, the second focus for data gathering in Hocking's (2001) schematic, relates to the purpose or contribution that the occupation serves for the client and others. Some suggested questions are as follows (p. 464):

> What functions are disrupted by the occupational challenges this person experiences and who is affected?

> In what ways does the physical environment support or impede the client from reaching the intended purpose of the occupation?

The third part of the schematic, form, is based on Clark et al.'s (1998) definition in which form refers to observable features of an occupation in its natural environment. Evaluation of form involves determining observable disruptions of performance and delineating occupational performance skills and environmental opportunities that facilitate performance. Some of the sample questions that Hocking provides include these (Hocking, 2001, p. 465):

> What actions are required to complete the occupation successfully?
>
> What performance standards will apply?
>
> Where and how often will the occupation occur?
>
> In what ways does the environment limit and facilitate performance?
>
> What outcomes might be observed?

Hocking (2001) stated that the way in which all of these questions are framed depends on the models that inform the therapist's clinical reasoning. The next step is to establish the type and extent of interference to performance. To do this, the therapist needs to know how the existing occupational form relates to what the person desires and needs. The therapist also identifies potential for change by considering questions such as these (p. 465):

> Does the individual have the ability to improve performance? How might the occupational context be modified to enhance performance?

If the cause of the limitation in occupational performance is not yet evident or more specific detail is needed, the therapist assesses occupational performance components. This assessment is congruent with models proposed by Baum and Law (1997), Mathiowetz (1993), and others.

Hocking (2001) listed and discussed three broad strategies for analyzing the occupational basis of assessments:

> a) determining whether the assessment actually measures some aspect of occupation, b) identifying what kind of occupation(s) the assessment involves and how clients might experience those occupations, and c) analyzing whether the occupations incorporated in the assessment are real or simulated and familiar or unfamiliar. (p. 466)

These are very important considerations when examining and implementing occupation-based and occupation-centered models of practice and theories. For example, the Canadian model of occupation and performance and the model of human occupation operationalize specific theories of occupational performance and provide guidelines.

Theory Validation and Research

Law (2000) stated, "A significant challenge in occupational therapy practice today is to ensure that our services are client-centered, focused on occupation, and supported by research evidence" (p. xi). Of all the occupation-centered models, the ones that have been the most researched and validated to date are the model of human of occupation and client-centered practice. Law (1998) concluded from her review of the literature that evidence supports client-centered occupational therapy practice (Law & Steinwender, 1996). Chapter 7 describes the research on the model of human occupation. Client-centered practice is a model for an approach to therapeutic intervention. It first emerged as a treatment method in psychology from the work of Carl Rogers (1939). Its use in OT involves respect for clients and their families and for their choices and decisions. The client participates as a full partner in therapy that is highly individualized and focuses on meaningful occupational performance (Law, 1998). Brown and Bowen (1998) found evidence in their study to suggest that current OT intervention is not consistent with consumer-oriented practice models such as occupation-centered practice.

Person–Environment–Occupation Fit

An important area for further theory development is the nature of person–environment–occupation fit. The following are possible research questions: What constitutes optimal occupational performance at different ages and in various contexts? What is the relationship between a person's perceptions of occupational performance and objective measures? Researchers (Law, 1993b; Peachey-Hill & Law, 2000; Rebeiro et al., 2001) have been working on validating environmental measures in terms of environmental factors that affect participation of children with disabilities, the effects of environmental sensitivity on occupational performance, transition to adulthood for adolescents with disabilities, and supportive work environments for people with persistent mental illness (Crist et al., 2000). Occupational therapists have used participatory action research with persons with disabilities to increase the awareness of their resources and strengths, and their abilities to effect and measure change (Cockburn & Trentham, 2002; Law, 1997). Thus, the field is expanding research methodologies using qualitative, especially participatory methods to study complex issues.

Because many of the occupation-centered models were established as a focus for research and practice frameworks in academic institutions, much of the research being carried out is with colleagues and doctoral students. For example, the OT doctoral planning committee at Texas Woman's University selected the concept of occupational adaptation as the focus for basic and applied research (Schkade & Schultz, 1992). Validation efforts are progressing through clinical application and research in a variety of settings, including Level II fieldwork (Dolecheck, & Schkade, 1999; Ford, 1995; Garrett & Schkade, 1995; J. P. Jackson & Schkade, 2001; Pasek & Schkade, 1996). Likewise, Dunn and her colleagues at the University of Kansas (Dunn et al., 1994; Dunn et al., 1998) developed the EHP model for multidisciplinary research and practice at their university. Thus, lines or themes of research become focused in academic settings based on research by the department or specific researchers.

Occupation, Health, and Well-being

Evidence is increasing that occupation is an important factor in health and well-being. Law and Steinwender (1996) presented an impressive review of research evidence concerning this relationship. Perhaps the most convincing study to date is that of independent-living older adults by Clark et al. (1997). Other research studies are supporting contextually relevant occupation-based and occupation-centered interventions in a wide variety of clinical settings (Brown & Bowen, 1998; George, Wilcock, & Stanley, 2001; Lin, Wu, Tickle-Degnen, & Coster, 1997; Thomas et al., 1999; Toth-Fejel, Toth-Fejel, & Hedricks, 1998). Many studies are case examples (Deshaies, Bauer, & Berro, 2001;

Rebeiro et al., 2001). Gray (1998) demonstrated how theory informs practice and vice versa in her case analysis that used multiple theoretical perspectives on occupation and neurodevelopmental theory and application. She addressed the difficulty of maintaining occupation as the center of therapeutic intervention. George et al. (2001) found evidence from their qualitative study that supported occupation-centered interventions with an emphasis on "doing" for stroke clients with emotional changes. They reaffirmed the necessity for therapists to take the time to engage clients in narratives so as to learn the meaning of occupation to each person and the best method to facilitate successful occupational engagement.

Yerxa (1998a) explored how other disciplines view the relationship between engagement in occupation and different aspects of health. She stated, "Occupational therapists and occupational scientists need to reaffirm that engagement in occupation, rather than being trivial, is an essential mediator of healthy adaptation and a vital source of joy and happiness in one's daily life" (p. 417). To achieve this goal, much more needs to be done to learn how adaptive skills are developed and how the "just right challenge" facilitates an adaptive response. Further research is needed to determine more about the characteristics of occupation that are most powerful in promoting health and well-being.

Knowledge generated in occupational science has been used to inform clinical reasoning and clinical practice (Wilcock, 1998). The transformative nature of occupations through the use of narrative analyses and occupational storymaking illustrate how people make sense of their lives and use occupation to resolve crises (Clark, 1993; Clark et al., 1996; Polkinghorne, 1996; Price-Lackey & Cashman, 1996). Volume 52, Issues 5 and 6, and Volume 54, Issue 3, of the *American Journal of Occupational Therapy* contain many articles emanating from occupational science that relate to clinical practice.

Another example of the contribution of occupational science to practice is Farnworth's (2000) exploration of time use and leisure occupations of young offenders to inform OT practice with such groups. Also, Ludwig (1997) developed a theoretical model of how routine—that is, the temporal context of occupations—facilitates well-being in older women. She (1998) found that older women tend to use routine less than they did when they had dependent children and husbands, and she discussed the implications of this for practice.

Occupational scientists have studied the form of occupation, that is, what people do in relation to time, space, and place. These studies have involved time studies, time logs, and observation. Creative qualitative methodologies, such as experience-sampling procedures, are helping to tap and illuminate some of the complex issues and relationships between the person, context, and occupational form (Larson, 1996; Primeau, 1998).

Wilcock (1993, 1998) expanded the concept of how occupation serves health and well-being in individuals to that of a public health model. This model incorporates occupational patterns characteristic of particular cultures or social groups and their effect on the health of towns, cities, neighborhoods, and other environments.

Occupation and Identity

The meaning of occupation is concerned with how meaning influences occupational engagement and performance, as well as how occupations are symbolic of higher social and cultural meanings. Studies of the human as an occupational being with an identity and sense of self fall within this category.

Narratives are useful in studying the relationship between occupation and identity. Braveman and Helfrich (2001) explored the usefulness of the construct of occupational identity as measured by the OPHI–II through the evolving narratives of three men with AIDS who were participating in a vocational rehabilitation program. Narratives were used to demonstrate what the construct of occupational identity could add to a traditional work history or functional capacity evaluation. In this framework, occupational identity aids in understanding how an event such as the onset of disability is framed by a person and how it affects the person's view of his or her past, current, and future self. Narratives have been found to provide unifying identities to people's lives when they form past, present, and future actions into a meaningful and coherent story (Polkinghorne, 1996). Narrative analysis has been used as a method to understand individuals' occupational choices (Larson, 1996). Narrative analysis also is a means for researchers and therapists to make systematic observations and to validate interpretations about people's lives as they interact collaboratively to create new meanings and life stories. Identities are reaffirmed, rebuilt, and bridged to provide coherence to clients' sense of self (Clark, 1993; Hasselkus, 1990, 1993; Mattingly, 1998). Kielhofner et al. (2001) conceptualized the term *occupational identity* as a means of defining the self and as a guide for future action. The relationship of occupational identity to occupational performance requires further study. Volume 17, Issue 2, of the *Occupational Therapy Journal of Research* centers on narrative and storytelling as methods for enhancing researchers and practice.

Clark (1993) and Price-Lackey and Cashman (1996) illustrated how the recursive relationship between engagement in occupation and meaningful interpretation of it in relation to an unfolding life story became therapeutic for two survivors of devastating injuries. These case studies illustrate how the occupational self emerges through childhood and helps a person to reemerge in a newly constructed self following a disabling accident. These studies support the central position of meaningful occupation in the therapeutic recovery process.

Definition of Terms and Taxonomies in Research

Christiansen (1994) referred to the use of classification, or taxonomies, as a fundamental step in the development of knowledge. He provided detailed reviews of taxonomies relevant to the study of occupation from a multidisciplinary perspective. He concluded that researchers who study occupation need to familiarize themselves with theoretical and methodological literature from the social and behavioral sciences. He made a very interesting comment when he stated, "It is possible that a workable and comprehensive classification system for occupational performance dysfunction may not be achievable until the complexities of human occupation and its relationship to health and well-being are better understood at a fundamental level" (p. 5).

Concepts are the basic elements of a theory and demarcate its phenomena. Clear or operational definitions are necessary to understand concepts. There are many varying viewpoints on and definitions of the term *occupation*. For example, AOTA (1995a) defined occupations as "the ordinary and familiar things that people do every day" (p. 1015). Yerxa et al. (1990) defined occupation as "specific 'chunks' of activity within the ongoing stream of human behavior which are named in the lexicon of the culture. . . . These daily pursuits are self initiated, goal directed (purposeful) and socially sanctioned" (p. 5). Definitions are usually developed for a specific purpose, such as the definitions of *occupation* for the profession of occupational therapy and for occupational science, respectively. Occupation is a complex and dynamic phenomenon that challenges the researcher to be comprehensive, yet simple, and not to limit the scope of practice of research too narrowly or to be too broad to be useful. Since 1999, the *Journal of Occupational Science* has included a section called "Occupational Terminology Interactive Dialog" to promote discussion around this central concept of occupational science and occupational therapy.

Pierce (2001b) wrestled with differentiating *activity* and *occupation* as two different core concepts of occupational therapy that offer "a rich set of theoretical relations for exploration" (p. 138). Other theorists do not differentiate or use various methods to separate these two concepts (Golledge, 1998). AOTA has dealt with the definition issue in several documents (AOTA, 1994, 1995a, 1995b). *Purposeful activity* and *meaning* have also received considerable attention as essential conceptual definitions that need differentiation to clarify concepts for research, discussion, discourse, and application to frameworks for practice (AOTA, 1983; Breines, 1984; Cynkin, 1995; Fisher, 1998; Gray, 1997; Nelson, 1988, 1996; Trombly, 1995; Yerxa, 1998a).

Definition debates generally revolve around issues such as what gives meaning to life, how meaning is constructed through occupation or activity, how to view of human beings (e.g., as active agents who construct meaning through their daily occupations), whether and how activity and occupation are related to each other (e.g., occupation fits into a hierarchy of activity), and what role context plays (e.g., environmental effects including sociocultural and temporal). The difference between *subjectivity* and *objectivity* is also important. Simply stated, *subjectivity* refers to the position that emphasizes the individual's own interpretation of occupation and what that engagement signifies to him or her (i.e., the insider's perspective), whereas *objectivity* refers to an external, or outsider's, perspective of observable objective reality.

Models have been developed that define *occupation* within a theoretical context. Most of those models have been discussed in chapters in this book, such as the model of human occupation (Chapter 7), lifestyle performance model (Chapter 2), occupational behavior (Chapter 6), and the models described in this chapter.

Nelson (1988) developed a model of occupation with two dimensions: occupational form and occupational performance. He defined *occupational form* as the structure of the activity, *occupational performance* as the doing process of the activity, and *occupation* as a "dynamic relationship between occupational form and occupational performance" (p. 633). His work reasoned about the reciprocal relationship between occupation and human adaptation. He emphazied that occupation needs to be considered as a complex dynamic of individuals and their purposive behavior within environmental contexts that have meaning and that change over time.

The discussion of definitions has important political implications for the occupational therapy profession (Pierce, 2001a). It is essential for therapists to be aware of how their own definitions of important terms fit with the definitions provided by various models. When the field defines terms such as *activity, occupation, therapeutic activity, purposeful activity,* it also sets a claim with boundaries that establish the domain of concern. In the final draft of the ICIDH–2, the World Health Organization (2001) defined disability as barriers to participation in activity, *activity* as "the execution of a task or action by an individual" (p. 9), and *participation* as "involvement in a life situation" (p. 9). The ICIDH–2 system also recognizes the importance of contextual factors for health and their effect on activity and participation.

Conclusions

One important factor to consider when examining occupation-based and occupation-centered approaches is their fit with the profession's philosophical assumptions and domain of concern. Although occupational therapists may legitimately focus on a performance component, the acquisition of skills is normally accomplished in an integrated manner through engagement in occupation—that is, daily ordinary tasks of living that comprise work, play, and leisure. Occupation-centered and occupation-based approaches are consistent with OT's core values.

More studies and applications in practice are needed to examine the meaning of occupations in the natural contexts in which they occur and where individuals determine what is meaningful or purposeful for them. In spite of attempts to define and identify meaning in specific activities, the only way to determine meaning is from each person. Meaning cannot be learned from observing form and performance. It has to be revealed by the individual, and even then it is interpreted from the therapist's (an outsider's) viewpoint. The need to consider the subjective experience of the individual and the complexities of the environment that influence behavior has led to the increased use of qualitative methods of inquiry. Occupation-centered and occupation-based theoretical models enhance understanding of the relationships among occupation, the individual, context, and its power in individuals' lives. Participatory action research includes participants as collaborators, which is in harmony with client-centered practice models and evidence-based practice that empowers the consumer.

Occupational therapy curricula also need to have occupation as a "keystone," according to Yerxa (1998b). She stated that "implementing an occupation-centered curriculum could create a more integrated profession in which practice, ideas, scholarship, and education nurture and support one another, increasing the autonomy of both the occupational therapy profession and recipients of its services" (p. 365). She provided recommendations for such a curriculum. Wood and her colleagues (2000) described how their graduate curriculum centered on occupation. Nielson (1998) also wrote about transitioning the academic culture to occupation-centered education.

Future Directions

Scholars and leaders in the profession of occupational therapy envision great potential for OT's future. The overall consensus is that there will be closer collaboration between groups of scholars, researchers, educators, and clinicians, which will lead to stronger theoretical and practice models. These models will be used in practice and provide a language and evidence to articulate OT's focus on occupation and patterns of engagement in occupation. Therapists will be asked even more to communicate the purpose of intervention to meet increasing consumer demands that evaluation and treatment be relevant and efficacious. There is a refreshing air of optimism and excitement about infusing occupation into practice and recognizing the power of the ordinary occupations of daily living that give life meaning and purpose.

> We are entering an exciting period of occupational therapy history. Perhaps at no other time since the inception of our profession have global health care trends been as congruent with our core values and beliefs as they are today. Our core values and beliefs—a profound respect for the doing and experiencing person; a view of the individual as greater than the sum of anatomical, physiological, and behavioral components; the belief that human action is dynamically interdependent with the social and physical environment; and a commitment to collaborative working relationships with clients—have not always been manifest in our practice. . . . Today, however, prospects are auspicious for the manifestation of occupational therapy's core values and beliefs in practice, research, and health care policy. (Tickle-Degnen, 2001, p. xvii)

Future directions will depend on the extent to which these practice models and theories permit therapists to measure treatment efficacy and outcome and to clearly articulate and explain OT to consumers and third-party payers. Occupation-based and occupation-centered frameworks have the potential to consolidate OT's professional identity, core knowledge, and methods of making a difference, and connect the field more deeply with societal needs, quality of life, and well-being.

Winnie Dunn, in her discussion during the workshop, published in *Infusing Occupation Into Practice* (Crist et al., 2000), stated,

> I think that focusing on the doing can result in changes. . . . You can focus on the occupation and have other person–variable changes as a result because of the person having access to the activity. So that relationship is something that would be very appropriate to study and might help us get away from always focusing on these component goals when, in fact, the goal is for them to be doing. (p. 142)

Law commented in the same workshop (Crist et al., 2000) on the need to have OT's models, terminology, and assessments congruent with the disablement classifications proposed by the World Health Organization (2001). She emphasized the importance of organizing models around positive concepts of occupational engagement instead of in terms of limitations and deficits.

Wood (1998a) wrote,

> It is . . . increasingly accepted that intentional, meaningful, contextually relevant, socioculturally attuned, and appropriately challenging activity—what occupational therapists have always called therapeutic occupation—is an essential and irreducible mechanism of adaptation. I consequently have no doubt but that occupational therapy's theoretical knowledge and pragmatic expertise could be invaluable in addressing the exceedingly complex challenges of daily living that lie ahead. (p. 323)

Wood (1998b) subsequently voiced concern over the continued viability of occupational therapy as a result of the encroachment of other professions, physical therapy in particular, on the domain of occupational therapy, especially in the areas of functional occupational outcomes and daily occupations.

Pierce (2001a) stated that the knowledge of occupation in the field of OT is increasing dramatically, while at the same time the health care system is increasingly valuing functional or occupational outcomes. She stated, "A potential time of congruence is approaching if occupational therapy can expeditiously translate an expanding knowledge of occupation into powerful occupation-based practice" (p. 249).

Pierce (2001a, 2001b) and Wood (1998a) feel that in these times when other fields are impinging on occupation and competing for OT's domains of practice, OT professionals must use occupation in the "most powerful therapeutic ways possible. We must consistently target functional occupational patterns as outcomes. And we must be eloquent about our unique clinical perspective" (Pierce, 2001a, p. 249). To connect basic research on occupation into practice, Pierce encourages the use of an occupation-based practice language, and research such as that by Coster (1998) using top-down approaches. More practice demonstrations are needed. She also encourages educators to teach students so that graduates will be able to explain why their occupation-based interventions are effective and designed for a specific person and goals. This training will enable students and practitioners to be more articulate about why occupation-centered approaches are effective. This is an ethical and pragmatic imperative for evidence-based practice in the 21st century (Holm, 2000).

Yerxa (1994) wrote,

> My most audacious dream is that the 21st century will begin the millennium of occupation. Occupation, as engagement in self-initiated, self-directed, adaptive, purposeful, culturally relevant, organized activity, speaks to my assumptions about the future in compelling ways. . . . In fact, authentic occupational therapy cannot take place unless the patient becomes his or her own agent of competency via education. (p. 587)

From studies such as the well-elderly research study by Clark et al. (1997), researchers may also find that preventive programs in OT may reduce morbidity and the effects of disability. The field can enlighten the medical model about the health-promoting effects of ordinary occupation and infuse it into practice and then move beyond the medical model to natural settings that provide contextual relevance. The field will increase therapists' skills in enriching contexts to maximize meaningful and competent occupational performance.

Baum (2000) wrote,

> Occupational therapy as a profession has a unique opportunity to serve as a flagship in this changing health care environment. Revisiting some of the fundamental tenets of the profession has uncovered new insights about the value of occupation, its contribution to the quality of life, and the role of the individual in its pursuit. These insights impose new requirements on the occupational therapy process: (a) a focus that emphasizes individual strengths and the capability of the client to participate in—and guide—the rehabilitation process, and (b) changes in how and where the profession is practiced. Effecting these changes can place occupational therapy at the forefront of developments in the health care community because the new perspective and approach of our discipline coin-

cide exactly with the emerging health care system paradigm that has as its concern the health of the population. (p. 12)

Baum (2000) also addressed another important issue:

Maintaining that disparity between the academic preparation of students and what they encounter as they enter fieldwork can only limit the potential of the strength of this profession to define the core and scope of its practice, limit its ability to influence public policy decision, weaken the evidence of its therapeutic interventions, and make it difficult to attract and retain occupational therapists and occupational therapy assistants in the profession. (p. 13)

Wilcock (2001) described her vision of occupational science's place in a global world. She stated,

I am an occupational therapist and an occupational scientist and my job is to consider the occupational consequences of any situation and to enable occupational health to the best of my ability; to fight for people's occupational rights and occupational health. (p. 416)

These forward thinkers see occupational therapists working more to decrease the risk of disablement and to promote occupational health and well-being. Consumers will include family, community, and agencies and institutions, in addition to the individual.

References

American Occupational Therapy Association. (1983). Position paper: Purposeful activity. *American Journal of Occupational Therapy, 37,* 805–806.

American Occupational Therapy Association. (1994). Uniform terminology for occupational therapy. *American Journal of Occupational Therapy, 48,* 1047–1055.

American Occupational Therapy Association. (1995a). Position paper: Occupation. *American Journal of Occupational Therapy, 49,* 1015–1018.

American Occupational Therapy Association. (1995b). Position paper: Occupational performance. *American Journal of Occupational Therapy, 49,* 1019–1021.

American Occupational Therapy Foundation. (2000, Fall). Proceedings of Habits I Conference. *Occupational Therapy Journal of Research, 20,* (Suppl. 1).

American Occupational Therapy Association. (2002a). Occupational therapy practice framework: Domain and process. *American Journal of Occupational Therapy, 56,* 609–639.

American Occupational Therapy Association. (2002b). Proceedings of Habits 2 Conference. *Occupational Therapy Journal of Research, 22* (Suppl. 1).

Barris, R. (1982). Environmental interactions: An extension of the model of human occupation. *American Journal of Occupational Therapy, 36,* 637–644.

Barris, R., Kielhofner, G., Levine, R. E., & Neville, A. M. (1985). Occupation as interaction with the environment. In G. Kielhofner (Ed.), *A model of human occupation; Theory and application* (pp. 42–62). Baltimore: Williams & Wilkins.

Bass-Haugen, J. B., & Mathiowetz, V. (1995). Contemporary task-oriented approach. In C. A. Trombly (Ed.), *Occupational therapy for physical dysfunction* (4th ed.). Baltimore: Williams & Wilkins.

Baum, C. (2000). Occupation-based practice: Reinventing ourselves for the new millenium. *Occupational Therapy Practice, 5*(1), 12–15.

Baum, C. (2001). Editorial: A forum for occupation, participation and health. *Occupational Therapy Journal of Research, 21,* 71–72.

Baum, C. M., & Baptiste, S. (2002). Reframing occupational therapy practice. In M. Law, C. Baum, & S. Baptiste (Eds.), *Occupation-based practice: Fostering Performance and Participation* (pp. 3–15). Thorofare, NJ: SLACK.

Baum, C. M., & Law, M. (1997). Occupational therapy practice: Focusing on occupational performance. *American Journal of Occupational Therapy, 51,* 277–288.

Berger, P. L., & Luckman, T. (1966). *The social construction of reality.* New York: Doubleday.

Braveman, B., & Helfrich, C. A. (2001). Occupational identity: Exploring the narratives of three men living with aids. *Journal of Occupational Science, 8,* 25–31.

Breines, E. (1984). The issue is—An attempt to define purposeful activity. *American Journal of Occupational Therapy, 38,* 543–544.

Brown, C., & Bowen, R. E. (1998). Including the consumer and environment in occupational therapy treatment planning. *The Occupational Therapy Journal of Research, 18,* 44–62.

Canadian Association of Occupational Therapists. (1991). *Client-centered guidelines for the practice of occupational therapy.* Toronto: Author.

Canadian Association of Occupational Therapists. (1997). *Enabling occupation: An occupational therapy perspective.* Ottawa: Author.

Carlson, M., & Dunlea, A. (1995). Further thoughts on the pitfalls of partition: A response to Mosey. *American Journal of Occupational Therapy, 49,* 73–81.

Carpenter, L., Baker, G. A., & Tyldesley, B. (2001). The use of the Canadian Occupational Performance Measure as an outcome of a pain management program. *Canadian Journal of Occupational Therapy, 68,* 16–22.

Christiansen, C. (1994). Classification and study in occupation: A review and discussion of taxonomies. *Journal of Occupational Science, 1*(3), 3–17.

Christiansen, C. (1996). Three perspectives of balance in occupation. In R. Zemke & F. Clark (Eds.), *Occupational science: The evolving discipline* (pp. 431–451). Philadelphia: F.A. Davis.

Christiansen, C. H. (1999). Defining lives: Occupation as identity—An essay on competence, coherence, and the creation of meaning. Eleanor Clarke Slagle Lecture. *American Journal of Occupational Therapy, 53,* 547–558.

Christiansen, C., & Baum, C. (Eds.). (1991). *Occupational therapy: Overcoming human performance deficits*. Thorofare, NJ: SLACK.

Christiansen, C., & Baum, C. (1997). Person-environment-occupational performance: A conceptual model for practice. In C. Christiansen & C. Baum (Eds.), *Enabling function and well-being* (2nd ed.) (pp. 46–70). Thorofare, NJ: SLACK.

Clark, F. A. (1993). Occupation embedded in a real life: Interweaving occupational science and occupational therapy. Eleanor Clarke Slagle lecture. *American Journal of Occupational Therapy, 47,* 1067–1078.

Clark, F. (1997). Reflections on the human as an occupational being: Biological need, tempo, and temporality. *Journal of Occupational Science, 4,* 86–92.

Clark, F., Azen, S. P., Zemke, R., Jackson, J., Carlson, M., Mandel, D., et al. (1997). Occupational therapy for independent-living older adults: A randomized controlled trial. *Journal of the American Medical Association, 278,* 1321–1326.

Clark, F., Ennevor, B. L., & Richardson, P. L. (1996). A grounded theory of techniques for occupational storytelling and occupational story making. In R. Zemke & F. Clark (Eds.), *Occupational science: The evolving discipline* (pp. 373–392). Philadelphia: F.A. Davis.

Clark, F. A., Parham, D., Carlson, M. E., Frank, G., Jackson, J., Peirce, D., et al. (1991). Occupational science: Academic innovation in the service of occupational therapy's future. *American Journal of Occupational Therapy, 45,* 300–310.

Clark, F., Wood, W., & Larson, E. A. (1998). Occupational science: Occupational therapy's legacy for the 21st century. In M. E. Neistadt & E. B. Crepeau (Eds.), *Willard and Spackman's occupational therapy.* (9th ed., pp. 13–21). Philadelphia: Lippincott.

Clark, F., Zemke, R., Frank, G., Parham, D., Neville-Jan, A., Hedricks, C., et al. (1993). The issue is—Dangers inherent in the partition of occupational therapy and occupational science. *American Journal of Occupational Therapy, 47,* 184–186.

Cockburn, L., & Trentham, B. (2002). Participatory action research: Integrating community occupational therapy practice and research. *Canadian Journal of Occupational Therapy, 69,* 20–30.

Commission on Practice, American Occupational Therapy Association. (2002). Occupational therapy practice framework domain and process. *American Journal of Occupational Therapy, 56,* 609–639.

Coster, W. (1998). Occupation-centered assessment of children. *American Journal of Occupational Therapy, 52,* 337–345.

Creighton, C. (1992). The origin and evolution of activity analysis. *American Journal of Occupational Therapy, 46,* 45–48.

Crepeau, E. B. (1995). Rituals (Module 6). In C. B. Royeen (Ed.), *The practice of the future: Putting occupation back into therapy.* Bethesda, MD: American Occupational Therapy Association.

Crist, P., & Royeen, C. B. (Eds.). (1997). *Infusing occupation into practice: Comparison of three clinical approaches in occupational therapy.* Bethesda, MD: American Occupational Therapy Association.

Crist, P. A., Royeen, C. B., & Schkade, J. (Eds.). (2000). *Infusing occupation into practice.* (2nd ed.). Bethesda, MD: American Occupational Therapy Association.

Csikszentmihalyi, M. (1990). *Flow: The psychology of optimal experience.* Cambridge, UK: Cambridge University Press.

Cumming, E., & Kaplan, W. (1991). *The arts and crafts movement.* London: Thames and Hudson.

Cynkin, S. (1995). Activities. In C. Royeen (Ed.), *The practice of the future: Putting occupation back into therapy* (pp. 7–1 to 7–52). Bethesda, MD: American Occupational Therapy Association.

Deshaies, L. D., Bauer, E. R., & Berro, M. (2001, July 2). Occupation-based treatment in physical disabilities rehabilitation. *OT Practice,* pp. 13–17. Bethesda, MD: AOTA, Inc.

Dewey, J. (1922). *Human nature and conduct.* New York: Henry Holt.

Dolecheck, J., & Schkade, J. K. (1999). Effects on dynamic standing endurance when persons with CVA perform personally meaningful activities rather than nonmeaningful tasks. *Occupational Therapy Journal of Research, 19,* 40–53.

Dunn, W., Brown, C., & McGuigan, A. (1994). The ecology of human performance: A framework for considering the effect of context. *American Journal of Occupational Therapy, 48,* 595–607.

Dunn, W., McClain, L. H., Brown, C., & Youngstrom, M. J. (1998). The ecology of human performance. In M. E. Neistadt & E. B. Crepeau, (Eds.), *Willard and Spackman's occupational therapy* (9th ed., pp. 531–534). Philadelphia: Lippincott.

Dunn, W., McClain, L., Brown, C., & Youngstrom, M. J. (2003). The ecology of human performance. In M. E. Neistadt, E. Crepeau, E. Cohen, & B. Schell (Eds.), *Willard and Spackman's occupational therapy* (10th ed., pp. 223–227). Philadelphia: Lippincott.

Farnworth, L. (2000). Time use and leisure occupations of young offenders. *American Journal of Occupational Therapy, 54,* 315–325.

Fearing, V. G., & Clark, J. (2000). *Individuals in context:* A practical guide to client-centered practice. Thorofare, NJ: Slack, Inc.

Fearing, V., Law, M., & Clark, J. (1997). Occupational performance process model. *Canadian Journal of Occupational Therapy, 64,* 5–14.

Ferguson, M. C., & Rice, M. S. (2001). The effect of contextual relevance on motor skill transfer. *American Journal of Occupational Therapy, 55,* 558–565.

Fisher, A. (1992a). The foundation—Functional measures: Part 1. What is function, what should we measure, and how should we measure it? *American Journal of Occupational Therapy, 46,* 183–185.

Fisher, A. (1992b). The foundation—Functional measures: Part 2. Selecting the right test, minimizing limitations. *American Journal of Occupational Therapy, 46,* 278–281.

Fisher, A. (1998) Uniting practice and theory in an occupational framework. 1998 Eleanor Clarke Slagle Lecture. *American Journal of Occupational Therapy, 52,* 509–521.

Fisher, A., & Short-DeGraff, M. (1993). Nationally speaking—Improving functional assessment in occupational therapy: Recommendations and philosophy for change. *American Journal of Occupational Therapy, 47,* 199–200.

Florey, L. L. (1969). Intrinsic motivation: The dynamics of occupational therapy theory. *American Journal of Occupational Therapy, 23,* 319–322.

Ford, K. (1995, March). Occupational adaption in home health: An occupational therapists's viewpoint. *Home and Community Health Special Interest Section Newsletter,* pp. 3–4.

Frank, G. (1994). The personal meaning of self-care occupations. In C. Cristiansen (Ed.), *Ways of living: Self-care strategies for special needs* (pp. 27–49). Rockville, MD: American Occupational Therapy Association.

Frederick, C. (1913). *The new housekeeping: Efficiency studies in home management.* New York: Doubleday.

Freidson, E. (1994). *Professionalism reborn: Theory, prophecy, and policy.* Chicago: University of Chicago Press.

Friedland, J. (1998). Looking back—Occupational therapy and rehabilitation: An awkward alliance. *American Journal of Occupational Therapy, 52,* 373–380.

Garrett, S., & Schkade, J. K. (1995). Occupational adaptation model of professional development as applied to level II fieldwork. *American Journal of Occupational Therapy, 49,* 119–126.

George, S., Wilcock, A., & Stanley, M. (2001). Depression and lability: The effects on occupation following stroke. *British Journal of Occupational Therapy, 64,* 455–461.

Gibson, J., & Schkade, J. K. (1997). Effects of occupational adaptation treatment with CVA. *American Journal of Occupational Therapy, 51,* 523–529.

Gilbreth, F. B. (1911). *Motion study.* New York: Van Nostrand.

Gilbreth, F. B., & Gilbreth, L. M. (1920). *Motion study for the handicapped.* London: Routledge.

Gilbreth, L. (1927). *The homemaker and her job.* New York: Appelton.

Gilbreth, L. M. (1943). The place of motion study in rehabilitation work. *Occupational Therapy and Rehabilitation, 22,* 61–64.

Gitlin, L., Corcoran, M., & Leinmiller-Eckhardt, S. (1995). Understanding the family perspective: An ethnographic framework for providing occupational therapy in the home. *American Journal of Occupational Therapy, 49,* 802–809.

Golledge, J. (1998). Distinguishing between occupation, purposeful activity, and activity: Part 1. Review and explanation. *British Journal of Occupational Therapy, 61,* 100–105.

Gray, J. (1997). A phenomenological perspective on occupation. *Journal of Occupational Science: Australia, 4,* 5–17.

Gray, J. (1998). Putting occupation into practice: Occupation as ends, occupation as means. *American Journal of Occupational Therapy, 52,* 354–364.

Hasselkus, B. R. (1990). Ethnographic interviewing: A tool for practice with family caregivers for the elderly. *Occupational Therapy Practice, 2,* 9–16.

Hasselkus, B. R. (1993). Death in very old age: A personal journey of caregiving. *American Journal of Occupational Therapy, 45,* 708–724.

Helfrich, C., Kielhofner, G., & Mattingly, C. (1994). Voliltion as narrative: Understanding motivation in chronic illness. *American Journal of Occupational Therapy, 48,* 311–317.

Hocking, C. (2001). The issue is—Implementing occupation-based assessment. *American Journal of Occupational Therapy, 55,* 463–469.

Holm, M. B. (2000). Our mandate for the new millennium: Evidence-based practice, 2000 Eleanor Clark Slagle Lecture. *American Journal of Occupational Therapy, 54,* 575–585.

Holm, M. B., Rogers, J. C., & Stone, R. G. (1998). Treatment of performance contexts. In M. E. Neistadt & E. B. Crepeau (Eds.), *Willard and Spackman's occupational therapy,* (9th ed., pp. 471–517). Philadelphia: Lippincott.

Jackson, J., Carlson, M., Mandel, D., Zemke, R., & Clark, F. (1998). Occupation in Lifestyle Redesign: The well-elderly study occupational therapy program. *American Journal of Occupational Therapy, 52,* 326–336.

Jackson, J. P., & Schkade, J. K. (2001). Occupational adaptation model versus biomechanical/rehabilitative models in the treatment of patients with hip fractures. *American Journal of Occupational Therapy, 55,* 531–537.

James, W. (1985). Habit. *Occupational Therapy in Mental Health, 5*(3), 55–67. (Reprinted from *Psychology, briefer course* [Chapter 10], 1892, New York: Holt).

Kielhofner, G. (1977). Temporal adaptation: A conceptual framework for occupational therapy. *American Journal of Occupational Therapy, 31,* 235–242.

Kielhofner, G. (Ed.). (1995). *A model of human occupation: Theory and application* (2nd ed.). Baltimore: Willilams & Wilkins.

Kielhofner, G. (Ed.). (2002). *A model of human occupation: Theory and application* (3rd ed.). Baltimore: Willilams & Wilkins.

Kielhofner, G., & Burke, J. P. (1977). Occupational therapy after 60 years: An account of changing identity and knowledge. *American Journal of Occupational Therapy, 31,* 675–689.

Kielhofner, G., Mallinson, T., Crawford, C., Nowak, M., Henry, A., & Walens, D. (1998). *A user's manual for the Occupational Performance History Interview* (Version 2.0, OPHI-II). Chicago: University of Illinois at Chicago.

Kielhofner, G., Mallinson, T., Forsyth, K., & Lai, J. (2001). Psychometric properties of the second version of the Occupational Performance History Interview (OPHI-II). *American Journal of Occupational Therapy, 55,* 260–267.

King, L. J. (1978). Toward a science of adaptive responses. 1978 Eleanor Clarke Slagle Lecture. *American Journal of Occupational Therapy, 32,* 429–437.

Kircher, M. A. (1984). Motivation as a factor of perceived exertion in purposeful versus nonpurposeful activity. *American Journal of Occupational Therapy, 38,* 165–170.

Larson, E. A. (1996). The story of Maricela and Miguel: A narrative analysis of dimensions of adaptation. *American Journal of Occupational Therapy, 50,* 286–298.

Law, M. (1993a). Evaluating activities of daily living: Directions for the future. *American Journal of Occupational Therapy, 47,* 233–237.

Law, M. (1993b). *Planning for children with physical disabilities: Identifying and changing disabling environments through participatory research.* Unpublished doctoral thesis, University of Waterloo, Waterloo, Ontario.

Law, M. (1997). Changing disabling environments through participatory research: A Canadian experience. In S. Smith, D. Williams, & N. Johnson (Eds.), *Nurtured by knowledge: Participatory action research* (pp. 184–204). New York: Aspen.

Law, M. (1998). Does client-centred practice make a difference? In M. Law (Ed.), *Client-centered occupational therapy* (pp. 19–27). Thorofare, NJ: Slack, Inc.

Law, M. (2000). Foreword. In V. G. Fearing & J. Clark, *Individuals in context: A Practical Guide to Client-Centered Practice* (p. xi). Thorofare, NJ: Slack, Inc.

Law, M., Baptiste, S., Carswell, A., McColl, M. A., Polataojko, H., & Pollock, N. (1998). *Canadian occupational performance measure manual* (3rd ed.). Toronto, Ontario: Canadian Association of Occupational Therapists.

Law, M., Baum, C. M., & Baptiste, S. (2002). *Occupation-based practice: Fostering performance and participation.* Thorofare, NJ: Charles B. Slack.

Law, M., Baum, C., & Dunn, W. (Eds.). (2001) *Measuring occupational performance: Supporting best practice in occupational therapy.* Throrofare, NJ: Slack, Inc.

Law, M., Cooper, B., Strong, S., Stewart, D., Rigby, P., & Letts, L. (1996). The person–environment–occupation model: A transactive approach to occupational performance. *Canadian Journal of Occupational Therapy, 63,* 9–23.

Law, M., Cooper, B. A., Strong, S., Stewart, D., Rigby, P., & Letts, L. (1997). Theoretical contexts for the practice of occupational therapy. In C. Christiansen & C. Baum (Eds.),

Occupational therapy: Enabling function and well-being (2nd ed., pp. 72–102). Thorofare, NJ: Slack, Inc.

Law, M., & Steinwender, S. (1996, June). *Occupation, health, and well-being: A review of research evidence.* Paper presented at the Canadian Association of Occupational Therapists Conference, Ottawa, Ontario.

Lawton, M. P. (1982). Competence, environmental press, and the adaptation of older people. In M. P. Lawton, P. G. Windley, & T. O. Byerts (Eds.), *Aging and the environment: Theoretical approaches* (pp. 33–59). New York: Springer.

Letts, L., Law, M., Rigby, P., Cooper, B., Stewart, D., & Strong, S. (1994). Person-environment assessments in occupational therapy. *American Journal of Occupational Therapy, 48,* 608–618.

Letts, L., Rigby, P., & Stewart, D. (2003). *Using environments to enable occupational performance.* Thorofare, NJ: SLACK.

Lin, K., Wu, C., Tickle-Degnen, L., & Coster, W. (1997) Enhancing occupational performance through occupationally embedded exercise: A meta-analytic review. *Occupational Therapy Journal of Research, 17,* 25–47.

Ludwig, F. M. (1997). How routine facilitates wellbeing in older women. *Occupational Therapy International, 49*(3) 213–228.

Ludwig, F. M. (1998). The unpackaging of routine in older women. *American Journal of Occupational Therapy, 52,* 168–175.

Ma, H., Trombly, C. A., & Robinson-Podolski, C. (1999). The effect of context on skill acquisition and transfer. *American Journal of Occupational Therapy, 53,* 138–144.

Madigan, M. J., & Parent, L. H. (1985). Preface. In G. Kielhofner (Ed.), *A model of human occupation: Theory and practice* (pp. vii-ix). Baltimore: Williams & Wilkins.

Maslow, A. (1954). *Motivation and personality.* New York: Harper & Row.

Mathiowetz, V. (1993). Role of physical performance component evaluation in occupational therapy functional assessment. *American Journal of Occupational Therapy, 47,* 225–230.

Mathiowetz, V., & Bass Haugen, J. (1994). Motor behavior research: Implications for therapeutic approaches to central nervous system dysfunction. *American Journal of Occupational Therapy, 48,* 733–745.

Mattingly, C. (1998). *Healing dramas: The narrative structure of experience.* Cambridge, UK: Cambridge University Press.

Mattingly, C., & Fleming, M. (1994). *Clinical reasoning: Forms of inquiry in a therapeutic practice.* Philadelphia: F.A. Davis.

Meyer, A. (1922). The philosophy of occupational therapy. *Archives of Occupational Therapy, 1,* 1–10.

Mosey, A. C. (1992). The issue is: Partition of occupational science and occupational therapy. *American Journal of Occupational Therapy, 46,* 851–853.

Mosey, A. C. (1993). Partition of occupational science and occupational therapy: Sorting out some issues. *American Journal of Occupational Therapy, 47,* 851–853.

Murphy, S., Trombly, C. A., Tickle-Degnen, L., & Jacobs, K. (1999). The effects of keeping an end-product on intrinsic motivation. *American Journal of Occupational Therapy, 53,* 153–158.

Nelson, D. (1988). Occupation: Form and performance. *American Journal of Occupational Therapy, 42,* 633–641.

Nelson, D. (1996). Therapeutic occupation: A definition. *American Journal of Occupational Therapy, 50,* 775–782.

Nielson, C. (1998). The issue is—How can the academic culture transition to occupation-centered education? *American Journal of Occupational Therapy, 52,* 386–387.

Pasek, P. B., & Schkade, J. K. (1996). Effects of a skiing experience on adolescents with limb deficiencies: An occupational adaptation perspective. *American Journal of Occupational Therapy, 50,* 24–31.

Peachey-Hill, C., & Law, M. (2000). Impact of environmental sensitivity on occupational performance. *Canadian Journal of Occupational Therapy, 67,* 304–313.

Peirce, C. S. (1957). *Essays in the philosophy of science.* Philadelphia: Bobbs-Merrill.

Peloquin, S. M. (1996). Moral treatment: Contexts considered. In R. P. Cottrell (Ed.), *Perspectives on purposeful activity: Foundation and future of occupational therapy* (pp. 39–46). Bethesda, MD: American Occupational Therapy Association. (Reprinted from 1989 *American Journal of Occupational Therapy, 43,* pp. 537–544).

Pierce, D. (2001a). Occupation by design: Dimensions, therapeutic power, and creative process. *American Journal of Occupational Therapy, 55,* 249–259.

Pierce, D. (2001b). Untangling occupation and activity. *American Journal of Occupational Therapy, 55,* 138–146.

Polkinghorne, D. E. (1996). Transformative narratives: From victimic to agentic life plots. *American Journal of Occupational Therapy, 50,* 299–305.

Price-Lackey, P., & Cashman, J. (1996). Jenny's story: Reinventing oneself through occupation and narrative configuration. *American Journal of Occupational Therapy, 50,* 306–314.

Primeau, L. (1998). Orchestration of work and play in families. *American Journal of Occupational Therapy, 52,* 188–195.

Quiroga, V. (1995). *Occupational therapy: The first 30 years 1900–1930.* Bethesda, MD: American Occupational Therapy Association.

Rebeiro, K. L., & Cook, J. V. (1999). Opportunity, not prescription: An exploratory study of the experience of occupational engagement. *Canadian Journal of Occupational Therapy, 66,* 176–187.

Rebeiro, K. L., Day, D. G., Semeniuk, B., O'Brien, M. C., & Wilson, B. (2001). Northern initiative for social action: An occupation-based mental health program. *American Journal of Occupational Therapy, 55,* 493–500.

Reilly, M. (1962). Occupational therapy can be one of the great ideas of 20th century medicine. 1962 Eleanor Clarke Slagle Lecture. *American Journal of Occupational Therapy, 16,* 1–9.

Rocker, J. D., & Nelson, D. L. (1987). Affective responses to keeping and not keeping an activity product. *American Journal of Occupational Therapy, 41,* 152–157.

Rogers, C. R. (1939). *The clinical treatment of the problem child.* Boston: Houghton Mifflin.

Royeen, C. B. (Ed.). (1994). *AOTA self-study series—The practice of the future: Putting occupation back into therapy.* Rockville, MD: American Occupational Therapy Association.

Schkade, J. K., & McClung, M. (2001). *Occupational adaptation in practice: Concepts and cases.* Thorofare, NJ: SLACK.

Schkade, J. K., & Schultz, S. (1992). Occupational adaptation: Toward a holistic approach to contemporary Practice. Part I. *American Journal of Occupational Therapy, 46,* 829–837.

Schkade, J. K., & Schultz, S. (1993). Occupational adaptation: An integrative frame of reference. In H. Hopkins & H. Smith (Eds.), *Willard and Spackman's occupational therapy* (8th ed., pp. 529–531). Philadelphia: Lippincott.

Schultz, S., & Schkade, J. K. (1992). Occupational adaptation: Toward a holistic approach to contemporary Practice. Part 2. *American Journal of Occupational Therapy, 46,* 917–926.

Schultz, S., & Schkade, J. K. (1994, September). Home health care: A window of opportunity to synthesize practice. *Home and Community Health Special Interest Section Newsletter,* pp. 1–4.

Schultz, S., & Schkade, J. K. (1997). Adaptation. In C. Cristiansen and C. Baum (Eds.), *Enabling function and well-being* (pp. 457–481). Thorofare, NJ. SLACK.

Schultz, S., & Schkade, J. K. (2003). Occupational adaptation. In M. E. Neistadt, E. B. Crepeau, E. Cohen, B. Schell (Eds.), *Williard and Spackman's occupational therapy* (10th ed., pp. 220–223). Philadelphia: Lippincott.

Sewell, L., & Singh, S. (2001). The Canadian Occupational Performance Measure: Is it a reliable measure in clients with chronic obstructive pulmonary disease? *British Journal of Occupational Therapy, 64,* 305–310.

Shannon, P. (1977). The derailment of occupational therapy. *American Journal of Occupational Therapy, 31,* 169–172.

Slagle, E. C., & Robeson, H. A. (1941). *Syllabus for training of nurses in occupational therapy.* Utica, NY: State Hospital Press.

Spencer, J., Daybell, P. J., Eschenfelder, V., Khalaf, R., Pike, J. M., & Woods-Petitti, M. (1998). Contrasting perspectives on work: An exploratory qualitative study based on the concept of adaptation. *American Journal of Occupational Therapy, 52,* 474–484.

Spencer, J., Krefting, L., & Mattingly, C. (1993). Incorporation of ethnographic methods in occupational therapy assessment. *American Journal of Occupational Therapy, 47,* 303–309.

Steinbeck, T. M. (1986). Purposeful activity and performance. *American Journal of Occupational Therapy, 40,* 529–534.

Stewart, D., Letts, L., Law, M., Cooper, B., Strong, S., & Rigby, P. (2003). The person-environment-occupation model. In M. E. Neistadt, E. Crepeau, E. Cohen, & B. Schell (Eds.), *Willard and Spackman's occupational therapy* (10th ed., pp. 227–234). Philadelphia: Lippincott.

Strong, S., Rigby, P., Law, M., Cooper, B., Letts, L., & Stewart, D. (1999). Application of the person-environment-occupation model: A practical tool. *Canadian Journal of Occupational Therapy, 66,* 122–133.

Thibodeaux, C. S., & Ludwig, F. M. (1988). Intrinsic motivation in product-oriented and nonproduct-oriented activities. *American Journal of Occupational Therapy, 42,* 169–175.

Thomas, J. J. (1996). Materials-based, imagery-based, and rote exercise occupational forms: Effect on repetitions, heart rate, duration of performance, and self-perceived rest period in well-elderly women. *American Journal of Occupational Therapy, 50,* 783–789.

Thomas, J. J., Wyk, S. V., & Boyer, J. (1999). Contrasting occupational forms: Effects on performance and affect in patients undergoing Phase II cardiac rehabilitation. *The Occupational Therapy Journal of Research, 19,* 187–202.

Tickle-Degnen, L. (2001). Foreword. In M. Law, C. Baum, & W. Dunn (Eds.), *Measuring occupational performance: Supporting best practice in occupational therapy* (p. xvii). Thorofare, NJ: SLACK.

Toth-Fejel, G. E., Toth-Fejel, G. F., & Hedricks, C. A. (1998) Case report—Occupation-centered practice in hand rehabilitation using the experience sampling method. *American Journal of Occupational Therapy, 52* 381–385.

Trombly, C. A. (1993). The issue is—Anticipating the future: Assessment of occupational function. *American Journal of Occupational Therapy, 47,* 253–257.

Trombly, C. A. (1995). Occupation: Purposefulness and meaningfulness as therapeutic mechanisms. 1995 Eleanor Clarke Slagle Lecture. *American Journal of Occupational Therapy, 49,* 960–972.

University of Southern California, Department of Occupational Therapy. (1989). Proposal for a Ph.D. degree in occupational science. Unpublished manuscript.

White, R. W. (1971). The urge to competence. *American Journal of Occupational Therapy, 25,* 271–274.

Wilcock, A. (1993). A theory of the human need for occupation. *Occupational Science, 1*(1), 17–24.

Wilcock, A. (1998). *An occupational perspective of health.* Thorofare, NJ: Charles B. Slack.

Wilcock, A. (2001). Occupational science: The key to broadening horizons. *British Journal of Occupational Therapy, 64,* 412–417.

Wood, W. (1998a). Nationally speaking—The genius within. *American Journal of Occupational Therapy, 52,* 321–325.

Wood, W. (1998b). Nationally speaking—It is jump time for occupational therapy. *American Journal of Occupational Therapy, 52,* 403–411.

Wood, W., Nielson, C., Humphry, R., Coppola, S., Baranek, G., & Rourk, J. (2000). A curricular renaissance: Graduate education centered on occupation. *American Journal of Occupational Therapy, 54,* 586–597.

World Health Organization. (2001). *ICIDH-2: International classification of functioning, disability, and health.* Geneva, Switzerland: Author. Retrieved August 20, 2003, from http://www.who.int/icidh

Yerxa, E. J. (1992). Some implications of occupational therapy's history for its epistemology, values, and relation to medicine. *American Journal of Occupational Therapy, 46,* 79–83.

Yerxa, E. J. (1994). Dreams, dilemmas, and decisions for occupational therapy practice in a new millenium: An American perspective. *American Journal of Occupational Therapy, 48,* 586–589.

Yerxa, E. J. (1998a). Health and the human spirit for occupation. *American Journal of Occupational Therapy, 52,* 412–418.

Yerxa, E. J. (1998b). Occupation: The keystone of a curriculum for a self-defined profession. *American Journal of Occupational Therapy, 52,* 365–372.

Yerxa, E. J., Clark, F., Frank, G., Jackson, J., Parham, D., Pierce, D., Stein, C., et al. (1990). An introduction to occupational science: A foundation for occupational therapy in the 21st century. *Occupational Therapy in Health Care, 6*(4), 1–15.

Yoder, R. M., Nelson, D. L., & Smith, D. A. (1989). Added-purpose versus rote exercise in female nursing home residents. *American Journal of Occupational Therapy, 43,* 581–586.

Zemke, R. (1995). Habits. (Module 5). In C. B. Royeen (Ed.), *The practice of the future: Putting occupation back into therapy* (pp. 247–276). Bethesda, MD: American Occupational Therapy Association.

Analysis of the Theories 10

Kay F. Walker

Theory analysis provides a means to examine the unique features of a theory and, when applied to several theories in a field, can be used to identify major theoretical endeavors of that field. Because a theory is an attempt to explain, predict, or clarify phenomena, analysis of several theories in a profession serves to illuminate the field's major theoretical efforts. By analyzing the occupational therapy (OT) theories reviewed in this book as well as other OT theories, one can see how writers have explained and described occupational therapy.

Theory analysis seeks basically to answer five questions:

1. How was the theory developed?
2. Who developed the theory?
3. What is the theory?
4. How is the theory used?
5. How has the theory been tested?

In this chapter, I address each of these questions in an analysis of the works of the theorists Claudia Allen, Jean Ayres, Gail Fidler, Gary Kielhofner, Lela Llorens, Anne Mosey, Mary Reilly, and the occupation-based theorists discussed in Chapter 9. To provide a more comprehensive look at contemporary OT theory, I also briefly review theories that have been developed in recent years for OT practice in adult physical dysfunction.

Theory analysis may include the evaluation of theory through the use of checklists (Chinn & Jacobs, 1983), methods for selection (McKenna, 1997; Walker & Neuman, 1996), models (Meleis, 1997), or frameworks (Duldt & Giffin, 1985). A list of items to consider in theory critique is provided in Appendix 10.A. Use of this list may help therapists to select theory for practice, students to analyze theory for learning, and writers to synthesize theory for theory development. However, in this chapter, I compare OT theories and do not discuss their relative merits and flaws. The purpose of this final chapter is not to assess the theories, but rather to review and contrast them for their contribution to the contemporary status of theory in occupational therapy.

How the Theory Evolved: Processes of Theory Development

How does a theory begin? What is the impetus for the theorist to formulate the theory? Do clinical questions, research findings, the need for theory in an area, or the desire for explanations of the profession drive the writer? What about the role of research in the theory's development? Is the theory validated through research? Is the theory the work of an individual, or does it reflect the combined efforts of several like-minded persons? In this section, I review processes and elements of theory development and comment on a developing academic discipline.

Theory Development Processes

Theory development is a process of expressing ideas and applying and examining those ideas. Ideas are expressed as concepts, assumptions, propositions, constructs, premises, postulates, suppositions, and beliefs that are organized as conceptual models, frames of reference, and theories (see Appendix 10.B for terms and definitions related to the study of theory). However, theory, as I will examine it here, refers to a systematic organization of ideas that are subject to real-world application and review. In plain language, theory refers to the ideas behind what theorists do and how they use and test those ideas. Thus, in OT, theorists look at ideas about occupational therapy (theory), the clinical use of those ideas (practice), and the empirical testing of those ideas (research). In the following subsections, I examine the relationship of theory, practice, and research in OT theory in terms of three processes of OT theory development modified from Meleis (1997): the theory–practice–theory process, the practice–research–theory process, and the theory–theory–research/practice process (other processes are defined in Appendix 10.B). These processes yield new formulations of ideas and are distinguishable from *theory refinement processes* of an existing OT theory, which are often undertaken by people other than the original author. Theory refinement is addressed later in this chapter in the section on dissemination, validation, and further development.

Theory–Practice–Theory Process

In the theory–practice–theory process, the theorist selects preexisting theory from a field other than OT—thus referred to as "pre-OT theory"—and systematically applies it to OT practice to evolve "primary" OT theory (i.e., new theoretical formulations for occupational therapy). The theory–practice–theory process is used when the answers to clinical questions cannot be found in existing OT theoretical formulations. Although non-OT theories may help to explain or predict phenomena in occupational therapy, they lack direct applicability to OT practice and thus need to be rearticulated and reinterpreted within an OT perspective. The theory–practice–theory process can be identified in Fidler's, Mosey's, Llorens's, Reilly's, and Allen's work, as well as the theory base for practice in adult physical dysfunction (see top third of Figure 10.1).

Troubled by the lack of sound explanations for OT, the individual theorists looked to other theoretical bases for relevant principles. Reilly was concerned about reductionistic thinking that leads the clinician to ignore the importance of patient skills and competence in social role development and performance. She proposed a view of OT that emphasized social psychology perspectives. Fidler sought to develop a rationale for what her patients were doing in OT and whether it was helpful. She embraced the psychoanalytic theory base, the prevailing interpretation of mental illness at the time. Mosey, who was a student of Fidler, was inspired by Fidler's questioning of clinical practice theory definitions. Mosey drew upon a combination of biology, psychology, and sociology pre-OT theories. Early in her career,

Theory
Developmental

Cognitive development
Psychoanalytic
Biology, psychology, sociology
Social psychology

Cognitive, educational psychology

Neurobehavior
Motor learning

Practice
Pediatrics

→ **Practice** →
Pediatrics, OT process

Psychosocial dysfunction

Adult physical dysfunction

→ **Research** →
Factor analysis
Instrument development

Theory
Llorens—Developmental framework

Allen—Cognitive levels
Fidler—Communication process for psychiatry
Mosey—Frames of reference
Reilly—Occupational behavior

Abreu—Quadraphonic approach
Toglia—Multicontext treatment
Arnadottir—Cognitive deficits and daily activities
Farber—Model of neurorehabilitation
Sabari—Activity–based intervention

Theory
Ayres—Sensory integration theory

(continues)

Figure 10.1. Theory development processes.

THEORY →	THEORY →	RESEARCH / PRACTICE →
Reilly—Occupational behavior Systems theory	Kielhofner and Burke—Model of human occupation Christiansen and Baum— Person–environment–occupational performance	Qualitative and quantitative studies Instrument development
Various OT models	Dunn, Brown, and McGuigan—Ecology of human performance	OT practice
Environmental psychology	Fearing and Clark— Occupational performance process Howe and Briggs— Ecological Systems Model Law, Cooper, Strong, Stewart, Rigby, and Letts— Person–environment–occupation	
Adolph Myer	Schkade and Schultz— Occupational adaptation	Adaptive response
Various OT models Medical and social sciences	Trombly—Occupational functioning model Holmes, Rogers, and Stone— Environmental competence model Rousseau, Potvin, Dutil, and Falta— Model of competence	Adult physical dysfunction
Motor behavior Occupation- and client-centered OT models	Bass-Haugen, Mathiowetz, and Finn— Contemporary task-oriented approach	Adult physical dysfunction

Figure 10.1. *Continued.*

Allen was influenced by Fidler's and Mosey's work, but saw OT being relegated to a nonscientific fringe service as psychiatry moved to treatment through medication and neurobiological explanations of mental illness. She based her work on theories of cognitive development. Llorens realized early in her clinical career that therapists could readily demonstrate the value of OT, but could not explain its value. She systematically applied developmental pre-OT theories of Gesell, Piaget, Havighurst, Erickson, and Freud to OT practice to formulate her developmental frame of reference. These OT theorists all identified a need to clarify therapy rationale, and because OT theory was yet to be articulated, they looked beyond the field for relevant theory. They found new ways to apply existing theory from other fields to explain and conceptualize the rationale for OT practice.

The conceptual basis for OT practice in pediatrics reflects this theory–practice–theory process. Over the years, models for practice have adopted concepts and drawn upon the knowledge base of neurodevelopment, biomechanics, information processing, psychosocial development, adaptation and coping, behaviorism, cognitive development, and other development theories (Case-Smith, 2001; Dunn, 2000; Kramer & Hinojosa, 1993). This process parallels Llorens's application of developmentally based theory to occupational therapy.

Models for OT practice in adult physical dysfunction also reflect the theory–practice–theory process. Neural-based, biomechanical, and rehabilitative pre-OT conceptualizations (Trombly & Radomski, 2002; Williams & Pedretti, 2001) are applied to OT evaluation and treatment in physical disabilities. Neural-based pre-OT theories of Margaret Rood, Berta and Karl Bobath, Signe Brunnstrom, and Margaret Knott and Dorothey Voss, developed by physical therapists as pragmatic clinical applications of neuroscience and neurophysiology, are used in occupational therapy. Farber (1982) synthesized these treatment rationales in her model of neurorehabilitation for persons with central nervous system dysfunction. Toglia (1991) drew from cognitive psychology and educational psychology to prescribe the multicontext treatment approach to address generalization in cognitive rehabilitation of persons with brain injury. Similarly, Abreu's (1999) quadraphonic approach is a cognitive model for holistic rehabilitation in brain injury. Arnadottir (1990) applied theories of neurobehavior to assess how cognitive–perceptual deficits interfere with the performance of daily activities. Sabari (1991) applied motor learning concepts to activity-based intervention.

Remedial approaches based on pre-OT biomechanical knowledge of joint and muscle function and work have been applied in OT to address muscle strength, joint motion, and endurance for performing purposeful activities. Similarly, compensatory approaches based on rehabilitation philosophy and medical, physical, and social sciences have been applied in OT adaptations of task and environment to maximize functional capacities. Theoretical and practical knowledge from anatomy, neuroscience, kinesiology, physical science, muscle physiology, and medicine have been combined with OT principles of activity analysis, self-care, and functional adaptation to provide a rich array of techniques for OT intervention in physical disabilities.

Practice–Research–Theory Process

In the practice–research–theory process, clinical practice questions drive the generation of hypotheses, and research findings drive the refinement of theory. The theorist conducts research aimed at answering questions and refuting or validating hypotheses, and uses research findings to develop and modify theory. This is the process used by Ayres in the development of sensory integration theory.

To formulate explanations and pose testable hypotheses about sensory integrative dysfunction, Ayres identified patient problems as the most challenging and motivating factor. She formulated her own ideas and consulted neuroscience and neurobehavioral literature, designed and implemented research to develop standardized tests and sensory integration constructs, and synthesized the results of these studies to examine and modify theory, reflecting on her findings within the context of children's problems as well as the scientific literature.

Theory–Theory–Research/Practice Process

The theory–theory–research/practice process uses existing pre-OT as well as derived or primary OT theory to build new OT theory, which is then tested through research and applied in clinical practice. This process is available to theorists when the field has developed sufficient primary theory—that is, theory developed by and for the field—so that the theorist can incorporate it in constructing new theory. This process is increasingly possible in OT because of the theory ground-breaking not only by the field's founders (see Chapter 1) but also by the theorists reviewed in this book, the Eleanor Clark Slagle lecturers (see Appendix 10.C), and a host of occupational therapists concerned with the ideas of the profession.

Kielhofner's work is an example of the theory–theory–practice/research process. He and Burke used Reilly's occupational behavior paradigm (primary OT theory) and systems theory (pre-OT theory) to develop the model of human occupation (new OT theory). Kielhofner and colleagues continue to apply and test this model through clinical practice and research.

The occupation-centered frameworks and some frameworks for adult physical dysfunction also reflect the theory–theory–research/practice process in that they base their models on existing OT models *and* non-OT theory; they apply their models to practice and, to some extent, test the models through research. What distinguishes these authors who engage in the theory–theory–practice/research process from the theory–practice–theory group discussed previously is that the former clearly incorporate existing OT models and frames of reference, not just general OT concepts. These occupation-based models include the ecological systems model (Howe & Briggs, 1982), person–environment–occupational performance (Christiansen & Baum, 1997), ecology of human performance (Dunn, Brown, & McGuigan, 1994), occupational performance process (Fearing & Clark, 2000), intervention process model (Fisher, 1998), person–environment–occupation model (Law et al., 1996), and occupational adaptation (Schkade & Schultz, 1992). Models for OT practice in physical dysfunction also reflect the theory–theory–research/practice process. Trombly's (2002) occupational functioning model draws from medical and social sciences as well as extant OT practice models and advocates cognitive–perceptual, biomechanical, and motor learning approaches to treatment. Bass-Haugen, Mathiowetz, and Flinn (2002) base their contemporary task-oriented approach on motor behavior theory as well as occupation- and client-centered OT models. Other models emphasize competence within one's environment and the role of assistive devices (Holm, Rogers, & Stone, 1998) and universal accessibility

(Rousseau, Potvin, Dutil, & Falta, 2002). This theory–theory–research/practice process yields views of occupation as the core concept of the profession and the clinical application, measurement instruments, and research to examine that concept.

Common Elements of Theory Development

Identification of three processes used to build theory in OT reveals several important common elements among the theorists reviewed. First, these OT theories emanate from a concern for OT practice. As a practice profession, occupational therapy seeks to identify the unique theoretical underpinnings of services for patients and clients. Second, the pioneering efforts of Reilly, Fidler, Llorens, Mosey, and Allen bridged pre-OT and OT theory, making it possible for a second generation of OT theory to evolve. Third, research to test and validate OT practice and to build a body of knowledge for the profession is under way. The incorporation of research in theory building that characterizes the works of Ayres and Kielhofner is being increasingly emphasized. Examining the processes by which theories are built illustrates common clinical practice concerns among the theorists, the ways in which theories build upon theories, and the relationship of research to contemporary OT theory development.

Occupational Science: A Developing Academic Discipline

The discussion of theory building in occupational therapy would be incomplete without reference to occupational science, a developing academic discipline. Established by Elizabeth Yerxa in 1989 at the University of Southern California (F. A. Clark et al., 1991; Yerxa et al., 1990), this discipline is based on concepts and philosophies of occupational therapy, including Reilly's occupational behavior, and focuses on the form, function, and meaning of human occupation. Theory development in an academic discipline may take several of the process pathways discussed in this chapter (see Appendix 10.B), can be expected to generate several theories, and can contribute to a delineated branch of study recognized by the academic community. Occupational science (OS) is a developing social science discipline that seeks to generate knowledge about human occupation that will be a resource to anyone seeking this information. The relationship of OS to OT may be thought of as similar to sociology and social work, psychology and counseling psychology, and anthropology and forensic anthropology; the academic discipline provides an available knowledge base for professional practice.

As an academic discipline, however, occupational science seeks to develop knowledge of humans as occupational beings, knowledge that may or may not be directly applicable in the practice profession of occupational therapy (Ottenbacher, 1996). Similarly, findings from a specific research project, occupational science based or otherwise, may contribute to the understanding of a phenomenon, yet not be directly applicable to a given clinical situation. The mutual embracing between the OS academic discipline and the OT profession is generally evident in OT publications, research programs, and curriculum models. How this OS–OT pairing should and could affect theory and research for the practice of occupational therapy stimulated discourse on the theory–research–practice processes (F. A. Clark et al., 1993; Kielhofner, 2002a; Mosey, 1992b, 1993).

Who Developed the Theory: Historical Context Analysis

Historical Context Theory Analysis Method

Another way to analyze theory development is to explore the individual theorist's own historical context. This method of theory analysis

- Assumes that a theorist's background influences his or her career development and hence theory development.

- Answers the question, "What are the social, political, and professional forces that may have shaped the writer and thus, to some extent, the writings?"

- Views statements of theoretical positions as reflecting individualized perceptions that have been shaped by the person's life experiences, the prevailing social climate and

national events, and professional issues of the time in which
the person lived.

- Examines a theory against a backdrop of the theorist's life
  and times and reveals important influences that contributed to the person the theorist became and therefore
  to the theory that was developed.

Next, I look at parallel streams of events in the national
area, the world of occupational therapy, and the individual theorist's lives. Although I review the biographical sketches of the
seven individual theorists included in this book within the context of national and professional events, I do not go the next step
to connect the historical events and their possible impact on the
assumptions made by the theorists that were imparted to the
theory they developed. Methodology for this type of analysis is
available in qualitative approaches in the social sciences. The
reader who enjoys looking at developments from a historical perspective may find this section useful to begin a full-scale historical theory analysis. On the other hand, readers who are not as
interested in this type of review can scan Tables 10.1 to 10.6 for
a briefer review of the historical analysis.

1910 to 1950 (Table 10.1)

1910 to 1950—National Events

During the years 1910 to 1950, the United States was involved
in World War I (WWI) (1917–1918) and World War II (WWII)
(1939–1945); the 19th amendment to the Constitution was rati-
fied, ensuring women's voting rights (1920); and citizens
suffered through the stock market crash (1929) and the Great
Depression (1930–1939). In 1947, the polio epidemic threatened
the lives and health of many Americans (Hopkins, 1988; Reed &
Sanderson, 1999).

1910 to 1950—Occupational Therapy

The OT profession was established in 1917, and its growth was
influenced by the two world wars. During the period 1910 to
1950, educational training developed from nondegree training
courses to master's degree programs, a journal was established,

Table 10.1

Historical Perspectives 1910 to 1950

National Events	Theorists	
World War I (1914–1918)	**Fidler**	Born 1916, Spencer, IA
19th Amendment ratified (1920)		Oldest of 4 children
Stock market crash (1929)		Debating team, sports in high school
Great Depression (1930–1939)		BA degree education and psychology (1938)
World War II (1939–1945)		Aide in state mental hospital
Polio epidemic (1947)		U of Pennsylvania OT certificate (1942)
		White Institute of Psychiatry and Psychology (1947–1951)
		First publication, AJOT (1948)
Occupational Therapy Events		
	Reilly	Born 1916, Boston, MA
National Association for the Promotion of Occu-		Strict girls' school
pational Therapy formed (1917)		Boston U OT certificate 1940
		U.S. Army Medical Department (1941–1955)
Reconstruction aides trained for WWI Journals:		First paper, OT and Rehabilitation (1943)
Archives of Occupational Therapy (1922), *Occu-*		
pational and Rehabilitation (1925), *American*	**Ayres**	Born 1923, California farm
Journal of Occupational Therapy (AJOT; 1947)		Childhood illness
		First publication, AJOT (1949)
War emergency courses for WWII		
	Llorens	Born 1933, Shreveport, LA
Educational standards (1923)		Pre–Civil Rights era
More occupational therapists in psychiatry in	**Mosey**	Born 1938, Minneapolis, MN
1937 but increase in those working in physical		3rd of 7 children
disabilities with WWII		
	Allen	Born 1942, Oregon farm
Registration examination (1939)	**Kielhofner**	Born 1949, Missouri farm

the populations treated in OT changed, and individuals who would go on to make major theoretical contributions to OT were born.

By the time the United States entered WWI, the National Society for the Promotion of Occupational Therapy had been organized, with its membership numbering 47 physicians, social workers, nurses, artists, and teachers. The country's involvement in WWI provided an impetus for expansion of occupational therapy as OT reconstruction aides were trained to work with the wounded soldiers. In the next few years, training programs were designed, training manuals written, and in 1922 a journal, *Archives of Occupational Therapy,* was started. With the increase in the number of training programs for occupational therapists came the establishment of educational standards (1923) and, by 1939, the registration examination.

WWII greatly stimulated the growth of the field and influenced the direction of OT treatment. In 1937, there were twice as many occupational therapists in psychiatric settings as in general hospital and orthopedic facilities, but the wartime need for OT in the treatment of the injured soldier resulted in increased development of treatment techniques in physical disabilities. The number of OT programs increased from 5 to 18 from 1940 to 1945, and the population of therapists nearly doubled between 1941 and 1946. OT graduate education began with the establishment of the first OT master's degree program in 1947 at the University of Southern California (Hopkins, 1988; Reed & Sanderson, 1999).

1910 to 1950—The Theorists

Both Fidler and Reilly were born in 1916, the year before the United States entered WWI and before occupational therapy was organized as a profession. The independent and goal-oriented nature of the careers of these two women was becoming more socially acceptable by the time Fidler and Reilly were growing up. Women had secured the right to vote and, because of the wars, had been initiated into previously male vocations, such as military nursing and civilian assembly line work. In addition, early school experiences seem to have fostered the independence of both Fidler and Reilly. Fidler's high school sports and debating team activities provided outlets for independent expression, and Reilly's early schooling in a strict scholastic girl's school contributed to her lifelong interest in scholarly pursuits. As college graduates in the late 1930s, Fidler and Reilly found OT training through the established 1-year certificate programs.

Early employment experiences influenced the directions of Fidler's and Reilly's careers. Fidler's first job was in psychiatry, setting her lifelong focus on mental health occupational therapy. Her first publication in 1948 concerned psychological evaluation of OT activities. After 1 year of working with children, Reilly worked for 14 years in the U.S. Army Medical Department in physical disabilities, and she coauthored her first publication there in 1943 (Light & Reilly, 1943). Her enduring concern with the nature of the profession was evidenced in this first publication in which she addressed the relationship of occupational therapy to physical therapy.

Ayres was born in 1923, and thus was influenced by national and professional forces similar to those affecting Fidler and Reilly. However, Ayres's childhood on a farm in California during the Depression years, her battles with childhood illnesses, and her struggles with family issues seem to have been key elements in the development of her characteristic determination and independence. She obtained her OT education from the University of Southern California (USC) in 1945 at the time when Margaret Rood was developing the country's first OT master's degree there. This academic climate that promoted advanced degrees may have influenced Ayres's use of scientific research methodology for theory development, and Rood's neurophysiologic theories may have promoted Ayres's use of neuroscience in her theory. Ayres's first OT job was in a psychiatric setting, where she published her first journal article in 1949 on the use of crafts with persons undergoing electroshock therapy (ECT).

Born in 1933, Llorens grew up before the Civil Rights movement, a time when racial segregation was the norm. Llorens's personal situation and her father's goal-oriented childrearing practices seem to have been major contributing factors to her ambitions to surpass the usual limited expectations for Black females and to achieve independent career success.

Mosey was born in 1938 and grew up in a large Irish family where she was the third of seven children. Claudia Allen was born in 1941 and grew up on a farm in Oregon. Kielhofner, the youngest of the seven theorists, was born in 1949 into an extended farm family. By the time Kielhofner was born, Fidler and Reilly were experienced therapists; Reilly, Fidler, and Ayres had each published an article in OT journals; Llorens was completing high school; and Mosey was in middle school. While Kielhofner was still a youngster, these other authors would go on to develop theories that he would later study before developing his own theory.

1950 to 2002

1950 to 2002—National Events

Major events in the United States in the mid-20th century included in the early 1950s involvement in the Korean War and, in the 1960s, the Civil Rights movement, protests against U.S. involvement in the Vietnam War, the Great Society of the Johnson administration that provided federal funding for social and health programs, the establishment of Medicare, and the first walk on the moon. The 1970s saw the Watergate scandal, the modern-day women's movement, concern with ecology, and the passage of the Education for All Handicapped Children Act of 1975. Inflation, cutbacks in federal spending, the "information age," and corporate health care characterized the 1980s. The 1990s and the beginning of the 21st century saw the explosion of communication via the Internet, cellular phones, and e-mail. Headlines included disturbing events of the Gulf War, Waco Texas Massacre, Oklahoma City bombing, Columbine shootings, U.S. presidential scandal, and the attack on the World Trade Center in New York City on September 11, 2001. As health care reform was implemented, the effects were felt at all levels of health care. The Americans with Disabilities Act of 1990 and the Individuals with Disabilities Education Act Amendments of 1991 provided further benefits to adults and children with disabilities.

1950s—OT Events and the Theorists (Table 10.2)

During the 1950s, improved OT techniques for physical disabilities were developed through federally funded rehabilitation programs. The focus shifted from acute care, such as bedside

Table 10.2

Historical Perspective 1950–1960

National Events	Theorists	
National Events	**Theorists**	
Korean War begins (1951)	**Fidler**	*Introduction to Psychiatric Occupational Therapy* (Fidler & Fidler, 1954)
Vocational Rehabilitation Act Amendments of 1954		Coordinator AOTA Mental Health Institute (1952–1955)
Federal money for health professions training		Coordinator AOTA Psychiatric Study Project (1955–1957)
		Instructor, U Pennsylvania; Department of Mental Health (1955–1957)
		Supervision workshops, Columbia U
Occupational Therapy Events	**Reilly**	UCLA Neuropsychiatric Institute (1959–1968)
Shift from acute to chronic care as medicine controls polio, tuberculosis, etc.		Intrinsic motivation theory of B. Smith
World Federation of Occupational Therapists formed (1952)	**Ayres**	MA degree OT, USC (1954)
		USC faculty (1954–1968)
Therapeutic use of self in OT psychiatry	**Llorens**	BS degree OT, Western Michigan U (1953)
Improved rehab techniques		Lafayette Clinic Pediatric Psychiatry, influence of research team (1958–1968)
	Mosey	
	Allen	
	Kielhofner	

therapy for the injured soldier, to more chronic care as the war ended and medical science conquered such diseases as tuberculosis and polio. The World Federation of Occupational Therapists was formed. Occupational therapy in psychiatry focused on the therapeutic use of self, and Fidler's psychodynamic and psychoanalytic theories for OT in psychiatry were developed. Fidler and her husband Jay (a psychiatrist) coauthored the book *Introduction to Psychiatric Occupational Therapy*, published in 1954. Her leadership in mental health OT was recognized in her appointment as coordinator of American Occupational Therapy Association's (AOTA's) Psychiatric Study Project 1955–1957 (Hopkins, 1988).

During the 1950s, the other theorists were involved in formative experiences that influenced the direction of their careers and theory development. From 1959 to the mid-1960s, Reilly was at the University of California at Los Angeles (UCLA) Neuropsychiatric Institute, where her mentor, B. Smith, influenced her thinking on intrinsic motivation. Ayres completed her master's degree in OT in 1954, worked with children with cerebral palsy, and was appointed to the USC faculty. Completing her OT education in 1953, Llorens worked in pediatric psychiatry at the Lafayette Clinic, where, over the course of the next 10 years, she was involved in teaching, research, and clinical roles with colleagues and mentors who were influential in her career development. In the late 1950s, Mosey was in college, where she was influenced by Marvin Lepley, an early mentor; Allen was finishing high school; and Kielhofner was in grade school.

1960s—OT Events and the Theorists (Table 10.3)

In the 1960s, the number of occupational therapists did not keep up with the demands for OT services, and other disciplines absorbed roles created by the shortage of occupational therapists. Group techniques and object relationships were developed for mental health OT, occupational therapy in community-based settings was emphasized, and the American Occupational Therapy Foundation (AOTF) was established in 1965 to promote research.

OT theory developed further with the emergence of Reilly's occupational behavior theory, Ayres's sensory integration theory, and Llorens's developmental theory (Hopkins, 1988). Their contributions to theory development were recognized as each of the

Table 10.3
Historical Perspective 1960–1970

National Events

Civil Rights movement
Kennedy, Johnson administrations
Vietnam War
Medicare

Occupational Therapy Events

OT shortages; roles absorbed by other professions
OT in the community
Group techniques and object relations in OT psychiatry
Entry MA at USC (1964)
AOTA established for business;
AOTF established for research (1965)
Theory: Reilly-occupational behavior
Ayres-sensory integration
Llorens-developmental

Theorists

Fidler	*Occupational Therapy: A Communication Process in Psychiatry* (Fidler & Fidler, 1963)
	ECS Lecture (1965)
	Directorships: NY State Neuropsychiatric Institute, Activities Therapy; NYU and Columbia U OT MA
Reilly	ECS Lecture (1961)
	USC OT faculty, graduate director, & program chair
Ayres	Postdoctoral work Brain Research Institute (1964–1965)
	ECS Lecture (1963)
	AOTA Award of Merit (1965)
	PhD, USC (1961)
	USC special ed faculty (1966–1977)
Llorens	First publication, AJOT (1960)
	Instructor Wayne State U (1960–1968)
	MA degree Wayne State U (1962)
	Developing Ego Functions (Llorens & Rubin 1967)
	OT consultant (1968–1971)
	ECS Lecture (1969)
Mosey	BS degree OT, U Minnesota (1961)
	NY Neuropsychiatric Institute (1962–1966)
	MA degree OT, NYU (1965)
	Instructor OT Columbia U (1966–1968)
	PhD, NYU (1968)
	First publication, AJOT (1968)
	Occupational Therapy: Theory and Practice (1968)
Allen	BS degree OT, San Jose State U (1963)
	Jobs in pediatrics and adult psychiatry in Pennsylvania (1968)
	MS degree OT, NYU (1968)
Keilhofner	Monastic college for 2 years
	Vietnam conscientious objector
	Hospital recreation job

Note. ECS = Eleanor Clarke Slagle.

three, as well as Fidler, was awarded Eleanor Clarke Slagle Lectureships in the 1960s. Reilly was honored as the Eleanor Clarke Slagle (ECS) Lecturer in 1961 and gave the lecture in which she stated her often-quoted OT premise: "Man, through the use of his hands, as they are energized by mind and will, can influence the state of his own health" (Reilly, 1962, p. 2). In 1963, Ayres lectured on perceptual motor development. Fidler's (1966) lecture was on the teaching-learning process. In 1969, Llorens (1970) presented her developmental framework of occupational therapy in her Eleanor Clarke Slagle Lecture.

Fidler was professionally productive during the 1960s. She published a book, *Occupational Therapy: A Communication Process in Psychiatry* (Fidler & Fidler, 1963), directed professional education at New York State Neuropsychiatric Institute, and coordinated the master's program in mental health OT both at New York University (NYU) and Columbia University.

Mosey was in school during the 1960s, completing her undergraduate OT degree in 1961, master's degree in 1965, and doctorate in 1968. She was influenced by Fidler, who was at the Neuropsychiatric Institute during the 4 years Mosey worked there and who was also director of the OT master's program at NYU when Mosey was a student there.

Allen completed her OT education in 1963 and was married that same year. She held her first OT jobs in pediatrics and adult psychiatry and in 1968 completed her master's degree. During these years, she studied and observed the functional problems of persons with chronic disorders, which were later to become the focus of her theory development.

In 1960, Llorens published her first article; in 1962 she completed her master's work; and in 1967 she coauthored the book, *Developing Ego Functions in Disturbed Children* (Llorens & Rubin, 1967). During the 1960s, Ayres completed her doctoral work and engaged in postdoctoral studies at the Brain Research Institute, confirming her interest in the neurosciences. In the mid-1960s, Reilly served as chairperson and graduate faculty member at USC. Kielhofner's classical and rigorous scholarly background in a Catholic seminary high school fueled his ability and interest in writing. He completed high school and began college during the 1960s.

1970s—OT Events and the Theorists (Table 10.4)

In the 1970s, accountability was the watchword in health care, and the AOTA adopted documents that addressed quality care in OT: (a) standards for practice in mental health, developmental disabilities, physical disabilities, and home health; (b) guidelines for administration and supervision; (c) a statement on referral; (d) revised essentials for accredited curricula; (e) a code of professional ethics; (f) an official definition of occupational therapy; and (g) uniform terminology guidelines. Occupational therapists were licensed in New York in 1976, and other states soon developed licensure laws. Specialization was recognized with the adoption of special interest sections in mental health, physical disabilities, developmental disabilities, sensory integration, and geriatrics. In OT theory, Mosey's emphasis on frames of reference for OT practice gained national recognition (Hopkins, 1988).

Two of Mosey's major works, *Three Frames of Reference for Mental Health* (1970) and *Activities Therapy* (1973), addressed the need for a frame of reference to guide practice, a need in keeping with the widespread concern that the field have standards, ethics, and defined practice guidelines. Mosey taught her theories to OT graduate and undergraduate students at NYU, where she also chaired the OT program for 8 years during the 1970s.

In the 1970s, Fidler's publications addressed broad professional issues and reflected the concerns encountered in her work experiences as associate executive director of AOTA for 5 years, adjunct faculty to several universities, and consultant to hospitals and a state mental health agency.

The establishment of sensory integration as one of AOTA's special interest sections reflected the impact that Ayres had on the field in the 1970s. During this decade, Ayres served as an OT faculty member at USC and established the Ayres Clinic, training and teaching students in sensory integration therapy. Her research efforts were funded through grants from a private foundation. She authored two books during the 1970s, *Sensory Integration and Learning Disorders* (1972a) and *Sensory Integration and the Child* (1979).

Llorens continued to develop her framework for OT practice in her book *Application of a Developmental Theory for Health*

Table 10.4
Historical Perspective 1970–1980

National Events	Occupational Therapy Events
Watergate	Accountability in health care
Women's movement	AOTA practice standards
Ecology issues	OT licensure
P.L. 94–142 Education for all Handicapped Children Act (1975)	Specialty sections
	Mosey's frames of reference for OT practice

Theorists

Fidler	Reilly	Ayres	Llorens	Mosey	Allen	Kielhofner
Associate Director AOTA (1971–1975)	*Play as Exploratory Learning* (1974)	*Sensory Integration and Learning Disorders* (1972)	U Florida faculty (1971–1976)	*Three Frames of Reference for Mental Health* (1970)	Moved to California (1973)	BA degree psychology, St. Louis U (1971)
Adjunct appointments to several universities	Retired (1977)	Sensory Integration Tests	*Consultation in the Community* (1973)	NYU OT chair (1972–1980)	USC faculty	MS degree OT, USC (1975)
Consultant to hospitals, state mental health agency		USC OT faculty (1976–1988)	U Florida Chair (1976–1982)	*Activities Therapy* (1973)	Chief OT at Los Angeles County, USC Medical Center	Neuropsychiatric Institute, Los Angeles (1975–1979)
		Private founation research money	PhD Walden U (1976)			First publication, AJOT (1976)
		Ayres Clinic opened	*Application of Developmental Theory* (1976)			USC OT faculty (1977–1979)
						DPH degree USC (1979)
						Virginia Commonwealth U OT faculty (1979–1984)

and Rehabilitation (1976) and, reflecting the national trend for developing OT consultancy roles, edited the book *Consultation in the Community: Occupational Therapy in Child Health* (1973). She completed her doctoral degree during this decade and served as OT faculty member and then chair at the University of Florida.

In 1974, Reilly's book, *Play as Exploratory Learning*, was published; it was the culmination of the work–play theory of occupational behavior that she and her students had been developing for the three previous decades. Allen moved to California in 1973 and held a joint position as faculty at USC and OT director at USC Medical Center. Allen's focus on cognition and neurobiology contrasted with Reilly's occupational behavior theory that prevailed in the USC academic program. Although Allen was influenced by Reilly, she simultaneously brought a different perspective to the faculty discussions. By the time Reilly retired from her faculty position at USC in 1977, she had influenced the thinking of many students over the years, most notably Gary Kielhofner. Kielhofner completed his bachelor's degree in psychology in 1971. In 1975, he received his master's degree in occupational therapy at USC, where the mentoring relationship he enjoyed with Mary Reilly was a major determining factor in the development of his theoretical formulations. Kielhofner went on to publish several papers, earn his doctoral degree, and serve as OT faculty member in two universities in the 1970s.

1980s—OT Events and the Theorists (Table 10.5)

The 1980s were characterized by an increased emphasis on research, study of OT personnel shortages (AOTA, 1985b), national training initiatives, increases in graduate education, entry-level role delineation concerns, political action, and human occupation theory. The AOTF's research initiatives included grants for OT research and sponsorship of (a) the research forum at the AOTA national conferences, (b) the publication *Occupational Therapy Journal of Research*, and (c) the honorary Academy of Research. The AOTA initiated continuing education courses, including *TOTEMS: Training Occupational Therapy Management in Schools* (1979); *PIVOT: Planning and Implementing Vocational Readiness in Occupational Therapy* (1985c);

Table 10.5
Continued Historical Perspective 1980–1990

National events	**Llorens**
Corporate health care	San Jose State U OT chair (1982–1993)
Inflation	OT Sequential Client Care Record
Federal money cutbacks	AOTA Award of Merit (1986)
Information age	A. Jean Ayres Award (1988)
	Introduction to Research (Oyster et al., 1987)
	AOTF Meritorious Service Award (1989)
Occupational Therapy Events	**Mosey**
	Occupational Therapy: Configuration of a Profession (1981)
Research emphasis	ECS Lecture (1985)
OT doctoral degrees	*Psychosocial Components of Occupational Therapy* (1986)
AOTA Training programs: TOTEMS, SCOPE, ROTE, PIVOT	**Allen**
Governmental representation	Chief of OT Psychiatry Los Angeles/USC Medical Center
Role delineation	USC faculty
Kielhofner et al.—model of human occupation	Medical reviewer for allied health for Blue Cross of California
	Occupational Therapy for Psychiatric Diseases (1985)
	ECS Lecture (1987)
	Cognitive Disabilities: Expanded Activity Analysis (Earhart & Allen,1988)
	Allen Cognitive Level Test Manual (1990)
Theorists	**Kielhofner**
Fidler	*Health Through Occupation* (1983)
AOTA Award of Merit (1980)	*Psychosocial Occupational Therapy* (Barris, Kielhofner, & Watts, 1983)
Consultancies NYU, New Jersey Mental Health Hospitals	Charter member AOTF Academy of Research (1984)
CEO Hagadorn Center for Geriatrics	Boston U OT faculty (1984–1986)
Reilly	*A Model of Human Occupation* (1985)
Charter member AOTF Academy of Research (1983)	U of Illinois OT chair (1986–present)
Article on client vs. patient (1984)	A. Jean Ayres Award (1988)
Ayres	
Charter member AOTF Academy of Research (1983)	
Retires from Ayres Clinic (1984)	
Developmental Dyspraxia and Adult Onset Apraxia (1985)	
AOTF A. Jean Ayres Award created (1987)	
Died, December 16, 1988	
Sensory Integration and Praxis Tests (1989)	

Note. ECS = Eleanor Clarke Slagle

ROTE: Role of Occupational Therapy with the Elderly (1986a); and SCOPE: Strategies, Concepts, and Opportunities for Program Development and Evaluation (1986b). In 1987, Professional and Technical Role Analysis (PATRA) (AOTA, 1988) was begun as a follow-up to the AOTA 1981 role delineation study (Bullock et al., 1981). The AOTA Government and Legal Affairs Division successfully lobbied the passage of legislation affecting occupational therapy, such as Medicare amendments to provide increased funding for OT services.

The number of master's programs slowly but steadily increased in the 1980s (AOTA, 1985a), and the field resolved the debate of master's level entry into OT by encouraging (not mandating) the development of OT graduate education programs. Two students graduated from the OT doctoral program at NYU in 1984, initiating the doctoral degree as the terminal degree in OT (AOTA, 1985a).

In 1980, occupation was officially adopted as the major concern of occupational therapy (Hopkins, 1988). This event coincided with increasing interest in the human occupation model of Kielhofner and Burke, and Kielhofner's emergence as a leader in theory development for occupational therapy. Having completed his doctorate in 1979, Kielhofner held faculty positions at Virginia Commonwealth University and Boston University and became chair at the University of Illinois. In addition to journal publications, his first three books described the human occupation model. In 1983, Kielhofner edited Health Through Occupation and coauthored Psychosocial Occupational Therapy (Barris, Kielhofner, & Watts, 1983); in 1985, he edited A Model of Human Occupation. Kielhofner's contributions to the field were recognized by his appointment in 1984 for charter membership in the AOTF Academy of Research and in 1988 as the recipient of the AOTF A. Jean Ayres Award for his contributions to theory.

In the mid- and late 1980s, Allen emerged as a new OT theorist. She published Occupational Therapy for Psychiatric Diseases in 1985 and coauthored Cognitive Disabilities: Expanded Activity Analysis with Earhart in 1988. In 1987 she was awarded the Eleanor Clarke Slagle Lectureship for her work in cognitive disabilities and chronic disorders; her address was titled "Activity: Occupational Therapy's Treatment Method." Her work roles included chief of OT psychiatry at USC Medical Center, USC faculty, and medical reviewer for allied health for Blue Cross of California.

From 1980 to 1990, the other theorists continued to be recognized nationally for their contributions to the field. They were productive in various ways, continuing to develop their theories, to pursue work activities, and, in some cases, to begin to gear down or refocus their pursuits as they approached retirement age. Fidler served as a consultant and administrator to mental health facilities and, in 1980, received the AOTA Award of Merit.

Reilly was named to the Academy of Research in 1983. Although she had withdrawn from the field, she expressed her opinions about the use of the terms *client* versus *patient* in a 1984 article.

Mosey and Llorens continued their careers in academia. Mosey published *Occupational Therapy: Configuration of a Profession* in 1981 and *Psychosocial Components of Occupational Therapy* in 1986. She was named the 1985 Eleanor Clarke Slagle Lecturer and advocated multiple principles to address existing and expanding practice areas in her lecture: "A Monistic or a Pluralistic Approach to Professional Identity?" Llorens became chair at San Jose State University in 1982, the year that her book, *Occupational Therapy Sequential Client Care Record Manual*, was published. She was awarded the AOTA Award of Merit in 1986, the AOTF A. Jean Ayres Award in 1988, and the AOTF Meritorious Service Award in 1989. Llorens coauthored a book on research (Oyster, Hanten, & Llorens, 1987) and wrote about OT for elders (1988).

Occupational therapy suffered the loss of one of its greatest theorists upon Jean Ayres's death on December 16, 1988. Despite her long illness, Ayres had continued to be productive. She retired from the Ayres Clinic in 1984 to complete the Sensory Integration and Praxis Tests, published in 1989. Eulogized in several ways after her death, she was also recognized before her death. In 1983, she was named to the AOTF Academy of Research, and in 1987, the AOTF created the A. Jean Ayres Award for outstanding research in her honor. Her last written work, published posthumously in 1991, was a coauthored chapter (Ayres & Marr, 1991) in the book *Sensory Integration Theory and Practice* (Fisher, Murray, & Bundy, 1991). The 2002 revision of this comprehensive text (Bundy, Lane, & Murray, 2002) continues Ayres's tradition of inquiry, critical literature analysis, and theorizing about how the brain processes sensation for human functioning.

1990s—OT Events and the Theorists (Table 10.6)

The increase in federal and third-party funding created a critical demand for occupational therapists, and despite the looming health care reimbursement reform that was to burst this employment boom, there was an explosion of OT schools. By the turn of the century, employment opportunities had shifted, school enrollments had declined, and the AOTA mandate for entry-level postprofessional education by 2006 led to a gradual decrease in numbers of OT educational programs.

Meanwhile, the number of OT doctoral programs was growing. The USC doctoral program in occupational science began in 1989 with the intent to develop research and theory in the science of occupation in health and dysfunction (Brown, 1991). Texas Woman's University opened the first OT doctoral program in a public university in 1993 (AOTA, 1993) and this, together with existing doctoral programs at NYU, Boston University, and USC, brought to four the number of OT doctoral programs in the nation at that time. By 2002, the number had increased to 13 doctoral programs including PhD, OTD, and ScD degrees, many with a multidisciplinary base.

In his book, *Conceptual Foundations of Occupational Therapy*, Kielhofner (1992) reviewed numerous frameworks for OT and revised this content in 1997. In 1995 and again in 2002, he updated *A Model of Human Occupation* (Kielhofner, 1995, 2002b). He had numerous publications during this decade (see Chapter 7) and developed centers in the United States and elsewhere for research and practice related to the model.

Allen coauthored a text on OT treatment of cognitive diseases (Allen, Earhart, & Blue, 1992) and published the Allen Cognitive Level Test (1990), the Allen Diagnostic Module (Earhart, Allen, & Blue, 1993), and Cognitive Levels 0 and 0.8 (Allen, 2000). She also authored journal articles, book chapters, and monographs during this decade. She continued as chief of OT psychiatry at USC Medical Center and medical reviewer for Blue Cross of California, and she lectured at OT schools.

In 1990, Fidler accepted an offer to help an OT professional education program through difficult times and became interim

Table 10.6

Historical Perspective 1990–2002

National events	**Reilly**
Communication explosion: Internet, cellular phones, e-mail	Continued separation from profession
Amendments to ADA 1990, IDEA 1991	Occupational science as academic discipline founded on Reilly's concepts of occupational behavior
Health care reform implemented	**Ayres**
Gulf War	Others continue research, test development, and clinical application of Ayres's theory of sensory integration
World Trade Center bombing 9/11/2001	**Llorens**
	Retired San Jose State U chair and interim associate academic vice president
Occupational Therapy Events	Continued publishing and involvement in professional activities
Employment boom shifted by end of decade	**Mosey**
Rapid, then slowed proliferation of OT schools	*Applied Scientific Inquiry in the Health Professions* (1992, 1996)
Postprofessional entry education required by 2006	*Psychosocial Components of Occupational Therapy* (1996)
Refinement of models of occupation; group efforts	**Allen**
Occupational science	Chief of OT Psychiatry, Harbor UCLA Medical Center
	Lecturer at OT schools
	Medical reviewer for Allied Health for Blue Cross of California
	Allen Cognitive Level Test Manual (1990)
	Occupational Therapy Treatment Goals for the Physically and Cognitively Disabled (Allen, Earhart, & Blue, 1992)
	Allen Diagnostic Module (Earhart, Allen, & Blue, 1993)
	Cognitive Levels 0 and 0.8 (2000)
Theorists	**Kielhofner**
Fidler Consultancies NYU, NY Mental Health	Centers for MOHO research and practice in U.S. and other nations
CEO Hagdorn Center for Geriatrics	U of Illinois OT chair (1986–present)
Scholar in residence, College Misericordia	*Conceptual Foundations of Occupational Therapy* (1992, 1997)
Recapturing Competence (Fidler & Bristow, 1992)	*Model of Human Occupation* (1995, 2002)
Lyfe-Style Performance: From Profile to Conceptual Model (1996)	
Activities: Reality and Symbol (Fidler & Velde, 1999)	
Lifestyle Performance: A Model for Engaging the Power of Occupation (Velde & Fidler, 2001)	

Note. ADA = Americans with Disabilities Act; IDEA = Individuals with Disabilities Education Act.

program director there. Throughout the decade, she continued to be involved in professional activities through presentations at institutes and workshops and to express her ideas in articles and books. She wrote about the impact of occupational therapists' beliefs and values on the profession (1990), the changes in mental health practice (1991), and the future of OT (2000) and community practice (2001). She coauthored books on geropsychiatric rehabilitation (Fidler & Bristow, 1992), activities (Fidler & Velde, 1999), lifestyle performance (Velde & Fidler, 2001), and the lifestyle performance model (Fidler, 1996).

Mosey's work in the 1990s focused on scientific inquiry and differentiating applied and basic scientific inquiry (1992a, 1996a). She advocated applied inquiry in OT to address practice questions in contrast to basic inquiry to generate new theory and knowledge, exploring these issues in two editions of her book on epistemology in health professions published by AOTA (1992a, 1996a). In addition, she expressed her controversial views on separating OT inquiry from occupational science (1992b, 1993). Mosey also published the second edition of her 1986 book, *Psychosocial Components of Occupational Therapy* (1996b).

Llorens published chapters on developmental theory for OT (1991), consultation (1992a, 1992b), and elders (McCormack, Llorens, & Glogoski, 1991). She also authored articles on research utilization (1990), health promotion (Ross, Washington, & Llorens, 1990), self-esteem (Bolding & Llorens, 1991), stroke (Shiotsuka, Burton, Pedretti, & Llorens, 1992), activity analysis (Llorens, 1993), ethnogeriatrics (Llorens, Umphred, Burton, & Glogoski-Williams, 1993), and students with disabilities (Llorens, Burton, & Still, 1999).

In the past decade, these theorists remained actively involved in the profession, although Fidler, Mosey, and Llorens were in or approaching retirement. Reilly remained apart from the field. Allen's work centered on her model, and Kielhofner continued to be extremely productive in publishing and funded research. The 1990s saw an explosion of group-generated, occupation-centered models, reviewed in Chapter 9, that are a departure from the solo efforts of individual leaders in first-generation OT theory development.

What the Theory Is: Premises, Scope, and Complexity

In this section, I address the question, What is the theory? by reviewing the major premises and the scope and complexity of each theory. Essentially, I analyze theory content.

Premises

A review of the premises of the seven individual theorists discussed in this book is presented in Table 10.7. This review addresses the primary idea, conjecture, supposition, or position proffered by each theorist and the key terms used in the theory. From this review of premises and key terms, similarities among the premises regarding human occupation and environmental influences can be identified.

Table 10.7

Theorists' Premises and Terminology

Theorist	Premises	Terminology
Allen	Persons with disabilities will engage in activities to the extent that they have the cognitive capacity to do so. The degree of thought used to guide one's actions can be inferred by observing one's interactions with materials, objects, and people.	Cognitive levels Cognitive disabilities
	OT adjusts activities so that they can be accomplished by persons with disabilities.	
Ayres	Learning occurs in the brain, and learning disabilities reflect neural dysfunction.	Sensory integration Tactile defensiveness Developmental dyspraxia Vestibular and bilateral integration dysfunction
	Sensory integration supports neural functioning, and sensory integration dysfunction reflects neural dysfunction.	
	Body senses and subcortical functions are important for visual, auditory, and cortical functions.	
	Sensory integration therapy employs movement for its sensory-generating effects.	*(continues)*

Table 10.7 *Continued.*

Theorist	Premises	Terminology
Fidler	Purposeful activity and "doing" are the core of OT. Activity is a communication process for nonverbal communication and expression. Object relationships are used for exploration and mastery of the environment.	Object relation OT is a communication process Doing is becoming
Kielhofner	Humans are occupational beings who interact as open systems with the environment through the subsystems: volitional (personal causation, values, and interests); habituation (roles and habits); performance (motor, process, and communciation/interpersonal skills). Humans interact with the environment in input–throughput–feedback processes. OT identifies and remedies problems in performance, habituation, and volitional subsystems to enhance occupational role functioning.	Model of human occupation Work–play continuum Occupational roles
Llorens	Humans develop chronologically and simultaneously in all areas of development. OT is a facilitation process for achievement and mastery of life tasks at various life stages. OT activities and interpersonal relationships are used to facilitate development.	OT is a developmental process
Mosey	OT treatment process recapitulates ontogenesis of development. Three frames of reference are useful in mental health OT: analytic, acquisitional, and developmental. Activities therapies use action-oriented interaction to promote mental health. Therapists should have a frame of reference for practice.	Recapitulation of ontogenesis Biopsychosocial model Activities Therapy Epistemology Scientific inquiry

(continues)

Theorist	Premises	Terminology
Reilly	Humans are occupational beings who have an intrinsic need to act upon and master their environment.	Occupational behavior
	Occupational roles provide social meaning and belonging.	Work–play continuum
	Play is a precursor to occupational role and is important through life.	Occupational roles
	OT uses occupations to restore abilities for role performance.	

Human Occupation

The most obvious similarity among these theorists' premises is the focus on the importance of activities, tasks, and occupations for human functioning. Humans are not idle creatures; they are active, moving, stimulus-seeking beings who act on, interact with, and seek to alter their surroundings. Taking a broad viewpoint, Reilly (1962) portrayed humans as occupational beings who have an intrinsic need to act on and master their environment and to do so in ways that are in keeping with social role expectations. Meaning as a social being is derived through successful role performance whereby the individual is able to develop those skills necessary to meet role demands. One is satisfied with life and feels reinforced by one's society when one can perform in expected ways.

Building on Reilly's work, Kielhofner (1985) proposed that humans are occupational beings who interact as open systems with the environment. As open systems, humans are active, goal-directed, purposeful creatures who take in information and energy from the environment (intake), use this information or energy for self-maintenance or to initiate further interaction with the environment (throughput), act or produce interaction with the environment (output), and monitor and alter responses on the basis of feedback from the environment.

Contemporary occupation-centered models propose that "through their occupations, people develop their self-identity and derive a sense of fulfillment" (Christiansen & Baum, 1997, p. 48) and they interact with context to select and perform tasks (Dunn, et al., 1994). Law et al. (1996) differentiate activity as the "basic unit of a task," task as a "set of purposeful activities," and occupation as "groups of self-directed functional tasks and activities in which a person engages over the lifespan" (p. 16).

Although the early writings of Fidler, Mosey, Llorens, and Allen focused more narrowly on "activity," their theories have elements of what the field has come to know as the broader concept of occupation. Fidler posited that purposeful activity is the core of occupational therapy (Fidler & Fidler, 1978). Like Fidler, Mosey described activity therapies as those therapies that provide action-oriented interaction to help the patient with mental illness. Activities, according to Llorens (1976), facilitate human growth and development by enabling one to explore the environment, establish relationships, acquire knowledge, and adapt successfully to one's world. Concerned that activities are undervalued in OT and that their therapeutic value is hard to explain to those outside of OT, Allen (1987) sought to provide a philosophical framework to emphasize the value of activities as therapeutic. Convinced that humans engage in activity for a purpose and that humans use thoughts to guide activities, she proposed the levels of thought required to guide one's behavior in engaging in an activity. She used activities to explain cognitive deficits: "Disability is understood within the context of doing an activity" (Allen, 1987, p. 565). Although Ayers did not elaborate activity postulates, she (1972a) described children's gross motor play activities in terms of sensory integrative properties and the organizing effects of movement in human neural functioning.

In summary, Fidler said that "doing is becoming," Mosey advocated action-oriented interactions, Llorens described activity in the OT process of facilitating developmental progression, Allen focused on the levels of thought necessary to perform activities, Ayres focused on the importance of movement for neutral integration, Reilly and Kielhofner described the occupational nature of humans, and newer occupation-centered models emphasized the influence of the environment on occupational performance.

Environment

The theorists reviewed in this book agree that, through action on and interaction with the environment, humans grow and develop those skills and abilities that enable them to be competent members of a society and to gain a sense of self and social worth. According to Fidler, through interaction with objects in the environment, humans respond to an innate drive to explore and master their environment (Fidler & Fidler, 1963). Through action-oriented experiences, humans test skills; clarify relationships; develop and integrate sensory, motor, cognitive, and psychological functions; become socialized to cultural norms and roles; and gain competence as social beings. The skills one develops through "doing" help one become competent in self-care, provide intrinsic gratification, and afford one the means to care for others. Skill development is influenced by both the environment and the individual's biological makeup (Fidler, 1996; Fidler & Fidler, 1978; Fidler & Velde, 1999).

Mosey (1973) stated that humans, through engagement in activity, learn to perform life tasks necessary to meet their own needs and the demands of living in their community. Interaction with the nonhuman environment enables the individual to acquire the skills necessary for the performance of life tasks. Mosey defined life tasks as requiring not only the performance of manual skills but also interpersonal relationships, work roles, and recreation.

In Llorens's (1970) outline of 10 premises for the OT process, she stated that humans naturally develop and master skills, abilities, and relationships simultaneously and chronologically across all areas of development. This development is fostered by the interaction of the individual's genetic makeup and the environment.

Allen (1987) stated, "Human functioning is the process of engaging in purposeful motor actions within a context of material objects and people" (p. 565). Interaction of individual and environment is seen in her recommendations for adjusting the task parameters to enable the individual to perform. By defining what the patient needs to do to accomplish everyday tasks and what the therapist needs to do to adapt the task, Allen described cognitive levels needed for normal task performance within one's environment.

To Ayres (1972a), learning occurs in the brain and is dependent on neural processes to take in information through the senses and integrate and process that sensory information. The body senses (tactile, proprioceptive, kinesthetic, and vestibular) are integrated with the visual and auditory systems. Neural mechanisms that support sensory integration contribute to the development of cortical, conscious processes. Thus, Ayres considered the body senses and neural developmental processes to be important for competent interaction with the environment.

Reilly (1974) emphasized the performance of social role in the environment, particularly occupational roles. Occupational roles develop in childhood through play, chores, and schooling as the child acquires the adaptive skills and interactive skills needed to be a competent adult worker. Play and social recreation are important throughout life because they promote manipulatory and social skills necessary for role performance and provide socially accepted outlets for aggression.

In the model of human occupation, Kielhofner (1985) proposed that the human open system includes three hierarchical subsystems: volitional, habituation, and performance. The volitional subsystem addresses the human drive for competence and mastery and includes motivation and belief in one's ability to act (personal causation) and the development of interests and values. In the habituation subsystem, one develops habits and roles for efficient coping with daily life experience. Underlying the habituation subsystem is the performance subsystem, which includes motor, process, and communication skill development through symbolic, neurologic, and musculoskeletal components. These subsystems interact with the environment in an input–throughput–output feedback process, as noted previously, to bring about occupational role functioning.

In summary, these theorists proposed that human–environment interaction is the mechanism for the development of skills to master the environment and perform as competent members of a society. Fidler said that one becomes competent through doing. Mosey offered her organization of various frames of reference for conceptualizing skill development through engagement in occupations. Llorens described interaction with the environment as crucial for human development. Allen defined the cognitive levels necessary to perform ordinary activities. Ayres posed the relationship of learning to effective interaction with the environment through sensory systems and motor functioning. To Reilly, interaction with the environment in a play–work continuum was necessary for role skill development. Kielhofner viewed humans as open systems interacting with the environment for adaptive functioning. Occupation-centered models emphasize human adaptation in the context of the human and nonhuman environment. Assessment determines challenges presented by the environment, as well as the environmental resources. Intervention address the individual and his or her occupational functioning within the environment. Outcomes are expressed in terms of occupational performance and optimal contexts supportive of performance.

Scope and Complexity

The review of *scope* addresses the range and focus of the theories. Does each theory apply to all of occupational therapy or to only a part? Is it specific to one clinical area, or does it address the entire field? Does it seek to explain the profession as a whole or to focus on one aspect of the profession? Is the theory a closed theory, or does it allow for expansion and further development? The review of *complexity* explores the number of concepts in each theory, the intensity of study needed to understand the theory, its implications, and the internal consistency of the theory.

Scope

The theorists reviewed in this book address the entire range of population ages, settings, and disabilities seen in OT practice, although the scope of each theory differs. Fidler's contribution to the body of knowledge in the field is perhaps most appropriately viewed in terms of various constructs for OT practice. She provided theoretical formulations for psychoanalytically based OT in psychiatry and expanded these to include new knowledge through the years. In addition, her work influenced Mosey and Llorens.

In scope, Mosey has helped articulate the wholeness of OT and its parts by presenting frameworks for viewing the profession and what therapists are using and doing. She provided (a) frameworks for structuring and thinking about the OT profession and its knowledge (1968, 1970, 1992a); (b) a taxonomy for identifying the elements of the profession (1981); and (c) therapy approaches for OT in mental health (1973, 1986).

Allen provided depth in a focused area of study: the level of cognition needed to perform tasks. She identified six levels of thinking that one uses and analyzed numerous ordinary tasks in terms of these levels. Allen described the cognitive requisites for performing a task, revealing the level of cognitive deficits that exists when an individual is unable to perform a task at a given level. Thus, her work is applicable across disability areas and diagnoses in adults because it focuses on cognitive ability, regardless of the cause of the patient's problem.

The scope of Llorens's work has included all of OT, but has been most applicable to pediatrics which focuses on developmental processes during childhood. Llorens (1976) provided a way to conceptualize OT practice, to explain what OT is, and to be able to teach this to students. Because her work is a point of view for the field and embodies beliefs about the field, it could be considered a paradigm. However, Llorens presented her work more as the process of OT practice than as a paradigm for the profession.

Sensory integration theory (Ayres, 1972a) focused on children with learning disabilities who have no demonstrable neurological deficits but are having difficulty learning. However, Ayres's principles for understanding sensory and motor functioning and for treatment have been used with several patient populations.

Reilly's work (1962) is considered a paradigm because she attempted to articulate the idea underlying the field of OT. She imposed order on multidisciplinary information to proclaim the particular features of the profession. Reilly's paradigm provides her grand-scale perception of the exciting uniqueness of OT.

Going beyond Reilly, Kielhofner (1985) provided a comprehensive model for addressing the complexity of the occupational aspects of humans in a clinical situation. This model includes a framework for evaluation, treatment, and research.

The group-generated occupation-centered models for the profession elaborate on OT's central concern: the occupational nature of humans. These models present prescriptive guidelines on occupational therapy's domain of concern, delineating the areas of human functioning that occupational therapists should address in practice.

Complexity

Fidler's work has been most valuable in articulating the constructs of object relationships, doing and becoming, competence, and mastery. She proposed the lifestyle performance model

(1996) as a complex and cogent theoretical framework that interrelates person, environment, and task for planning and implementing intervention. Criticisms regarding the clarity and applicability of the model and its overlap with similar models (Hocking & Whiteford, 1997) were countered by rebuttal in support of the framework (Velde, Gerney, Trompetter, & Amory, 1997). Fidler (2000) expressed concern for the larger issue of professional development: "I can envision an occupational scientist, an occupationalist who will have a number of options for specialized study, research, and practice across a broad spectrum of opportunities" (p. 101).

Mosey progressively expanded and modified her theoretical contributions in a continued quest for a model for the profession. A prolific writer, Mosey's work has been complex, although her ideas have been presented in a logical and orderly way. Whereas terminology in her synthesis works was sometimes awkward, perhaps due to the difficulty of clearly presenting distillations of the ideas of other theorists, terminology in her recent works has been clearly defined and used consistently. She has developed original ideas as her perceptions have been refined through her relentless examination of ideas underlying OT theory.

Allen described six cognitive levels from first-hand observations of how humans are able or unable to do tasks. Her rationale, definitions, task analyses, evaluations, and treatment applications provide a comprehensive yet practical way for therapists to think about the patient's or client's thinking.

Llorens provided 10 premises for OT practice that are succinctly stated, comprehensive, and internally consistent. She has continued to refine the application of these concepts in later works.

Ayres's complex theory of sensory integration requires knowledge of neuroscience and thoughtful study of the theory for thorough understanding. Her reliance on neuroscience literature requires the reader to have a background in neurophysiology and neuropsychology. Concepts are consistently and logically presented, building on one another. Terminology is well developed and used consistently throughout.

Although Reilly's ideas were simply and consistently presented, an understanding of her theory requires thoughtful study and careful reading of her writings and that of her students. Because the theory is a macroview of the profession, some readers may find it difficult to bring it from the realm of the theoretical to the practical.

Kielhofner's work on the model of human occupation demonstrated his belief in the need for a comprehensive theory for occupational therapy that could be developed through research. Thorough study is necessary to grasp the model in its complexity. His development of new meanings for existing terms and his introduction of new terms into the field have led to some confusion and concern (Labovitz & Miller, 1986).

In summary, these seven theorists demonstrate a heroic commitment to writing the ideas that form the basis for the profession and the principles that guide OT intervention. Fidler presented constructs for OT practice; Mosey, conceptual frameworks for the profession, for OT practice in mental health, and for theory building; Allen, analyses of the cognitive ability needed to perform tasks; Llorens, a conceptualization of the OT practice process; Ayres, a research-based theory for OT practice in pediatrics; Reilly, a paradigm; and Kielhofner, a comprehensive practice model. The theories are intricate and complex in their own ways and are deserving of careful study for appreciation of the depths of knowledge offered.

The group-generated, occupation-centered models are both simple and elegant in their complexity. They seek to explain the complicated individual–occupation–environment processes in understandable definitions, diagrams, and formats.

How the Theory Is Used: Clinical Application

Use of a theory is examined in its clinical application—that is, the assessment and intervention approaches derived from the theories (see Table 10.8). These OT theorists advocated the therapeutic use of occupations to restore, regain, or renew skills. To Fidler (Fidler & Fidler, 1963), OT in psychiatry was a communication process involving the psychodynamics of activities and therapeutic relationships. By engaging in activities, patients come to express their emotions and thoughts, learn to interact effectively with the nonhuman environment, and develop skills. Fidler's clinical contributions include her prescriptive use of

Table 10.8

Clinical Applications of Theory

Theorist	Evaluation	Treatment	Patient Population and Setting
Allen	Allen Cognitive Level Test Routine Task Inventory Cognitive Disabilities Expanded Activity Analysis	Activities adjusted to cognitive level of person with disability Daily living skills	Developed for adult mental health and expanded to adult physical dysfunction
Ayres	Southern California Sensory Integration Tests Postrotary Nystagmus Test Sensory Integration and Praxis Tests Ayres's clinical observations	Sensory integrative therapy with tactile, proprioceptive, vestibular, and kinesthetic emphasis Use of scooter boards, net hammock, and suspended swings	Children with learning disabilities in schools and community clinics
Fidler	Projective Diagnostic Battery Object History Play History Lifestyle Performance Profile Patient questionnaires	Activity analysis Prescriptive use of activities Task groups Nonverbal communication	Adult psychiatry in institutional and community settings
Kielhofner	Observation, history, interview, and projective assessments	Therapy principles for treatment planning	Applicable to all age and disability groups and settings, but roots are in psychosocial dysfunction

(continues)

Table 10.8 *Continued.*

Theorist	Evaluation	Treatment	Patient Population and Setting
Llorens	Developmental Analysis, Evaluation and Intervention Schedule Sequential Client Care Record	Age-appropriate activities Interpersonal relationships	All developmental age groups, disabilities, and settings
Mosey	Survey instruments: Group interaction, self-care, childcare work, and recreation Activity configuration Questionnaires based on Fidler's	Use of groups Body image treatment Activities therapy	Adult and adolescent psychiatry in institutional and community settings
Reilly	Observation, history, and interview techniques	Use of arts, crafts, toys, games, and leisure activities	Applicable to all age and disability groups and settings, but focuses on adults in the community

activities, suggestions for the use of task groups, and use of activities in nonverbal communication and object relations work in mental health (Fidler & Fidler, 1954, 1963). Fidler constructed clinical observation tools for use in psychosocial evaluation (Projective Diagnostic Battery, Object History, Play History) and across populations (Lifestyle Performance Profile, 1982).

Mosey (1970) regarded clinical practice as the scientific application of theory and provided practical guidelines for the use of activity in therapy. She described the use of work-related, recreational, and creative tasks for improving psychosocial functioning. She promoted activities therapy as a way to use everyday interactions and activities to help persons function in the broader community. The use of five types of groups (1973), treatment of distorted body image (1969), and guidelines for activities therapy in mental health (1973) comprise the specific treatment approaches she introduced. Mosey developed survey instruments for group interaction, self-care, childcare work, and recreation. She also devised an activity configuration for analysis of time spent in various activities throughout the day and questionnaires based on Fidler's work (1973).

According to Llorens (1976), activities and relationships that are in keeping with the patient's age and life roles can be used to facilitate development. Her early work was in child psychiatry, although her developmental model is applicable across age and dysfunction categories. Llorens (1970, 1976) described OT as a facilitation process that assists the individual to achieve and master the tasks of living presented at various life stages. The therapist functions as an enculturation agent to bridge the gap between the patient's functioning level and the level that is socially age expected. Occupational therapy can facilitate the closure of developmental gaps and prevent further dysfunction through the judicious analysis, selection, and use of activities and interpersonal relationships. Llorens's framework (1976) for practice that spanned infancy through adulthood and aging advocated testing, evaluation, and observation to determine the developmental level of the patient. Her Sequential Client Care Record (1982) was a method for case documentation of evaluation and treatment processes, and her Development Analysis, Evaluation and Intervention Schedule (1976) was a guide to case analysis using a developmental framework.

In contrast to these theories that began in mental health OT, Ayres (1972a) developed her sensory integrative therapy for children with learning disabilities. Sensory integrative therapy uses carefully selected motor and sensory activities applied in a developmental sequence to elicit increasingly adaptive sensory and motor responding. Ayres devoted a substantial portion of her work to the development of standardized testing instruments for use in OT evaluation of children with learning disabilities. Her tests include the Southern California Sensory Integration Tests (1972b), the Southern California Postrotary Nystagmus Test (1975), and the Sensory Integration and Praxis Tests (1989). These tests initiated psychometric testing in OT, requiring therapists' adherence to strict standard administration and scoring procedures. Equipment and devices such as the scooter board ramp, suspended hammock, swings, and bolsters emphasized bodily sensations of tactile, proprioceptive, kinesthetic, and vestibular systems; required sufficient clinical space to safely accommodate this large, moving equipment; and gave a new look to OT pediatric clinics.

Allen (1987) selected disability as the focus of study and developed taxonomies of cognitive levels to delineate what is missing or lost from normal functioning in persons with disabilities. She described ways to adjust activities to a level that enables persons with disabilities to use their remaining capacities to achieve some degree of functioning. Allen's methods for evaluating human cognitive levels include the Allen Cognitive Level Test (Allen, 1990), which is used in conjunction with an interview to screen for the level of cognition the individual used in learning leather lacing, and the Routine Task Inventory (Allen et al, 1992), which involves detailed observations of the level of cognition used in performing daily living skills. Allen emphasized the therapist's clinical observations as crucial for effective use of these evaluation instruments.

According to Reilly (1974), disease states run counter to the development of life role skills and result in role dysfunction and dissatisfaction. Occupational therapy promotes life satisfaction and self-actualization through the restoration of abilities needed for occupational role functioning. Reilly (1974) advocated the case method approach for patient treatment. She recommended direct observations, testing, interview, and history taking for evaluation and clinical problem solving and to accommodate individual patient variations. Evaluation results were examined to identify patterns of success and failure, learning style, and level of function, and to provide data for formulating an action plan.

Occupational therapy, according to Kielhofner (1985), addresses breakdowns in the human–environment open system interaction by identifying occupational role dysfunction and providing remediation at the subsystem level (performance, habituation, or volition) required to restore or enhance occupational role functioning. Although initially applied primarily in psychosocial areas (Barris et al., 1983), Kielhofner's (1985) framework can be used to conceptualize OT evaluation and treatment across patient categories. Assessment instruments related to Kielhofner's model of human occupation (MOHO) are described on the MOHO Clearinghouse Web site (http://www.uic.edu/ahp/OT/MOHOC/) and include observation, interview, and history taking tools.

The emphasis on client-centered intervention is explicit in contemporary occupation-centered theories. Christiansen and Baum (1997) described a collaborative therapy process that draws upon the skills of the client and the therapist engaging in a problem-solving process. Dunn et al. (1994) advocate therapy that is "embedded in real life" (p. 602) and that uses five intervention alternatives to establish or restore ability to perform, alter the context, adapt the task demands, prevent the development of maladaptation, or create contexts to promote adaptation. Law et al. (1996) say that occupational therapists will increase the number and scope of available interventions if the therapists think of clients in terms of individual occupational factors, as well as family, culture, community, economic, institutional, physical, and social factors. Schkade and Schultz (1992) emphasized helping the client to achieve internal adaptation in the therapy process.

An example of instrument development in other occupation-centered models is the Canadian Occupational Performance Measure (Law et al., 1994), designed to measure the client's perception of occupational performance. The Community Adaptive Planning Assessment is a tool for collaborative client–therapist planning and documentation (Spencer & Davidson, 1998).

Central Themes

Although the theorists discussed in this book present a variety of ideas and concepts that are enriched and embellished through their exploration of many issues in the profession, they repeatedly return to a few central themes: the view of humans as occupational beings; mastery of the environment through skill development; the ability of humans to affect their own state of health; the therapeutic value of tasks, activities, and occupations; and the influence of context and environment on occupational functioning. This work provides us with a working body of knowledge that can be confirmed through clinical practice and research, leading to refined theory building in occupational therapy.

How the Theory Is Tested: Dissemination, Validation, and Development of Theory by Others

Throughout their careers, the seven theorists discussed in Chapters 2 through 8 have consistently disseminated their ideas, hypotheses, and findings through writings, teachings, and presentations. They have also attempted to validate their theories and develop their ideas further through research and clinical application (see Table 10.9). Occupation-centered models and books, publications and conferences of these models are addressed more thoroughly in Chapter 9.

Dissemination

Estimating from the bibliographies in the preceding chapters of this text, the seven individual theorists discussed have written more than 25 books and nearly 300 articles and other scholarly writings. All of them have served as OT educators, and most have shared their ideas through workshops and presentations. Fidler has written 6 books and 27 articles and has disseminated her ideas through workshops, lectures, clinical teaching, supervision, and service to the AOTA. Mosey has written 6 books and 16 papers and has disseminated her concepts through OT graduate

Table 10.9

Theory Dissemination, Research, and Application/Development of Theory by Others

Theorist	Topics of Books and Articles	Topics of Presentations	Topics of Research	Application/ Development of Theory by Others
Allen	Cognitive disabilities Assessment of cognitive levels	Clinical teaching: Assessment	Cognitive levels	Assessment of cognitive levels
Ayres	Sensory integration theory SI dysfunction Testing and treatment	Workshops, OT education, Clinical teaching: Sensory integration treatment	Sensory integration Learning disabilities Autism, aphasia	Sensory Integration International Adult psychiatry Aphasia Mental retardation Cerebral palsy Hyperactivity Developmental disabilities
Fidler	OT psychiatry OT theory Activities Professional issues	Workshops, Clinical teaching: Group process OT psychiatry Program design Management Activities		

(continues)

Table 10.9 *Continued.*

	Topics of	Topics of	Topics of	Application/Development
Kielhofner	Human occupation theory and application	OT education, Workshops	Human occupation Psychosocial problems Adolescents Delinquency Elderly Adult mental retardation Assessment and instrument development	Learning disabilities Alcoholism Adults with mental retardation Spinal cord injury Elderly Assessment and instrument development
Llorens	Development theory for OT OT in child psychiatry Consultation in Community Black culture OT record system Cognitive–perceptual–motor dysfunction	OT education Workshops: Developmental theory	Emotional disturbance in children OT record system	
Mosey	OT theory OT psychiatry Activity	OT education, Workshops: Frames of reference Activity		
Reilly	Work–play continuum OT education OT profession	OT education: Play Work OT education OT profession		Roles, Play, Work Interests, Motivation Curriculum design Temporal adaptation Occupational behavior theory Assessment

education and workshops. Many of Llorens's 79 publications and much of her teaching in workshops and graduate and undergraduate OT programs reflect aspects of her developmental theory. Ayres published 3 books, 52 articles, 22 test instruments, and 4 professional films. She informed students and therapists about sensory integration theory through workshops and clinical training in her Ayres Clinic. Reilly's theories have been disseminated through her writings (16 articles and 1 book) and through numerous students' works. As a scholar, Reilly's goal was to enable students to learn to think critically; use logical thought processes; and develop qualitative, quantitative, and historical perspectives. Kielhofner, who has authored or coauthored 5 books and nearly 100 papers, is the most prolific writer of the theorists reviewed and is distinctive in extensive collaborative authorships. He also teaches in workshops and classrooms. Allen, the newest of the theorists reviewed, has published more than a dozen articles and 3 books and developed test instruments.

Validation

Validation efforts vary among these theorists: Some have validated their ideas empirically through years of clinical practice, some have conducted research, and some have stimulated others to do research. Fidler derived her ideas from, and tested them through, clinical practice. Although she has not conducted research, she advocated that occupational therapists study activities according to a standardizing process to search for the meaning of activity and its application in the field.

Similarly, Allen developed her taxonomy of cognition for task performance from her clinical practice. In the practice arena, she and colleagues have developed test instruments and conducted research.

Mosey advocated research to test theories and theoretical foundations, but has not conducted research herself. She proposed research as indirectly related to practice and to practice frames of reference. The role of research in theory building should be to contribute to the theoretical base and body of knowledge. Through their modification of the theoretical base, research findings then trickle down to frames of reference for practice. Thus, clinical practice is based on theoretical foundations that are modified by research.

Llorens's nearly two decades of clinical practice contributed to the formulation of her ideas for a developmental theory of occupational therapy. She conducted research in child psychiatry and the use of her OT record system, and promoted research through her leadership role in the AOTF. Her Sequential Client Care Record and case study methods are clinical research data-gathering tools, and she has coordinated their use with therapists in various states in the nation.

In the construction of sensory integration theory, Ayres spent more than two decades in research efforts. Her work included test instrument development and treatment efficacy studies with children with learning disabilities, autism, and aphasia.

The focus of OT research, according to Reilly, should be to study the nature of occupation from a developmental perspective. Thus, research should focus on achievement, creativity, aptitude, and interest patterns in relation to occupations and activities. Reilly's influence led to an established tradition of OT scholarly productivity that has endured at USC.

With the model of human occupation now well described, Kielhofner and his colleagues and students conduct research using the model. This research is aimed at the development of assessments and testing treatment based on the model.

Development of the Theory by Others

Further application, research, and development have occurred in sensory integration theory, occupational behavior theory, the model of human occupation, and cognitive disability theory. Ayres's sensory integration theory has spawned research efforts by clinicians and students, and therapists have applied the treatment principles to several patient populations, including those with learning disabilities, developmental disabilities, hyperactivity, aphasia, autism, cerebral palsy, and adult psychiatry. Corporate support of sensory integration theory, research, practice, and test certification in the United States and abroad is provided by Sensory Integration International, Pediatric Therapy Network, and Sensory Integration Resource Center.

Reilly's students were instrumental in researching and applying her theory through (a) the development of survey, interview, observation, and history tools; (b) the description of roles and occupational stages, the influence of interests and motivation, and the work–play continuum; and (c) sequences and variables for clinical practice for use with adolescents with delinquent behaviors, geriatric patients, and persons with physical disabilities, mild mental retardation, and psychiatric disorders. Reilly's occupational behavior conceptualizations contribute to formulations of occupational science (Yerxa et al., 1990) and to the study of play as occupation (Parham & Fazio, 1997). Her ideas about OT curricula have been incorporated into curriculum designs based on occupation (Levine, 1984). Reilly profoundly influenced Kielhofner's ideas.

Kielhofner's students and colleagues have researched the model of human occupation with several patient groups, including children with learning disabilities, persons with alcoholism, adults with retardation, persons with spinal cord injury, and the elderly. Other research efforts have addressed assessment and instrument development. Kielhofner is nationally and internationally recognized for his work on the model of human occupation and for publications too numerous to justly summarize here (see Chapter 7).

Although Allen's theory has received some research attention, Fidler's, Mosey's, and Llorens's theories have not been developed through an identifiable body of research or through an identified group of researchers. However, these theorists' works are cited in the literature when reference is made to basic ideas of occupational therapy and have been included in theory compilations (P. N. Clark & Allen, 1985; Kielhofner, 1992; Reed & Sanderson, 1999). Mosey's writings influenced others' writings on the use of groups in occupational therapy (Howe & Schwartzberg, 1995). Like Reilly, these theorists synthesized theory for OT practice and made it possible for Kielhofner and others to develop theory from within the field. All of these theorists generously shared their ideas through written and spoken communications. They have contributed their hypotheses and conceptualizations to the rest of the profession for use, examination, and improvement.

Conclusion

In considering theory for the practice of OT, does one adopt a theory based on the merit of its postulates, research, and clinical application, or are other factors involved? Other possible influences include the sociopolitical climate of the field; trends in occupational therapy; national association spotlight on the work; persona of the theorist as a leader in the field; publications in occupational therapy versus other journals; first-hand contact in workshops and presentations; and reading assignments in OT school. As the field grows and theories continue to proliferate, therapists may seek theories that reflect abiding concepts that undergird the profession (Wilcox, 2002), yet are useful for explaining, interpreting, and guiding contemporary OT practice, education, and research. From the array of ideas and viewpoints that are available now and that will be forthcoming in the future, discerning therapists may subject each theory to the questions put forth at the beginning of this chapter:

- How was the theory developed?
- Who developed the theory?
- What is the theory?
- How is the theory used?
- How has the theory been tested?

Whether a theory is focused and prescriptive, descriptive and researched, or grand and speculative (Meleis, 1997), the answers to these questions can help the therapist to determine applicability in the practice and research settings.

In this book, we have reviewed the rationales for the profession and the explanations of OT practice proposed by Fidler, Mosey, Llorens, Ayres, Reilly, Kielhofner, and Allen and by proponents occupation-based models for practice. These theories are being examined in OT practice and research. Much remains to be done to validate these theoretical formulations, as well as those beyond the scope of this book. Hudson's thoughts, as expressed in the *American Journal of Occupational Therapy* in 1954, on the nature of research, provide a challenge to each occupational therapist: "It is exciting to realize that we are all on a scientific frontier that has hardly been penetrated—that the opportunities for individual contribution to knowledge are endless" (Hudson, 1954, p. 150).

Appendix 10.A Outlines for Theory Critique and Theory Analysis

I. Outline for Theory Critique

   A. Structure and function—theoretical foundations of theory

      1. Clarity—precision, orderliness, consistent conceptual and operational definitions

      2. Consistency—congruence of components (assumptions, concepts, definitions)

      3. Simplicity/complexity—number of phenomena and their relationships

      4. Tautology/teleology—needless repetition (tautology) and use of new concepts to define existing ones (teleology)

   B. Diagram—visual, graphic representations enhance the written descriptions

      1. Clarity and accuracy in depicting concepts
      2. Logical representation
      3. Completeness
      4. Congruence with written explanations

   C. Circle of contagiousness—adoption of theory by others

      1. Influence of theory versus theorist
      2. Geographic spread
      3. Citations

   D. Usefulness

      1. Practice—sufficient directions for use in practice

         a. Client populations, problems
         b. Assessments
         c. Interventions
         d. Feasibility for adopting

      2. Research

         a. Generation of hypotheses, research questions
         b. Testability through research

3. Education

   a. Appropriateness for adoption as curriculum model
   b. Suitability for different student levels (undergraduate, graduate)

4. Administration

   a. Theoretical framework for practice guidelines
   b. Compatibility with institutional mission
   c. Rationale for quality control, patient classification systems

E. External components

   1. Congruence with personal, professional, and social values
   2. Value to humanity

II. Outline for Theory Analysis

A. Structure

   1. Assumptions
   2. Concepts
   3. Propositions

B. Functions—the consequences of the theory

   1. Focus of the theory
   2. Implications for the client–therapist relationship
   3. Problems identified
   4. Assessments developed and usable
   5. Intervention strategies explained

C. The theorist background and career

D. Paradigmatic origins of the theory

E. Internal dimensions

   1. Rationale
   2. System of relations
   3. Content
   4. Theory beginnings
   5. Scope
      a. Grand
      b. Single domain
      c. Mid-range

6. Goal
7. Context
8. Abstractness
9. Method of theory development

F. Critique

Note. Adapted from McKenna (1997), Meleis (1997), Walker and Newman (1996).

Appendix 10.B Terms and Definitions Related to the Study of Theory

Academic discipline. Body of knowledge derived through science in an area of inquiry; knowledge generation for the sake of knowledge.

Assumptions. Statements accepted as true based on philosophy and values but perhaps not tested; implicit (writer implies) and explicit (writer identifies).

Concept. Units of a theory; a word or collection of words expressing mental images of phenomena.

Concept, observable. Concept with a physical referent (e.g., "spoon," "computer," "ice").

Conceptual definition. Description of the concept or variable in general terms without reference to how it is measured.

Construct. Concept (e.g., "intelligence," "motivation," "depression") not directly observable via our senses; concept that is defined, inferred, or observed indirectly by test scores or behavioral observations.

Frame of reference. System of ideas in which other ideas are interpreted or assigned meaning.

Hypothesis. Statement of expected relationship between or among variables.

Model. Tentative description of a theory or system that accounts for all of its known properties; framework for applying a theory or system of ideas.

Model, practice. Integrated framework that is congruent with profession's theory or paradigm and that serves to guide practice; also guidelines for practice, therapeutic approach, and frame of reference.

Operational definition. Defines the concept or variable in terms of how it is measured and interpreted.

Paradigm. Prototype, exemplar, standard, pattern, model; broad constructs underlying and defining the scope of a discipline.

Phenomena. A condition, event, or activity.

Postulate. Assumed without proof of being self-evident or generally accepted; a basic principle.

Practice–research–theory process. Research aimed at answering questions and refuting or validating hypotheses, and research findings used to develop and modify theory.

Practice–theory process. Theory evolved from practice to describe and explain practice.

Pre-OT theory. Theory developed in other fields that may be adopted by occupational therapy (OT) to explain OT phenomena; also be termed non-OT theory.

Primary OT theory. Theory developed in and for occupational therapy.

Principle. Basic truth, law, or assumption; rule or law concerning phenomena, processes, or relationships between concepts.

Proposition. Describes relationship between concepts; also termed *principle* or *postulate proposition*.

Proposition, nonrelational. Statement about one concept that defines the concept.

Proposition, relational. Statement about two or more concepts that defines the relationship between or among concepts.

Research, applied. Addresses areas of knowledge to enhance humanity; connects research questions or hypotheses to theory for practice.

Research, basic. Pursuit of knowledge for knowledge's sake; not required to address functional problems or practical conditions.

Research, programmatic. Addresses specific problems in a specific setting; of practical, localized importance; action research (program evaluation).

Research–theory process. Research findings systematically organized into theory.

Theory. System of assumptions, accepted principles, rules of procedures devised to analyze, predict, and explain the nature or behavior of a specified set of phenomena; involves abstract reasoning. Distinguished from *experiment* or *practice*.

Theory, grand. Broad, philosophical theories of the nature, mission, or goals of the field.

Theory, mid-range. Based on research, applicable across a variety of areas of practice.

Theory–practice–theory process. Preexisting non-OT theory selected from other fields and systematically applied to OT practice to evolve primary OT theory.

Theory refinement. Further development of an existing OT framework; not a new theory but a modification or enhancement of the theory.

Theory–research process. Development of theory process in which specific theory is refuted or supported.

Theory–research–theory process. Theory guides research questions and is modified by research findings.

Theory, single domain. Focuses on a specific situation, population, or problem.

Theory–theory–practice/research process. Preexisting theory from outside the field as well as derived or primary theory to build new theory, which is then tested through research and applied in clinical practice.

Note. Adapted from McKenna (1997), Meleis (1997), and Walker and Newman (1996).

Appendix 10.C
Eleanor Clarke Slagle Lectures

1955 **Florence M. Stattel, MA, OTR, FAOTA**
Stattel, F. M. (1956). Equipment designed for occupational therapy. *American Journal of Occupational Therapy, 10*, 194–198.

1956 **June Sololov*, OTR, FAOTA**
Sokolov, J. (1957). Therapist into administrator: Ten inspiring years. *American Journal of Occupational Therapy, 11*, 13–19, 34.

1957 **Ruth Brunyate Wiemer, MEd, OTR, FAOTA**
Wiemer, R. B. (1958). Powerful levers in little common things. *American Journal of Occupational Therapy, 12*, 193–202.

1958 **Margaret S. Rood*, MA, OTR, RPT, FAOTA**
Rood, M. S. (1958). Everyone counts. *American Journal of Occupational Therapy, 12*, 326–329.

1959 **Lilian Berth Wegg, OTR, FAOTA**
Wegg, L. B. (1960). The essentials of work evaluation. *American Journal of Occupational Therapy, 14*, 65–69, 79.

1960 **Muriel Ellen Zimmerman, OTR, FAOTA**
Zimmerman, M. E. (1960). Devices: Development and direction. In *Proceedings of the 1960 Annual Conference*, pp. 17–24.

1961 **Mary Reilly, EdD, OTR, FAOTA**
Reilly, M. (1962). Occupational therapy can be one of the great ideas of 20th century medicine. *American Journal of Occupational Therapy, 16*, 1–9.

1962 **Naida Ackley*, OTR, FAOTA**
Ackley, N. (1962). The challenge of the sixties. *American Journal of Occupational Therapy, 16*, 273–281.

1963 **A. Jean Ayres*, PhD, OTR, FAOTA**
Ayres, A. J. (1963). The development of perceptual-motor abilities: A theoretical basis for treatment of dysfunction. *American Journal of Occupational Therapy, 17*, 221–225.

1964 **None**

1965 **Gail S. Fidler, OTR, FAOTA**
Fidler, G. S. (1966). Learning as a growth process: A conceptual framework for professional education. *American Journal of Occupational Therapy, 20*, 1–8.

1966 **Elizabeth June Yerxa, EdD, OTR, FAOTA**
Yerxa, E. J. (1967). Authentic occupational therapy. *American Journal of Occupational Therapy, 21*, 1–9.

*Deceased.

1967 Wilma L. West*, MA, OTR, FAOTA
West, W. L. (1968). Professional responsibility in time of change. *American Journal of Occupational Therapy, 22*, 9–15.

1968 None

1969 Lela Augustine Llorens, PhD, OTR, FAOTA
Llorens, L. A. (1970). Facilitating growth and development: The promise of occupational therapy. *American Journal of Occupational Therapy, 24*, 93–101.

1970 None

1971 Geraldine Louise Finn, MS, OTR, FAOTA
Finn, G. L. (1972). The occupational therapist in prevention programs. *American Journal of Occupational Therapy, 26*, 59–66.

1972 Jerry A. Johnson, EdD, MBA, OTR, FAOTA
Johnson, J. A. (1973). Occupational therapy: A model for the future. *American Journal of Occupational Therapy, 27*, 1–7.

1973 Alice C. Jantzen*, PhD, OTR, FAOTA
Jantzen, A. C. (1974). Academic occupational therapy: A career specialty. *American Journal of Occupational Therapy, 28*, 73–81.

1974 Mary R. Fiorentino*, MusB, OTR, FAOTA
Fiorentino, M. R. (1975). Occupational therapy: Realization to activation. *American Journal of Occupational Therapy, 29*, 15–21.

1975 Josephine C. Moore, PhD, OTR, FAOTA
Moore, J. C. (1976). Behavior, bias, and the limbic system. *American Journal of Occupational Therapy, 30*, 11–19.

1976 A. Joy Huss, MS, OTR, RPT, FAOTA
Huss, A. J. (1977). Touch with care or a caring touch. *American Journal of Occupational Therapy, 31*, 11–18.

1977 None

1978 Lorna Jean King, OTR, FAOTA
King, L. J. (1978). Toward a science of adaptive responses. *American Journal of Occupational Therapy, 32*, 429–437.

1979 L. Irene Hollis, OTR, FAOTA
Hollis, L. I. (1979). Remember? *American Journal of Occupational Therapy, 33*, 493–499.

1980 Carolyn Manville Baum, PhD, OTR/C, FAOTA
Baum, C. M. (1980). Occupational therapists put care in the health system. *American Journal of Occupational Therapy, 34*, 505–516.

---

*Deceased.

1981 **Robert Kendall Bing*, EdD, OTR, FAOTA**
Bing, R. K. (1981). Occupational therapy revisited: A paraphrastic journey. *American Journal of Occupational Therapy, 35*, 499–518.

1982 **None**

1983 **Joan C. Rogers, PhD, OTR/L, FAOTA**
Rogers, J. C. (1983). Clinical reasoning : The ethics, science, and art. *American Journal of Occupational Therapy, 37*, 601–616.

1984 **Elnora M. Gilfoyle, ScD (Hon), OTR, FAOTA**
Gilfoyle, E. (1984). Transformation of a profession. *American Journal of Occupational Therapy, 38*, 575–584.

1985 **Anne Cronin Mosey, PhD, OTR, FAOTA**
Mosey, A. C. (1985) A monistic or a pluralistic approach to professional identity? *American Journal of Occupational Therapy, 39*, 504–509.

1986 **Kathlyn L. Reed, PhD, OTR, FAOTA, MLIS, AHIP**
Reed, K. L. (1986). Tools of practice: Heritage or baggage. *American Journal of Occupational Therapy, 40*(9), 597–605.

1987 **Claudia Kay Allen, MA, OTR, FAOTA**
Allen, C. K. (1987). Activity: Occupational therapy's treatment method. *American Journal of Occupational Therapy, 41*, 563–575.

1988 **Anne Henderson, PhD, OTR, FAOTA**
Henderson, A. (1988). Occupational therapy knowledge: From practice to theory. *American Journal of Occupational Therapy, 42*, 567–576.

1989 **Shereen D. Farber, PhD, OTR, FAOTA**
Farber, S. D. (1989). Neuroscience and occupational therapy: Vital connections. *American Journal of Occupational Therapy, 43*, 637–646.

1990 **Susan B. Fine, MA, OTR, FAOTA**
Fine, S. B. (1991). Resilience and human adaptability: Who rises above adversity? *American Journal of Occupational Therapy, 45*, 493–503.

1991 **None**

1992 **None**

1993 **Florence Arcuri Clark, PhD, OTR, FAOTA**
Clark, F. A. (1993). Occupation embedded in a real life: Interweaving occupational science and occupational therapy. *American Journal of Occupational Therapy, 47*, 1067–1078.

1994 **Ann P. Grady, PhD, OTR, FAOTA**
Grady, A. P. (1995). Building inclusive community: A challenge for occupational therapy. *American Journal of Occupational Therapy, 49*, 300–310.

1995 **Catherine Anne Trombly, ScD, OTR/L, FAOTA**
Trombly, C. A. (1995). Occupation: Purposefulness and meaningful-
ness as therapeutic mechanisms. *American Journal of Occupational
Therapy, 49*, 960–972.

1996 **David L. Nelson, PhD, OTR, FAOTA**
Nelson, D. L. (1997). Why the profession of occupational therapy will
flourish in the 21st century. *American Journal of Occupational Therapy, 51*, 11–24.

1997 **None**

1998 **Anne G. Fisher, ScD, OTR, FAOTA**
Fisher, A. G. (1998). Uniting practice and theory in an occupational
framework. *American Journal of Occupational Therapy, 52*, 509–521.

1999 **Charles H. Christiansen, EdD, OTR, OT(C), FAOTA**
Christiansen, C. H. (1999). Defining lives—Occupation as identity:
An essay on competence, coherence, and the creation of meaning.
American Journal of Occupational Therapy, 53, 547–558.

2000 **Margo B. Holm, PhD, OTR/L, FAOTA, ABDA**
Holm, M. B. (2000). Our mandate for the new millennium: Evidence-
based practice. *American Journal of Occupational Therapy, 54*,
575–585.

2001 **Winifred Weise Dunn, PhD, OTR, FAOTA**
Dunn, W. (2001). The sensation of everyday life: Empirical, theoreti-
cal, and pragmatic considerations. *American Journal of Occupational
Therapy, 55*, 608–620.

2002 **None**

2003 **Charlotte B. Royeen, PhD, OTR, FAOTA**
Chaotic occupational therapy: Collective wisdom for a complex profession. *American Journal of Occupational Therapy, 57*.

2004 **Ruth Zemke, PhD, OTA, FAOTA**

References

Abreu, B. C. (1999). Evaluation and intervention with memory and learning impairments. In C. Unsworth (Ed.), *Cognitive and perceptual dysfunction: A clinical reasoning approach to evaluation and intervention* (pp. 163–207). Philadelphia: F.A.
Davis.

Allen, C. K. (1985). *Occupational therapy for psychiatric diseases: Measurement and
management of cognitive disabilities.* Boston: Little, Brown.

Allen, C. K. (1987). Activity: Occupational therapy's treatment method. *American Journal of Occupational Therapy, 41*, 563–575.

Allen, C. K. (1990). *Allen Cognitive Level Test manual.* Colchester, CT: S&S Worldwide.

Allen, C. K. (2000). *Cognitive levels 0 and 0.8*. (Available from Ivelisse Lazzarini, Edward and Margaret Doisey School of Allied Health Professions, St. Louis University, St. Louis, MO 63103)

Allen, C. K., Earhart, C. A., & Blue, T. (1992). *Occupational therapy treatment goals for the physically and cognitively disabled*. Rockville, MD: American Occupational Therapy Association.

American Occupational Therapy Association. (1979). TOTEMS: Training occupational therapy management in the schools. Rockville, MD: Author.

American Occupational Therapy Association. (1985a). *Education Data Survey*. Rockville, MD: Author.

American Occupational Therapy Association. (1985b). *Occupational therapy manpower: A plan for progress*. Rockville, MD: Author.

American Occupational Therapy Association. (1985c). *PIVOT: Planning and implementing vocational readiness in occupational therapy*. Rockville, MD: Author.

American Occupational Therapy Association. (1986a). *ROTE: Role of occupational therapy with the elderly*. Rockville, MD: Author.

American Occupational Therapy Association. (1986b). *SCOPE: Strategies, concepts, and opportunities for program development and evaluation*. Rockville, MD: Author.

American Occupational Therapy Association. (1988). *Professional and Technical Role Analysis*. Rockville, MD: Author.

American Occupational Therapy Association. (1993). TWU establishes PhD program in occupational therapy. *OT Week, 7*(1), 12.

Americans with Disabilities Act of 1990, 42 U.S.C. § 12101 *et seq.*

Arnadottir, G. (1990). *The brain and behavior: Assessing cortical dysfunction through activities of daily living (ADL)*. St. Louis, MO: Mosby.

Ayres, A. J. (1949). An analysis of crafts in the treatment of electroshock patients. *American Journal of Occupational Therapy, 3*, 195–198.

Ayres, A. J. (1963). The development of perceptual motor abilities as a theoretical basis for treatment of dysfunction. *American Journal of Occupational Therapy, 6*, 221–225.

Ayers, A. J. (1972a). *Sensory integration and learning disorders*. Los Angeles: Western Psychological Services.

Ayres, A. J. (1972b). *Southern California Sensory Integration Tests*. Los Angeles: Western Psychological Services.

Ayres, A. J. (1975). *Southern California Postrotary Nystagmus Test*. Los Angeles: Western Psychological Services.

Ayres, A. J. (1979). *Sensory integration and the child*. Los Angeles: Western Psychological Services.

Ayres, A. J. (1985). *Developmental dyspraxia and adult onset dyspraxia*. Torrance, CA: Sensory Integration International.

Ayres, A. J. (1989). *Sensory Integration and Praxis Tests*. Los Angeles: Western Psychological Services.

Ayres, A. J., & Marr, D. M. (1991). Sensory Integration and Praxis Tests. In A. G. Fisher, E. A. Murray, & A. C. Bundy (Eds.), *Sensory integration theory and practice* (pp. 203–229). Philadelphia: F.A. Davis.

Barris, R., Kielhofner, G., & Watts, J. H. (1983). *Psychosocial occupational therapy*. Laurel, MD: Ramsco.

Bass-Haugen, J., Mathiowetz, V., & Flinn, N. (2002). Optimizing motor behavior using the occupational therapy task-oriented approach. In C. A. Trombly & M. V. Radomski (Eds.), *Occupational therapy for physical dysfunction* (pp. 481–499). Philadelphia: Lippincott, Williams & Wilkins.

Bolding, D. J., & Llorens, L. A. (1991). The effects of habilitative hospital admission on self-care, self-esteem and frequency of physical care. *American Journal of Occupational Therapy, 45,* 796–800.

Brown, E. J. (1991, January 7). Occupational science: What will it mean to OT? *Advance for Occupational Therapists.*

Bullock, J., Cummings, M. J., Madigan, J., Masagatani, G., McGourty, L., Moulin, N., Prendergast, N., Ryan, S., Walker, J., Gray, M., Hays, C., & Presseller, S. (1981). Entry-level role delineation for OTRs and COTAs: Approved by Representative Assembly March 1981. *Occupational Therapy News, 35*(6), 1–9.

Bundy, A. C., Lane, S. J., & Murray, E. A. (Eds.). (2002). *Sensory integration theory and practice.* Philadelphia: F.A. Davis.

Case-Smith, J. (Ed.). (2001). Occupational therapy for children (4th Ed.). St. Louis: Mosby.

Chinn, P. L., & Jacobs, M. K. (1983). *Theory and nursing—A systematic approach.* St. Louis, MO: Mosby.

Christiansen, C., & Baum, C. (1997). Person–environment occupational performance: A conceptual model for practice. In C. Christiansen & C. Baum (Eds.), *Occupational therapy: Enabling function and well-being* (pp. 47–70). Thorofare, NJ: SLACK.

Clark, F. A., Parham, D., Carlson, M. E., Frank, G., Jackson, J., Pierce, D., Wolfe, R. J., & Zemke, R. (1991). Occupational science: Academic innovation in the service of occupational therapy's future. *American Journal of Occupational Therapy, 45,* 300–310.

Clark, F. A., Zemke, R., Frank, G., Parham, D., Neville-Jan, A., Hedricks, C., Fazio, L., & Abreu, B. (1993). Dangers inherent in the partition of occupational therapy and occupational science. *American Journal of Occupational Therapy, 47,* 184–186.

Clark, P. N., & Allen, A. S. (1985). *Occupational therapy for children.* St. Louis, MO: Mosby.

Duldt, B. W., & Giffin, K. (1985). *Theoretical perspectives for nursing.* Boston: Little, Brown.

Dunn, W. (2000). *Best practice occupational therapy in community service with children and families.* Thorofare, NJ: SLACK.

Dunn, W., Brown, C., & McGuigan, A. (1994). The ecology of human performance: A framework for considering the effect of context. *American Journal of Occupational Therapy, 48,* 595–607.

Earhart, C. A., & Allen, C. K. (1988). *Cognitive disabilities: Expanded activity analysis.* Colchester, CT: S&S Worldwide.

Earhart, C. A., Allen, C. K., & Blue, T. (1993). *Allen Diagnostic Module: Instruction manual.* Colchester, CT: S&S Worldwide.

Education for all Handicapped Children Act of 1975, 20 U.S.C. § 1400 *et seq.*

Farber, S. D. (1982). *Neurorehabilitation: A multisensory approach.* Philadelphia: Saunders.

Fearing, V. G., & Clark, J. (2000). *Individuals in context.* Thorofare, NJ: SLACK.

Fidler, G. S. (1948). Psychological evaluation of occupational therapy activities. *American Journal of Occupational Therapy, 1,* 284–287.

Fidler, G. S. (1966). Learning as a growth process: A conceptual framework for professional education. The Eleanor Clarke Slagle Lecture. *American Journal of Occupational Therapy, 20,* 1–8.

Fidler, G. S. (1982). The Lifestyle Performance Profile: An Organizing Frame. In B. Hemphill (Ed.) *The examination process in psychiatric occupational therapy* (pp. 43–47). Thorofare, NJ: Slack, Inc.

Fidler, G. S. (1990). Reflections on choice. *Occupational Therapy in Mental Health, 10,* 77–84.

Fidler, G. S. (1991). The challenge of change to OT practice. *Occupational Therapy in Mental Health, 11,* 1–11.

Fidler, G. S. (1996). Life-style performance: From profile to conceptual model. *American Journal of Occupational Therapy, 50,* 139–147.

Fidler, G. S. (2000). Beyond the therapy model: Building our future. *American Journal of Occupational Therapy, 54,* 99–101.

Fidler, G. S. (2001). Community practice: It's more than geography. *Occupational therapy in Health Care Community OT Education and Practice, 3* (3/4), 7–9.

Fidler, G. S., & Bristow, B. (1992). *Recapturing competence: A system's change for geropsychiatric care.* New York: Springer.

Fidler, G. S., & Fidler, J. W. (1954). *Introduction to psychiatric occupational therapy.* New York: Macmillan.

Fidler, G. S., & Fidler, J. W. (1963). *Occupational therapy: A communication process in psychiatry.* New York: Macmillan.

Fidler, G. S., & Fidler, J. W. (1978). Doing and becoming: Purposeful action and self-actualization. *American Journal of Occupational Therapy, 32,* 305–310.

Fidler, G. S., & Velde, B. P. (1999). *Activities: Reality and symbol.* Thoroughfare, NJ: SLACK.

Fisher, A. G. (1998). Uniting practice and theory in an occupational therapy framework. Eleanor Clarke Slagle Lecture. *American Journal of Occupational Therapy, 52,* 509–521.

Fisher, A. G., Murray, E. A., & Bundy, A. C., (Eds.). (1991). *Sensory integration theory and practice.* Philadelphia: F.A. Davis.

Hocking, C., & Whiteford, G. (1997). What are the criteria for development of occupational therapy theory? A response to Fidler's life style performance model. *American Journal of Occupational Therapy, 51,* 154–157.

Hopkins, H. L. (1988). An historical perspective on occupational therapy. In H. L. Hopkins & H. D. Smith (Eds.), *Willard and Spackman's occupational therapy* (7th ed., pp. 16–42). Philadelphia: Lippincott.

Holm, M. B., Rogers, J. C. & Stone, R. G. (1998). Treatment of performance contexts. In M. E. Neistadt & E. B. Chepeau (Eds.), Willard and Spackmans Occupational Therapy, (9th ed., pp. 471–517). Philadelphia: Lippincott.

Howe, M. C., & Briggs, A. K. (1982). Ecological systems model for occupational therapy. *American Journal of Occupational Therapy, 36,* 322–327.

Howe, M. C., & Schwartzberg, S. L. (1995). A functional approach to group work in occupational therapy (2nd ed.). Philadelphia: Lippincott.

Hudson, B. (1954). What is research? *American Journal of Occupational Therapy, 8,* 140–141, 150.

Individuals with Disabilities Education Act Amendments of 1991, 20 U.S.C. § 1400 *et seq.*

Kielhofner, G. (Ed.). (1983). *Health through occupation: Theory and practice of occupational therapy.* Philadelphia: F.A. Davis.

Kielhofner, G. (Ed.). (1985). *A model of human occupation: Theory and application.* Baltimore: Williams & Wilkins.

Kielhofner, G. (1992). *Conceptual foundations of occupational therapy.* Philadelphia: F.A. Davis.

Kielhofner, G. (Ed.). (1995). *A model of human occupation: Theory and application,* (2nd ed.). Baltimore: Williams & Wilkins.

Kielhofner, G. (1997). *Conceptual foundations of occupational therapy* (2nd ed.). Philadelphia: F.A. Davis.

Kielhofner, G. (2002a, June 27). *Challenges and directions for the future of occupational therapy.* Paper presented at the meeting of the World Federation of Occupational Therapy, Stockholm, Sweden.

Kielhofner, G. (Ed.). (2002b). *A model of human occupation: Theory and application* (3rd ed.). Baltimore: Lippincott, Williams & Wilkins.

Kramer, P., & Hinojosa, J. (1993). *Frames of reference for pediatric occupational therapy.* Baltimore: Williams & Wilkins.

Labovitz, D. R., & Miller, R. J. (1986). Commentary—Organization of knowledge in occupational therapy: A proposal and a survey of the literature. *Occupational Therapy Journal of Research, 6,* 85.

Law, M., Baptiste, S., Carswell, A., McColl, M. A., Polatajko, H., & Pollock, N. (1994). *The Canadian Occupational Performance Measure* (3rd ed.). Ottawa, Ontario: Canadian Association of Occupational Therapy.

Law, M., Cooper, B. A., Strong, S., Stewart, D., Rigby, P., & Letts, L. (1996). The person-environment–occupation model: A transactive approach to occupational performance. *Canadian Journal of Occupational Therapy, 63,* (1), 9–21.

Levine, A. E. (1984, May). *A design for an entry-level curriculum based on occupation.* Paper presented at the meeting of the American Occupational Therapy Association Commission on Education, Kansas City, MO.

Light, S., & Reilly, M. (1943). The correlation of physical therapy and occupational therapy. *Occupational Therapy and Rehabilitation, 22,* 171–175.

Llorens, L. A. (1960). Psychological testing in planning treatment goals. *American Journal of Occupational Therapy, 14,* 243–246.

Llorens, L. A. (1970). Facilitating growth and development: The promise of occupational therapy. Eleanor Clarke Slagle Lecture. *American Journal of Occupational Therapy, 24,* 93–101.

Llorens, L. A. (Ed.). (1973). *Consultation in the Community: Occupational therapy in child health.* Dubuque, IA: Kendall/Hunt.

Llorens, L. A. (1976). *Application of a developmental theory for health and rehabilitation.* Rockville, MD: American Occupational Therapy Association.

Llorens, L. A. (1982). *Occupational Therapy Sequential Client Care Record manual.* Laurel, MD: Ramsco.

Llorens, L. A. (Ed.). (1988). Health care for ethnic elders: The cultural context. In *Proceedings of Stanford Geriatric Education Center Conference.* (Available from Stanford Geriatric Education Center, 703 Welch Road, Palo Alto, CA 94305)

Llorens, L. A. (1990). Research utilization: A personal/professional responsibility. *Occupational Therapy Journal of Research, 10*(1), 3–6.

Llorens, L. A. (1991). Performance tasks and roles throughout the life span. In C. Christiansen & C. Baum (Eds.), *Occupational therapy: Overcoming human performance deficits* (pp. 45–66). Thorofare, NJ: Charles B. Slack.

Llorens, L. A. (1992a). Program consultation for children and adults. In E. Jaffe & C. F. Epstein (Eds.), *Occupational therapy consultation: Theory, principles and practice* (pp. 356–363). St. Louis, MO: Mosby.

Llorens, L. A. (1992b). Roles for occupational therapist consultation in higher education. In E. Jaffe & C. F. Epstein (Eds.), *Occupational therapy consultation: Theory, principles and practice* (pp. 496–500). St Louis, MO: Mosby.

Llorens, L. A. (1993). Activity analysis: Agreement between participant and observers on perceived factors in occupation components. *Occupational Therapy Journal of Research, 13*(3), 198–211.

Llorens, L. A., Burton, G., & Still, J. R. (1999). Achieving occupational role: Accommodations for students with disabilities. *Occupational Therapy in Health Care, 11*(4), 1–7.

Llorens, L. A., & Rubin, E. Z. (1967). *Developing ego functions in disturbed children: Occupational therapy in milieu.* Detroit: Wayne State University Press.

Llorens, L. A., Umphred, D. B., Burton, G. U., & Glogoski-Williams, C. (1993). Ethnogeriatrics: Implications for occupational therapy and physical therapy. *Physical and Occupational Therapy in Geriatrics, 11*(3), 59–69.

McCormack, G., Llorens, L., & Glogoski, C. (1991). The culturally diverse elderly. In J. Kiernat (Ed.), *Occupational therapy for the older adult: A clinical manual* (pp. 11–24). Gaithersburg, MD: Aspen.

McKenna, H. (1997). *Nursing theories and models.* New York: Routledge.

Meleis, H. I. (1997). *Theoretical nursing: Development and progress* (3rd ed.). Philadelphia: Lippincott.

Mosey, A. C. (1968). Recapitulation of ontogenesis: A theory for practice of occupational therapy. *American Journal of Occupational Therapy, 22,* 426–432.

Mosey, A. C. (1969). Treatment of pathological distortion of body image. *American Journal of Occupational Therapy, 23,* 413–416.

Mosey, A. C. (1970). *Three frames of reference for mental health.* Thorofare, NJ: Charles B. Slack.

Mosey, A. C. (1973). *Activities therapy.* New York: Raven Press.

Mosey, A. C. (1981). *Occupational therapy: Configuration of a profession.* New York: Raven Press.

Mosey, A. C. (1985). A monistic or a pluralistic approach to professional identity? Eleanor Clarke Slagle Lecture. *American Journal of Occupational Therapy, 39,* 504–509.

Mosey, A. C. (1986). *Psychosocial components of occupational therapy.* New York: Raven Press.

Mosey, A. C. (1992a). *Applied scientific inquiry in the health professions: An epistemological orientation.* Rockville, MD: American Occupational Therapy Association.

Mosey, A. C. (1992b). The issue is—Partition of occupational science and occupational therapy. *American Journal of Occupational Therapy, 46,* 851–853.

Mosey, A. C. (1993). Partition of occupational science and occupational therapy: Sorting out some of the issues. *American Journal of Occupational Therapy, 47,* 751–754.

Mosey, A. C. (1996a). *Applied scientific inquiry in the health professions: An epistemological orientation* (2nd ed.). Rockville, MD: American Occupational Therapy Association.

Mosey, A. C. (1996b). *Psychosocial components of occupational therapy* (2nd ed.). Philadelphia: Lippincott-Raven.

Ottenbacher, K. (1996). Academic disciplines: Maps for professional development. In R. Zemke & F. Clark (Eds.), *Occupational science: The evolving discipline* (pp. 329–330). Philadelphia: F.A. Davis.

Oyster, C. K., Hanten, W. P., & Llorens, L. A. (1987). *Introduction to research: A guide for the health science professional.* Philadelphia: Lippincott.

Parham, L. D., & Fazio, L. S. (Eds.). (1997). *Play in ocupational therapy for children.* St. Louis: Mosby-Year Book.

Reed, K. L., & Sanderson, S. R. (1999). *Concepts of occupational therapy* (4th ed.). Philadelphia: Lippincott.

Reilly, M. (1962). Occupational therapy can be one of the great ideas of 20th century medicine. The Eleanor Clarke Slagle Lecture. *American Journal of Occupational Therapy, 1,* 1–9.

Reilly, M. (Ed.). (1974). *Play as exploratory learning.* Beverly Hills, CA: Sage.

Reilly, M. (1984). The issue is—The importance of the client versus patient issue for occupational therapy. *American Journal of Occupational Therapy, 38,* 404–406.

Ross, H. S., Washington, W. N., & Llorens, L. A. (1990, March/April). Health promotion in a multicultural community. *Health Education.*

Rousseau, J., Potvin, L., Dutil, E., & Falta, P. (2002). Model of Competence: A conceptual framework for understanding the person–environment interation for persons with motor disabilities. *Occupational Therapy in Health Care, 16*(1), 15–36.

Sabari, J. S. (1991). Motor learning concepts applied to activity-based intervention with adults with hemiplegia. *American Journal of Occupational Therapy, 45,* 523–530.

Schkade, J. K., & Schultz, S. (1992). Occupational adaptation: Toward a holistic approach to contemporary practice. Part 1. *American Journal of Occupational Therapy, 46,* 829–837.

Shiotsuka, W., Burton, G., Pedretti, L., & Llorens, L. A. (1992). An examination of performance scores on activities of daily living between elders with right and left cerebrovascular accident. *Physical and Occupational Therapy in Geriatrics, 10*(4), 47–57.

Spencer, J. C., & Davidson, H. A. (1998). Community Adaptive Planning Assessment: A clinical tool for documenting future planning with clients. *American Journal of Occupational Therapy, 52,* 19–30.

Toglia, J. P. (1991). Generalization of treatment: A multicontext approach to cognitive perceptual impairment in adults with brain injury. *American Journal of Occupational Therapy, 45,* 505–516.

Trombly, C. A. (2002). Conceptual foundations for practice. In C. A. Trombly & M. V. Radomski (Eds.), *Occupational therapy for physical dysfunction* (5th ed., pp. 1–15). Philadelphia: Lippincott, Williams & Wilkins.

Trombly, C. A. & Radomski, M. V. (Eds.) (2002). *Occupational therapy for physical dysfunction* (5th ed.). Philadelphia: Lippincott, Williams & Wilkins.

Velde, B. S., Gerney, A., Trompetter, L., & Amory, M. A., (1997). Fidler's Life Style Performance Model: Why we disagree with Hocking and Whiteford's critique. *American Journal of Occupational Therapy, 52,* 784–787.

Velde, B. S., & Fidler, G. S. (2001). *Lifestyle performance: A model for engaging the power of occupation.* Thoroughfare, NJ: SLACK.

Walker, P. H., & Neuman, B. (Eds.). (1996). *Blueprint for the use of nursing models: Education, research, practice, and administration.* New York: NLN Press.

Wilcox, A. A. (2002). *Occupation for health: Volume 1. Journey from self health to prescription.* London: College of Occupational Therapists.

Williams, L., & Pedretti, L. W. (Eds.). (2001). *Occupational therapy practice skills for physical dysfunction* (5th ed.). St. Louis: Mosby Year Book.

Yerxa, E., Clark, F., Frank, G., Jackson, J., Parham, D., Pierce, D., Stein, C., & Zemke, R. (1990). An introduction to occupational science, a foundation for occupational therapy in the 21st century. *Occupational Therapy in Health Care, 1*(6), 1–17.

Index